Series Editor: Daniel K. Onion

SECOND EDITION

John A. Sutherland, MD, FACC
Arizona Heart Institute
Phoenix, Arizona

JONES AND BARTLETT PUBLISHERS
Sudbury, Massachusetts
BOSTON TORONTO LONDON SINGAPORE

World Headquarters
Jones and Bartlett
Publishers
40 Tall Pine Drive
Sudbury, MA 01776
978-443-5000
info@jbpub.com
www.jbpub.com

Jones and Bartlett
Publishers Canada
6339 Ormindale Way
Mississauga, ON L5V 1J2
CANADA

Jones and Bartlett
Publishers International
Barb House, Barb Mews
London W6 7PA
UK

Jones and Bartlett's books and products are available through most bookstores and online booksellers. To contact Jones and Bartlett Publishers directly, call 800-832-0034, fax 978-443-8000, or visit our website www.jbpub.com.

ISBN-13: 978-0-7637-3761-0
ISBN-10: 0-7637-3761-5

Library of Congress Cataloging-in-Publication Data
Sutherland, John, 1946–
The little black book of cardiology / John A. Sutherland. — 2nd ed.
p. ; cm.
Rev. ed. of: Blackwell's primary care essentials. Cardiology. © 2001.
Includes bibliographical references and index.
ISBN 0-7637-3761-5
1. Cardiology—Handbooks, manuals, etc. 2. Cardiovascular system —Diseases—Handbooks, manuals, etc. 3. Primary care (Medicine) —Handbooks, manuals, etc. I. Sutherland, John, 1946– . Blackwell's primary care essentials. Cardiology. II. Title.
[DNLM: 1. Cardiovascular Diseases—diagnosis—Handbooks.
2. Cardiovascular Diseases—therapy—Handbooks. WG 39 S966b 2006]
RC669.15.S88 2006
616.1′2—dc22

2005019335

6048

Production Credits
Executive Publisher: Christopher Davis
Production Director: Amy Rose
Associate Editor: Kathy Richardson
Associate Production Editor: Alison Meier
Associate Marketing Manager: Laura Kavigian
Manufacturing Buyer: Therese Connell
Composition: ATLIS Graphics
Cover Design: Anne Spencer
Cover Images: © Photos.com
Printing and Binding: Malloy, Inc.
Cover Printing: Malloy, Inc.

Printed in the United States of America
10 09 08 07 06 10 9 8 7 6 5 4 3

Contents

Preface

Gentle reader, you may believe . . . that I would want this book, the child of my brain, to be the most beautiful, gallant, and cleverest that one could imagine. But I could not transgress Nature's law wherein everything begets his like . . .

Cervantes, *Don Quixote*

Nothing, it seems, is destined to stand still in this world. In the five years since the first edition of *The Little Black Book of Cardiology* was published, I have noticed that the field of cardiovascular medicine has proven itself to be no exception to this principle. I would like this guidebook to maintain its clinical usefulness, and accordingly an updated version has become a necessity.

Happily, this book (and the series of which it is a part) continues to defy easy description. Certainly it makes no claim to be a comprehensive textbook, nor is it an abbreviated version of such a text. But it is also too dense and eclectic to serve as an introduction to cardiology. If I had to pick a single descriptive term for it, I think I would turn to the culinary arts rather than to medicine. The Indian kitchen has a wonderful rice dish known as *khitcherie;* the closest English translation is probably "hodge-podge." I think that describes this text. I have tried to include here the basic facts that a practitioner might need on the fly (such as drug dosages and protocols, and EKG interpretation criteria), as well as the guidelines for standard-of-care, evidence-based medicine that characterize the practice of cardiology in 2006. And then there are the myriad odd factlets that I have acquired as I have expanded my own understanding of cardiovascular disease. As in the first edition, one of this book's major strengths is the compulsive citation of references so that the reader can gain access to the literature to which this pocket helper can only point.

Virtually every chapter has been revised in this second edition. I have tried to address the clinically pertinent general literature of cardiology. Accordingly, many exciting but technical issues (stent characteristics and placement techniques, for example) are not addressed. Cardiac magnetic resonance imaging and genomics are both areas of active research and great promise, but because they are not ready for use in day-to-day clinical practice, I have—with regret—omitted discussion of them here. In short, this second edition remains a clinical resource for the here and now.

Once again, I am indebted to Dan Onion for starting and sustaining this project and for inviting me to become a participant in this series. Chris Davis and the staff at Jones and Bartlett have been everything an author could ask of an editor and publisher. I owe a special debt to Jake Tommerup, the proofreader with the patience of Job who has been willing to tackle the consequences of my two-finger typing skills without complaint. The Arizona Heart Institute and its founder and medical director Dr. Edward B. Diethrich continue to provide a clinical environment to which I owe my growth as a cardiologist.

At the end, it is always the same wish: I hope that you may find this book of use in helping to bring an end to suffering and to the causes of suffering.

John Sutherland, MD, FACC
Phoenix, Arizona

Medical Abbreviations

A_2	Aortic component of second heart sound
AAA	Abdominal aortic aneurysm
ABG	Arterial blood gas
ABI	Anke-brachial index
ac	Before meals
ACC	American College of Cardiology
ACE	Angiotensin-converting enzyme
ACS	Acute coronary syndrome
AECG	Ambulatory electrocardiogram
Afib	Atrial fibrillation
Aflut	Atrial flutter
AH	Atrial-Hi
AHA	American Heart Association
AI	Aortic insufficiency
AICD	Automatic internal cardioverter-defribrillator
AIR	Accelerated idioventricular rhythm
AMI	Anterior myocardial infarction
ANA	Antinuclear antibody
APC	Atrial premature contraction
aPTT	Activated partial thromboplastin time
AR	Aortic regurgitation
ARB	Angiotensin receptor blocker
ARDS	Adult respiratory distress syndrome
ARVD	Arrythomogenic right ventricular cardiomyopathy
AS	Aortic stenosis
ASA	Acetylsalicylic acid (aspirin)
asap	As soon as possible
ASHD	Atherosclerotic peripheral vascular disease
av	Arterial-venous
AV	Arterioventricular
AVNRT	Arterioventricular nodal reentrant tachycardia
AVR	Aortic Valve replacement
BBB	Bundle branch block
bid	Twice daily
BP	Blood pressure
BUN	Blood urea nitrogen
CA^{++}	Calcium
CABG	Coronary artery bypass graft surgery
CAD	Coronary artery disease

cAMP	Cyclic adenosine monophosphate
CBC	Complete blood count
CHF	Congestive heart failure
CK	Creatine kinase
cm	Centimeter
CMR	Cardiac magnetic resonance
CMV	Cytomegalovirus
CNS	Central nervous system
CO	Cardiac output
COPD	Chronic obstructive pulmonary disease
CPK	Creatine phosphokinase
CPP	Cranial perfusion pressure
CPR	Cardiopulmonary resuscitation
CRP	C-reactive protein
CT	Computed tomography
cTnl	Cardiac troponin
CVA	Cerebrovascular accident
CVD	Cardiovascular disease
CVP	Central venous pressure
CXR	Chest x-ray
d	Day(s)
DBP	Diastolic blood pressure
DC	Direct current
Ddx	Differential diagnosis
DIC	Disseminated intravascular coagulation
dL	Deciliter
DM	Diabetes mellitus
DOE	Dyspnea on exertion
DTS	Duke treadmill score
DVT	Deep venous thrombosis
dx	diagnosis
EBCT	Electron beam computed tomography
ECF	Extracorporeal fluid
echo	Echocardiogram
EECP	Enhanced external counterpulsation
EEG	Electroencephalogram
EF	Ejection fraction
EKG	Electrocardiogram
EMS	Emergency medical service
ER	Estrogen receptors; emergency room
ESD	End-systolic diameter
ESR	Erythrocyte sedimentation rate
ETOH	Ethyl alcohol
FBAO	Foreign body airway occlusion
FBS	Fasting blood sugar
Fe	Iron
fen/phen	Fenfluramine and phentermine
fx	Fracture
GCS	Glasgow Coma Score
GFR	Glomerular filtration rate
gi	Gastrointestinal
gm	Gram
GP	Glycoprotein
GTT	Glucose tolerance test
h/o	History of
HACEK	Haemophilus, Actinobacillus, Cardiobacterium, Eikenella, and Kingella species of bacteria

HCM	Hypertrophic cardiomyopathy
hct	Hematocrit
HCTZ	Hydrochlorthizide
HDL	High-density lipoprotein cholesterol
Hg	Mercury
hgb	Hemoglobin
His	Histidine
HIV	Human immune deficiency virus
HMG-COA	3-Hydroxyl-3-methylglutaryl-coenzyme A
HR	Heart rate
hr	hour(s)
hsCRP	High-sensitivity C-reactive protein
HT	Hypertension
HV	His-Ventricular
hx	History
IABP	Intraaortic balloon pump
IBD	Inflammatory bowel disease
ICD	Internal cardioverter-defibrillator
ICP	Intracranial pressure
ICU	Intensive care unit
IDDM	Insulin-dependent diabetes melitus
IE	Ineffective endocarditis
im	Intramuscular
in	Inch
INH	Isoniazid
INR	International normalized ratio
IRBBB	Incomplete right bundle branch block
ISA	Intrinsic sympathomimetic activity
ISDN	Isosorbide mononitrate
iv	Intravenous
IVS	Inferior vena cava
IWMI	Inferior wall myocardial infarction
J	Joule
JNC	Joint National Commission
JVD	Jugular venous distention
K	Potassium
kg	Kilogram
L	Left; liter
LA	Left atrium; long acting
LAD	Left anterior descending coronary artery
LAE	Left atrial enlargement
LAFB	Left anterior fascicular block
lb	Pound(s)
LBBB	Left bundle branch block
LCA	Left coronary artery
LCx	Left circumflex coronary artery
LDL	Low-density lipoprotein cholesterol
Li	Lithium
LICS	Left intercostals space
LIMA	Left internal mammary artery
LLSB	Lower left sternal border
LMCL	Left midclavicular line

LMW	Low molecular weight
LP	Lumbar puncture
Lp(a)	Lipoprotein(a)
LPFB	Left posterior fascicular block
LSB	Left sternal border
LV	Left ventricle
LVEF	Left ventricular ejection fraction
LVH	Left ventricular hypertrophy
LVOT	Left ventricular outflow tract
m	Meter
MAO	Monoamine oxidase
MAP	Mean arterial pressure
MAT	Multifocal atrial tachycardia
MCL	Mid-clavicular line
MET	Metabolic unit
mg	Milligram
Mg^{++}	Magnesium
μgm	Microgram
MI	Myocardial infarction
min	Minute(s)
mm	Millimeter
mon	Month(s)
MR	Mitral regurgitation
MRFIT	Multiple risk factor intervention trial
MRI	Magnetic resonance imaging
ms	Millisecond
MS	Mitral stenosis
mV	Millivolt
MVA	Mitral valve area
MVP	Mitral valve prolapse
MVR	Mitral valve replacement
Na^+	Sodium
NaCl	Sodium chloride (table salt)
ng	Nanogram
NG	Nasogastric
NIDDM	Non-insulin-dependent diabetes mellitus
nl	Normal
NO	Nitric oxide
NOS	Nitric oxide synthetase
npo	Nothing by mouth
NRMI	Nuclear magnetic resonance imaging
NS	Normal saline
NSAID	Nonsteroidal anti-inflammatory drug
NSR	Normal sinus rhythm
NYHA	New York Heart Association
O_2	Oxygen
OS	Opening snap
OT	Occupational therapy
oz	Ounce
P_2	Pulmonary component of second heart sound
PA	Pulmonary artery
PAD	Peripheral arterial disease
PAF	Paroxysmal atrial fibrillation
PAOP	Pulmonary artery occlusion pressure

PCI	Percutaneous intervention
PCP	*Pneumocystis carinii* pneumonia
PCWP	Mean pulmonary capillary wedge pressure
PDA	Patent ductus arteriosis
PE	Pulmonary embolus
PEA	Pulseless electrical activity
PEEP	Positive end-expiratory pressure
PET	Positron emission tomography
PMI	Point of maximal impulse of heart
PND	Paroxysmal nocturnal dyspnea
po	By mouth
prn	As needed
Protime	Protrombin time
PS	Pulmonary stenosis
PSA	Prostate-specific antigen
PSVT	Paroxysmal supraventricular tachycardia
PT	Physical therapy
pt(s)	Patient(s)
PTA	Percutaneous transluminal angioplasty
PTCA	Percutaneous transluminal coronary angioplasty
PTT	Partial thromboplastin time
PVC	Premature ventricular contraction
PVR	Peripheral vascular resistance
PVT	Prosthetic valve thrombosis
q	Each
qd	Once daily
qhs	Every night
qid	Four times daily
QP:QS	Pulmonary systemic blood flow ration
QTc	corrected QT interval
qv	Which see (Latin)
R	Right
RA	Rheumatoid arthritis; right atrium
RBBB	Right bundle branch block
RCA	Right coronary artery
RF	Rheumatic fever
RHC	Right heart catheterization
RICS	Right intercostals space
RSB	Right sternal border
RUQ	Right upper quadrant
RV	Right ventricle
RVEDP	Right ventricular end-diastolic pressure
RVG	Radionuclide ventriculogram
RVH	Right ventricular hypertrophy
RVOT	Right ventricular outflow tract
rx	Treatment
S. *aureus*	*Staphylococcus aureus*
s/p	Status post
S_1	First heart sound

S_2	Second heart sound
S_3	Third heart sound
S_4	Fourth heart sound
SA	Sinoatrial
SAM	Systolic anterior motion
SBP	Systolic blood pressure
sc	Subcutaneous
SCD	Sudden cardiac death
sec	Second(s)
si	signs
SIADH	Syndrome of inappropriate ADH
sl	Sublingual
SLE	Systemic lupus erythematosis
SMX-TMP	Sulfamethoxazole-trimethoprim
SPECT	Single positron emission computerized tomography
SSRI	Selective serotonin reuptake inhibitor
STEMI	ST-elevation myocardial infarction
SV	Supraventricular
SVC	Super vena cava
SVG	Saphenous vein graft
SVT	Supraventricular tachycardia
sx	Symptoms
T_3	Tiiodothyronine
T_4	Thyroxine
TAA	Transthoracic aortic aneurysm
tbc	Tuberculosis
tc	transcutaneous
TCA	Tricyclic antidepressants
TEE	Transesophageal echocardiogram
TENS	Transcutaneous electrical nerve stimulation
TG	Triglycerides
TIA	Transient ischemic attack
tid	Three times daily
TNG	Nitroglycerine
Tnl	Troponin I
TnT	Troponin T
TPA	Tissue-type plasminogen activator
TR	Tricuspid regurgitation
TSH	Thyroid-stimulating hormone
TTE	Transthoracic echocardiogram
TTP	Thrombotic thrombocytopenic purpura
TV	Transvenous
U	Unit(s)
UA	Urinalysis
US	Ultrasound
UTI	Urinary tract infection
VF/Vfib	Ventricular fibrillation
VLDL	Very low density lipoprotein
VQ	Ventilation-perfusion
VSD	Ventricular septal defect
VT	Ventricular tachycardia
VTE	Venous thromboembolism

WHO	World Health Organization	wt	weight
wk	Week(s)	yr	Year(s)
WPW	Wolff-Parkinson White syndrome		

Journals and Other Reference Abbreviations

AHA	American Heart Association
AHCPR	Agency for Health Care Policy Research
Am Hrt J	American Heart Journal
Am J Cardiol	American Journal of Cardiology
Am J Med	American Journal of Medicine
Ann EM	Annals of Emergency Medicine
Ann IM	Annals of Internal Medicine
Ann Thorac Surg	Annals of Thoracic Surgery
Arch IM	Archives of Internal Medicine
BMJ	British Medical Journal
Brit Hrt J	British Heart Journal
Cardiol Rev	Cardiology in Review
Circ	Circulation
Clin Cardiol	Clinical Cardiology
Clin Inf Dis	Clinical Infectious Disease
CV Res	Cardiovascular Research
Eur Heart J	European Heart Journal
Eur J Cardiothorac Surg	European Journal of Cardiothoracic Surgery
Framingham	Framingham Heart Study
J Am Coll Cardiol	Journal of the American College of Cardiology
J Am Soc Echocardiogr	Journal of the American Society of Echocardiography
J Cardiovasc Surg	Journal of Cardiovascular Surgery
J Nucl Surg	Journal of Nuclear Surgery
J Thorac Cardiovasc Surg	Journal of Thoracic and Cardiovascular Surgery
J Vasc Surg	Journal of Vascular Surgery
Jama	Journal of the American Medical Association

JNC-6, JNC-7	Joint National Committee on Prevention, Detection, Evaluation, and Treatment of High Blood Pressure
Lancet	Lancet
Mayo Clin Proc	Mayo Clinic Proceedings
Nejm	New England Journal of Medicine
NHLBI	National Heart, Lung, and Blood Institute
NIH	National Institutes of Health
Peds	Pediatrics
Prog Cardiovasc Dis	Progress in Cardiovascular Disease
Thorac Cardiovasc Surg	Thoracic and Cardiovascular Surgery

Study Acronyms

AVID	Antiarrhythmics vs Implantable Defibrillators
BARI	Bypass Angioplasty Revascularization Investigation
CAPTURE	C7E3 Fab Antiplatelet Therapy in Unstable Refractory Angina
CARE	Cholesterol and Recurrent Events
DANAMI	Danish Trial in Acute Myocardial Infarction
EPISTENT	Evaluation of Platelet IIb/IIIa Inhibitor for Stenting
ESSENCE	Efficacy and Safety of Subcutaneous Enoxaprin in Non-Q-Wave Coronary Events
FIRST	Flolan International Randomized Survival Trial
FRISC	Fragmin During Instability in Coronary Artery Disease Study
GISSI	Gruppo Italiano per lo Studio dello Streptochinasi nell'Infarto Miocardico
GUSTO	Global Use of Strategies to Open Occluded Coronary Arteries
HERS	Heart and Estrogen/Progestin Replacement Study
MADIT	Multicenter Automatic Defibrillator Implantation Trial
MUSTT	Multicenter Unsustained Tachycardia Trial Investigation
NHANES	National Health and Nutrition Examination Survey
OASIS	Organization to Assess Strategies in Acute Ischemic Syndromes
PEACE	Prevention of Events with Angiotensin-Converting Enzyme Inhibition
PIMI	Psychophysiologic Investigations of Myocardial Ischemia
PIOPED	Prospective Investigation of Pulmonary Embolism Diagnosis
PURSUIT	Platelet Glycoprotein IIb/IIIa in Unstable Angina
RITA	Randomized Intervention Treatment of Angina
SHEP	Systolic Hypertension in the Elderly Program
SOLVD	Studies of Left Ventricular Dysfunction
SPAF	Stroke Prevention in Atrial Fibrillation
TIMI	Thrombolysis in Myocardial Infarction
WISE	Women's Ischemia Syndrome Evaluation

Notice

We have made every attempt to summarize accurately and concisely a multitude of references. However, the reader is reminded that times and medical knowledge change, transcription or understanding error is always possible, and crucial details are omitted whenever such a comprehensive distillation as this is attempted in limited space. And the primary purpose of this compilation is to cite literature on various sides of controversial issues; knowing where "truth" lies is usually difficult. We cannot, therefore, guarantee that every bit of information is absolutely accurate or complete. The reader should affirm that cited recommendations are reasonable still, by reading the original articles and checking other sources including local consultants as well as recent literature before applying them.

Drugs and medical devices are discussed that may have limited availability controlled by the Food and Drug Administration (FDA) for use only in research study or clinical trial. The drug information presented has been derived from reference sources, recently published data, and pharmaceutical tests. Research, clinical practice, and government regulations often change the accepted standard in this field. When consideration is being given to use of any drug in the clinical setting, the clinician or reader is responsible for determining FDA status of the drug, reading the package insert, and prescribing information for the most up-to-date recommendations on dose, precautions, and contraindications and determining the appropriate usage for the product. This is especially important in the case of drugs that are new or seldom used.

Chapter 1

Protocols for Emergency Treatment

The following protocols represent the current ACLS guidelines published in Circ 2000;102:suppl I. Readers are strongly encouraged to study the comprehensive discussions of therapy that accompany the flowcharts in that volume; see also Nejm 2001;344:1304.

1.1 Basic Life Support for Adults

CPR Performed by 1 Rescuer

1. ***Assessment:*** Determine unresponsiveness (tap or gently shake pt and shout). If unresponsive, activate the EMS system.
2. ***Airway:*** Position pt and open the airway by the head tilt-chin lift or jaw-thrust maneuver.
3. ***Breathing:*** Assess breathing to identify absent or inadequate breathing.
   - If pt is unresponsive *with normal breathing* and spinal injury is not suspected, place pt in a recovery position, maintaining an open airway. If adult pt is unresponsive and *not breathing*, provide 2 initial breaths.
   - If you are unable to give initial breaths, reposition the head and reattempt ventilation. If you are still unsuccessful in making the chest rise with each ventilation after an attempt and reattempt, follow the unresponsive FBAO sequence.

- Be sure the pt's chest rises with each rescue breath you provide. Once you deliver the effective breaths, assess for signs of circulation.

4. ***Circulation:*** Check for signs of circulation; look for normal breathing, coughing, or movement and feel for a carotid pulse (take no more than 10 sec to do this). If there are no signs of circulation, begin chest compressions: 15 chest compressions at rate of ~100/min, depressing chest 1½ to 2 in (4 to 5 cm) with each. Then open the airway and deliver 2 breaths; begin 15 more compressions at 100/min.
5. ***Reassessment:*** After 4 complete cycles of 15 compressions and 2 ventilations, reevaluate pt, checking for signs of circulation. If there are no signs of circulation, resume CPR, beginning with chest compressions.
   - If signs of circulation are present, check for breathing. If breathing is present, place pt in a recovery position and monitor breathing and circulation. If breathing is absent but signs of circulation are present, provide rescue breathing at 10-12 times/min and monitor for signs of circulation every few min.
   - If there are no signs of circulation, continue compressions and ventilations in a 15:2 ratio. Stop and check for signs of circulation and spontaneous breathing every few min. Do not interrupt CPR except in special circumstances.

CPR Performed by 2 Rescuers

In 2-rescuer CPR, one person is positioned at the pt's side and performs chest compressions while the other remains at the pt's head, maintains an open airway, monitors the carotid pulse, and provides rescue breathing. Compression rate is 100/min; compression–ventilation ratio is 15:2 with a pause for ventilation of 2 sec after each compression until airway is secured.

- To determine whether victim has resumed spontaneous breathing and circulation, chest compressions must be stopped for 10 sec at approximately the end of the first min of CPR and every few min thereafter.

- Prolonged CPR is frequently associated with increases of serum PSA; therefore, PSA cannot be used for dx of adenocarcinoma of prostate during the first weeks after CPR (Circ 2000; 102:290).

1.2 Foreign Body Airway Occlusion

Finger Sweep and Tongue-Jaw Lift (should be used only in unresponsive/unconscious pt with complete FBAO): With pt face up, open pt's mouth by grasping both the tongue and lower jaw between the thumb and fingers and lifting the mandible (tongue-jaw lift). This maneuver alone may be sufficient to relieve an obstruction.

Insert index finger of other hand deeply into pt's throat to base of tongue. Use a hooking action to dislodge the foreign body and maneuver it into the mouth. It is sometimes necessary to use the index finger to push the foreign body against the opposite side of the throat to dislodge and remove it.

Relief of FBAO in a Responsive Pt Who Becomes Unresponsive: If you observe the pt's collapse and you know it is caused by FBAO, activate the emergency response system, and perform the tongue-jaw lift and finger sweep to remove object; open the airway and try to ventilate.

- If you cannot deliver effective breaths (the chest does not rise) even after attempts to reposition the airway, consider FBAO. Straddle the pt's thighs and perform the Heimlich maneuver (up to 5 times). Repeat the sequence of tongue-jaw lift, finger sweep, attempt (and reattempt) to ventilate, and Heimlich maneuver until the obstruction is cleared and the chest rises with ventilation or advanced procedures are available (ie, Kelly clamp, Magill forceps, cricothyrotomy) to establish a patent airway.

- To deliver abdominal thrusts to the unresponsive/unconscious pt, kneel astride the pt's thighs and place the heel of one hand against the pt's abdomen, in the midline slightly above the navel and well below the tip of the xiphoid. Place second hand directly on top of the first, and press both hands into the abdomen with quick upward thrusts.

Relief of FBAO in a Pt Found Unresponsive: Activate the emergency response system; open the airway and attempt to provide rescue breaths.

- If pt cannot be ventilated even after attempts to reposition the airway, straddle the pt's knees and perform the Heimlich maneuver (up to 5 times). After 5 abdominal thrusts, open the pt's airway using a tongue-jaw lift and perform a finger sweep to remove the object. Repeat the sequence of attempts (and reattempts) to ventilate, Heimlich maneuver, and tongue-jaw lift and finger sweep until the obstruction is cleared or advanced procedures are available to establish a patent airway.
- In either case, if the FBAO is removed and the airway is cleared, check breathing. If the pt is not breathing, provide slow rescue breaths and check for signs of circulation (pulse check and evidence of breathing, coughing, or movement). If there are no signs of circulation, begin chest compressions.

1.3 Universal ACLS Algorithm

- For adult cardiac arrest: initiate Basic Life Support (above); assess rhythm and check pulse.
- If rhythm VT/VF, attempt to defibrillate up to 3 times as needed; then continue CPR for at least 1 min after shocks

or

- If rhythm is anything else (ie, PEA or asystole), continue CPR for at least 3 min

and then

- Reassess and continue CPR and administer epinephrine 1 mg iv q 3-5 min as needed.
- As an alternative, pts with VT/VF rhythms refractory to initial shocks may receive vasopressin 40 U iv one time only as initial agent, followed by epinephrine as needed.
- Search for/treat potentially reversible conditions such as hypovolemia, hypoxia, metabolic disorders, hypothermia, tamponade, and tension pneumothorax (Circ 2000;102:I-144).

1.4 Asystole/Pulseless Electrical Activity Algorithm

- Assess pt; initiate basic CPR; confirm rhythm.
- Exclude and/or treat reversible causes (hypovolemia, hypoxia, acidosis, hyper- or hypokalemia, hypothermia, drug ingestion, cardiac tamponade, tension pneumothorax, acute coronary syndrome, pulmonary embolus).
- Transcutaneous pacing for asystole (routine use not recommended).
- $NaHCO_3$ 1 mEq/kg iv for hyperkalemia, tricyclic antidepressant or ASA overdose, prolonged arrest, or known acidosis.
- Epinephrine 1 mg iv q 3-5 min.
- Atropine 1 mg iv q 3-5 min as needed; maximum total dose 0.04 mg/kg (Circ 2000;102:I-151).

1.5 Bradycardia Algorithm

- Establish presence of bradycardia (HR < 60/min).
- Identify rhythm.
- If serious si/sx due to bradycardia present
  Atropine 0.5-1.0 mg iv
  Transcutaneous pacing
  Dopamine 5-20 μgm/kg/min iv
  Epinephrine 2-10 μgm/min iv

- If pt asymptomatic but Mobitz II second-degree block or complete heart block present, prepare for transvenous pacemaker placement; rx as above if sx develop (Circ 2000;102:I-156).

1.6 Tachycardia Overview Algorithm

- Determine if pt is hemodynamically stable and/or has sx.
  If pt is unstable or symptomatic, prepare for immediate cardioversion.
- Otherwise:

If rhythm is Aflut/Afib, assess LV systolic function, presence of WPW, and duration of arrhythmia and initiate anticoagulation.

If duration > 48 hr or unknown:

- Anticoagulation for 3-4 wk before cardioversion or iv heparin and TEE; may cardiovert if no thrombus seen. Control rate with β-blockers or slowing Ca^{++}-channel blockers if LV function normal; diltiazem, digoxin, or amiodarone if LV function abnormal.
- Anticoagulate minimum of 4 wk after cardioversion.

If duration < 48 hr:

- If LV systolic function normal, may consider use of amiodarone, flecanide, propafenone, procainamide, sotalol, or DC cardioversion; may also use these agents if WPW present but should avoid use of adenosine, digoxin, β-blockers, or slowing Ca^{++}-channel blockers.
- If LV systolic function impaired, use amiodarone or DC cardioversion; rx same if WPW present.

If rhythm is narrow complex tachycardia:

- Try to differentiate between PSVT, MAT, junctional tachycardia using EKG, vagal maneuvers, iv adenosine.
- Proceed according to Stable Narrow Complex Tachycardia Algorithm (p 8).

If rhythm is stable wide complex tachycardia of unknown type:

- Try to differentiate between aberrant conduction of SV rhythm using clinical data, EKG, esophageal lead.
- If SVT confirmed, proceed according to Stable Narrow Complex Tachycardia Algorithm (p 8).
- If VT confirmed, proceed according to Stable VT Algorithm (p 7).
- If uncertain, proceed with DC cardioversion or administration of amiodarone; procainamide also a choice if LV systolic function normal (EF > 40%, no clinical CHF) (Circ 2000;102:I-159).

PROTOCOLS FOR EMERGENCY TREATMENT

1.7 Ventricular Fibrillation/Pulseless VT Algorithm

- Initiate CPR.
- Shock up to 3 times (200, 200-300, and 360 J) as needed.
- If arrhythmia persists:

  Epinephrine 1 mg iv; repeat q 3-5 min

  or

  Vasopressin, 40 U iv (single dose, 1 time only)

  Defibrillate (360 J) within 30-60 sec
- If no success:

  Consider administration of amiodarone, lidocaine, Mg^{++}, or procainamide.

  Resume defibrillation at 360 J after each medication or after each min of CPR (Circ 2000;102:I-147).

1.8 Stable Ventricular Tachycardia Algorithm

- May proceed with immediate cardioversion

  or
- If rhythm is monomorphic VT:

  Administer lidocaine 0.5-0.75 mg/kg iv push (repeat in 5-10 min to maximum of 3 mg/kg in 1 hr) or amiodarone

150 mg iv over 10 min (may repeat q 10-15 min) and then cardiovert if LV function is poor.

Sotalol and procainamide are preferred agents if LV function is normal.

- If rhythm is polymorphic VT, check electrolytes.
  Administer Mg^{++}, isoproterenol, phenytoin, or lidocaine or use overdrive pacing if QT baseline interval is prolonged (suggests torsades de pointes).
  If QT normal, administer β-blockers, lidocaine, amiodarone, sotalol, or procainamide, or amiodarone or lidocaine followed by cardioversion if LV function abnormal (Circ 2000;102:I-163).

1.9 Stable Narrow Complex Tachycardia Algorithm

- Vagal stimulation or iv adenosine to assess arrhythmia.
- If rhythm is junctional tachycardia:
  Do not cardiovert.
  Administer amiodarone, β-blocker, or Ca^{++}-channel blocker if LV function normal; use amiodarone if LV function impaired.
- If rhythm is paroxysmal SVT:
  Choices (in order of preference) if LV function is normal: Ca^{++}-channel blocker, β-blocker, digoxin, cardioversion; may also consider amiodarone, sotalol, or procainamide.
  If LV function is impaired, choices (in order of preference) are digoxin, amiodarone, or diltiazem with avoidance of cardioversion.
- If rhythm is ectopic/multifocal atrial tachycardia, avoid cardioversion and administer amiodarone or slowing Ca^{++}-channel blocker; may also use β-blocker if LV function is normal (Circ 2000;102:I-162).

1.10 Acute Pulmonary Edema/Shock Algorithm

- Assess pt.
- If problem appears to be rate/rhythm related: Refer to appropriate arrhythmia algorithm.
- If problem appears to be acute pulmonary edema: Administer furosemide 0.5-1.0 mg/kg iv, morphine sulfate 2-4 mg iv, TNG 0.4 mg sl, O_2.
- If problem appears to be volume depletion: Administer fluids; consider blood transfusion, cause-specific interventions

and in either case

- Measure BP.
  If BP < 70 mm Hg, start norepinephrine 0.5-30 μgm/min iv.
  If BP 70-100 mm Hg, start dopamine 5-15 μgm/kg/min iv if si/sx shock present **or** dobutamine 2-20 μgm/kg/min if no si/sx shock present.
  If BP > 100 mm Hg, start TNG 10-20 μgm/min iv or consider nitroprusside 0.1-5.0 μgm/kg/min iv.
  Consider PA catheter, IABP, anigiography, or other studies (Circ 2000;102:I-189).

1.11 Suspected Stroke Algorithm

- Perform stroke screen: Look for facial droop, arm drift or weakness, abnormal speech.
- Obtain vital signs, EKG; check CBC, glucose, electrolytes, coagulation studies.
- Administer O_2.
- Full neurological exam, noncontrast CT scan.
- Lateral cervical spine film if pt is comatose or has hx of trauma.
- If CT scan shows intracerebral/subarachnoid hemorrhage: Reverse anticoagulants, treat bleeding disorders, treat HT in awake pts.

- If CT scan shows no hemorrhage: If suspicion of subarachnoid hemorrhage remains high, perform LP.
- Otherwise:
  Repeat neuro exam, checking for signs of variable/rapidly improving deficits.
  If no improvement, review fibrinolytic exclusions. If none present and sx onset < 3 hr, may consider thrombolytic rx (Circ 2000;102:I-205).

1.12 Antihypertensive Rx in Acute Stroke

In pts who are thrombolytic candidates, if systolic BP > 185 or diastolic BP > 110 mm Hg, apply 1-2″ topical TNG paste or administer labetolol (if not contraindicated) 10-20 mg iv push. Thrombolytic agents are contraindicated if BP does not respond.

During/after rx with thrombolytics:

- If diastolic BP > 140 mm Hg, start nitroprusside 0.5 μcg/kg/min iv.
- If systolic BP > 230 or diastolic BP 121-140 mm Hg, give labetolol 10-20 mg iv push over 1-2 min if not contraindicated. Repeat q 10 min (maximum 150 mg) or start infusion at 2-8 mg/min iv and consider nitroprusside if BP not controlled.
- If systolic BP 180-230 or diastolic BP 105-120 mm Hg, give labetolol 10-20 mg iv push over 1-2 min if not contraindicated. Repeat q 10 min (maximum 150 mg) or start infusion at 2-8 mg/min iv.

If pt ineligible for thrombolytic rx:

- If diastolic BP > 140 mm Hg, start nitroprusside 0.5 μgm/kg/min iv.
- If systolic BP > 230, diastolic BP 121-140, or MAP > 130 mm Hg, give labetolol 10-20 mg iv push over 1-2 min if not contraindicated; repeat q 10 min (maximum 150 mg).

- If systolic BP < 220, diastolic BP < 120, or MAP < 130 mm Hg, do not rx BP unless aortic dissection, acute MI, CHF, or hypertensive encephalopathy present.

1.13 Hypothermia Algorithm

Place pt supine, remove wet garments, and monitor cardiac rhythm and core temperature.

If pulse and respiration present:

- If core temperature 34-36°C, passive rewarming (blankets, warm room) and active external rewarming (warm packs, forced hot air, warm water bath).
- If core temperature 30-34°C, passive rewarming and active external rewarming of truncal areas only.
- If core temperature < 30°C, active internal rewarming (iv fluids at 43°C, warm humid O_2 at 42-46°C, peritoneal lavage, esophageal rewarming tubes, extracorporeal warming) until core temperature > 35°C.

If pulse or breathing absent:

- Initiate CPR; secure airway.
- Defibrillate up to 3 times (see VF/Pulseless VT Algorithm).
- Administer iv fluids at 43°C, warm humid O_2 at 42-46°C.
- If core temperature rises > 30°C, continue with VF algorithm but administer iv medications at longer than standard intervals. If core temperature remains < 30°C, continue CPR and active rewarming but withhold iv medications (Circ 2000;102:I-230).

Table 1.1 Electrolyte Imbalance

Condition	Causes	Si & Sx	Rx
Hyperkalemia ($K^+ > 5$ mEq/L)	Drugs (K^+-sparing diuretics, ACEIs, NSAIDs, potassium supplements) End-stage renal disease Muscle breakdown (rhabdomyolysis) Metabolic acidosis Hemolysis Tumor lysis syndrome Hypoaldosteronism (Addison disease, hyporeninemia) Type 4 renal tubular acidosis Other: hyperkalemic periodic paralysis	Weakness Ascending paralysis Respiratory failure EKG findings: • Peaked T waves (tenting) • Flattened P waves • Prolonged PR interval (1° heart block) • Widened QRS complex • Deepened S waves; merging of S and T waves • Idioventricular rhythm • Sine-wave formation • VF and cardiac arrest	*Mild* (5–6 mEq/L) • Diuretics: furosemide 1 mg/kg iv slowly • Resins: Kayexalate 15-30 gm in 50-100 mL 20% sorbitol po or by retention enema (50 gm Kayexalate) • Dialysis: peritoneal or hemodialysis *Moderate* (6-7 mEq/L) • $NaHCO_3$: 50 mEq iv over 5 min • Glucose + insulin: 50 gm glucose and 10 U regular glucose and 10 U regular insulin iv over 15-30 min • Nebulized albuterol: 10-20 mg over 15 min *Severe* (> 7 mEq/L with toxic EKG changes) • 10% $CaCl_2$: 5-10 mL iv over 2-5 min • $NaHCO_3$: 50 mEq iv over 5 min • Glucose + insulin: 50 gm glucose and 10 U regular insulin iv over 15-30 min • Nebulized albuterol: 10-20 mg over 15 min

			Furosemide: 40-80 mg iv Kayexalate enema Dialysis
Hypokalemia ($K^+ < 3.5$ mEq/L)	GI loss (diarrhea, laxatives) Renal loss (hyperaldosteronism, K^+-losing diuretics, carbenicillin, sodium penicillin, amphotericin B) Intracellular shift (alkalosis) Malnutrition	Weakness, fatigue, paralysis Respiratory difficulty Rhabdomyolysis Constipation, paralytic ileus Leg cramps EKG findings: • U waves • T-wave flattening • ST-segment changes • Arrhythmias Pulseless electrical activity or asystole	• K^+ administration: maximum iv K^+ replacement 10-20 mEq/hr with continuous EKG monitoring (more concentrated solution may be infused if central line is used; catheter tip should not extend into the RA) • If cardiac arrest imminent, give initial infusion of 2 mEq/min, followed by another 10 mEq iv over 5-10 min; document that rapid infusion is intentional in response to life-threatening hypokalemia • Estimates of total body deficit of K^+ range from 150 to 400 mEq for every 1 mEq decrease in serum K^+
Hypernatremia ($Na^+ > 145$ mEq/L)	Free water loss in excess of sodium loss (diabetes insipidus, hypernatremic dehydration)	Thirst Altered mental status Weakness Irritability Focal neurological deficits Coma, seizures	• Free water replacement: water deficit (L) = (plasma Na^+ concentration − 140)/140) × total body water (~50% of lean body wt in men; 40% in women)

Table 1.1 continued

Condition	Causes	Si & Sx	Rx
			• Administer fluid to lower serum Na^+ 0.5-1.0 mEq/hr; correction should be achieved over 48-72 hr • Replace fluid in asymptomatic pts by mouth or NG tube; if clinical status unstable, give D5/0.45 NaCl iv
Hyponatremia $Na^+ < 135$ mEq/L)	Thiazide diuretics Renal failure ECF depletion (eg, vomiting with continued water intake) Edematous states (CHF, cirrhosis with ascites, etc) Hypothyroidism Adrenal insufficiency "Tea and toast" diet Excessive beer drinking Uncontrolled diabetes mellitus SIADH (trauma, increased intracranial pressure, cancer, respiratory failure)	Frequently asymptomatic; $Na^+ < 120$ mEq/L may produce cerebral edema with nausea, vomiting, headache, irritability, lethargy, seizures, coma	• Restrict fluid intake • In asymptomatic pts, administer NaCl for maximum change of 10-15 mEq/L in first 24 hr (rapid correction can cause pontine myelinolysis) • For pt with neurological compromise, give 3% NaCl iv at 1 mEq/L/hr until neurological sx controlled; then correct at rate of 0.5 mEq/L/hr • Na^+ deficit in mEq = (desired $[Na^+]$ − Current $[Na^+]$) × 0.6 × body wt (kg) (use 0.5 for women); deficit/513 mEq = volume of 3% NaCl (L) needed

Hypermagnesemia $Mg^+ > 2.2$ mEq/L)	Renal failure Perforated viscus with continued intake of food Laxatives/antacids containing Mg^+	Muscular weakness, paralysis, ataxia Drowsiness, confusion Nausea/vomiting Vasodilation, hypotension Depressed level of consciousness, bradycardia, hypoventilation, cardiorespiratory arrest EKG abnormalities: • Increased PR and QT intervals • Increased QRS duration • Variable decrease in P = wave voltage • Variable degree of T-wave peaking • Complete AV block, asystole	• $CaCl_2$: 5-10 mEq iv; repeat if needed • Dialysis is the treatment of choice; if renal function normal and cardiovascular function adequate, iv saline diuresis with normal saline + furosemide, 1 mEq/kg; diuresis can also increase Ca excretion; development of hypocalcemia will make si/sx of hypermagnesemia worse
Hypomagnesemia $Mg^+ < 1.3$ mEq/L)	Bowel resection Pancreatitis Diarrhea Renal disease Starvation	Hypocalcemia Hypokalemia Muscular tremors, fasciculations, tetany Ocular nystagmus	• For severe/symptomatic hypomagnesemia, administer 1-2 gm iv $MgSO_4$ over 15 min • If torsades de pointes present, administer 2 gm $MgSO_4$ over 1-2 min

Table 1.1 continued

Condition	Causes	Si & Sx	Rx
	Drugs: • Diuretics • Pentamidine • Gentamicin • Digoxin Alcohol Hypothermia Hypercalcemia Diabetic ketoacidosis Hyperthyroidism Hypothyroidism Phosphate deficiency Burns Sepsis Lactation	Altered mentation Ataxia, vertigo Seizures Dysphagia EKG findings: • Prolonged QT and PR intervals • ST-segment depression • T-wave inversion • Flattening/inversion of precordial P waves • Widening of QRS • Torsades de pointes • Treatment-resistant VF • Worsening of digitalis toxicity	• If seizures present, administer 2 gm iv $MgSO_4$ over 10 min • Calcium gluconate administration (1 gm) usually appropriate; most pts with hypomagnesemia are also hypocalcemic • Replace Mg cautiously in patients with renal insufficiency
Hypercalcemia ($Ca^{++} > 10.5$ mEq/L)	Primary hyperparathyroidism Malignancy Acidosis will produce increase in ionized Ca^{++} level	Depression Weakness, fatigue Confusion, hallucinations, disorientation, hypotonicity, coma Dehydration	• In pts with adequate cardiovascular and renal function: 0.9% NaCl at 300-500 mL/hr until diuresis occurs; then iv NaCl at 100-200 mL/hr; monitor serum K^+, Mg^{++}

		Myocardial depression: decreased automaticity, arrhythmias, worsening digitalis toxicity Hypertension Hypokalemia Dysphagia Constipation Peptic ulcer Pancreatitis EKG findings: • Shorted QT interval • Prolonged PR and QRS intervals • Increased QRS voltage • T-wave flattening and widening • Notching of QRS • AV block; complete heart block; cardiac arrest	• Hemodialysis is rx of choice in pts with CHF or renal insufficiency • Chelating agents may be used for extreme conditions (eg, 50 mmol PO_4 over 8-12 hr or EDTA 10-50 mg/kg over 4 hr) • Use of furosemide (1 mg/kg iv) is controversial; use is required in CHF, but can foster reuptake of Ca^{++} from bone, thus worsening hypercalcemia
Hypocalcemia $Ca^{++} < 8.2$ mEq/L)	Toxic shock syndrome Abnormalities in serum Mg^{++}	Parasthesias, muscle cramps, carpopedal	• 10% calcium gluconate, 90-180 mg of elemental Ca^{++} iv over 10 min,

Table 1.1 continued

Condition	Causes	Si & Sx	Rx
	Tumor lysis syndrome Concentration of ionized Ca^{++} is pH-dependent: alkalosis reduces ionized Ca^{++}; total serum Ca^{++} dependent on serum albumin concentration (adjust total serum Ca^{++} by 0.8 mg/dL for every 1 g/m change in serum albumin)	spasm, stridor, tetany, seizures Hyperreflexia, positive Chvostek and Trousseau signs CHF Exacerbation of digitalis toxicity EKG findings: • QT-interval prolongation • Terminal T-wave inversion • Heart block • VF	followed by 540-720 mg of elemental Ca^{++} in 500-1000 mL D_5W at 0.5-2.0 mg/kg/hr (10-15 mg/kg); measure serum Ca^{++} every 4-6 hr • Abnormalities in Mg, K, and pH must be corrected simultaneously; untreated hypomagnesemia will make hypocalcemia refractory to therapy

(Circ 2000;102:I-217)

Chapter 2

Physical Examination

2.1 Examination of the Heart

Inspection/Palpation

Table 2.1 Physical Findings on Inspection/Palpation of the Chest

Location	Finding
Aortic area (2nd RICS)	Pulsation of aortic aneurysm Thrill from aortic stenosis Accentuated aortic valve closure (hypertension)
Pulmonary area (2nd-3rd LICS)	Pulsation of increased pressure/flow in PA Thrill from pulmonary stenosis Accentuated pulmonary valve closure (pulmonary hypertension)
RV area (lower half of sternum and subxyphoid area)	Sustained systolic lift from RV hypertrophy Thrill from VSD Prominent RV impulse in thin pts from fever, anxiety, anemia, hyperthyroidism, pregnancy
LV area (5th LICS just past midclavicular line)	Apical impulse • *Normal:* light tap or absent, lasts < half of systole, occupies one interspace • *Abnormal:* forceful, sustained up to S2, laterally displaced, diffuse (occupies > 1 interspace) Thrill of mitral disease Palpable S3
Epigastrium	Increased aortic pulse from aortic aneurysm or aortic regurgitation

Table 2.2 Findings on Palpation of Cardiac Impulse

Movement	Features
Normal	Within MCL 4th or 5th LICS
Hyperkinetic Apical Impulse Normal child Hyperdynamic states VSD PDA Aortic or mitral regurgitation	Exaggerated thrust at cardiac apex (coincident with S3, if present)
Sustained Apical Impulse Aortic stenosis Systemic hypertension	Maximal at apex; coincident with S4
Hyperkinetic RV Impulse ASD Pulmonary regurgitation	Maximal at LSB 3rd-4th LICS
Sustained RV Impulse Pulmonary hypertension Pulmonary stenosis	Maximal at LSB, 3rd-4th LICS
Ectopic LV Impulse Ventricular aneurysm	Maximal over mid-precordium

Auscultation of Heart Sounds

First Heart Sound (S1): Produced mostly by mitral valve closure; equal to/louder than S2 at apex, softer than S2 at base, synchronous with apical impulse, just precedes carotid impulse; accentuated with tachycardia (anxiety, exercise, anemia, hyperthyroidism, etc) and in mitral stenosis (mitral valve is still open widely at onset of ventricular systole); can be diminished in first-degree AV block; variable with heart block and very irregular heart rhythm (eg, Afib and other chaotic rhythms); splitting may be present and is usually best heard in tricuspid area (fifth LICS just lateral to sternum); differentiate split S1 from S4 or early systolic click by timing, variation, character of sounds

Second Heart Sound (S2): Usually louder than S1 at base; physiological splitting accentuated during inspiration, disappears during exhalation; wide and persistent splitting can be heard with early A2 (MR, VSD, WPW), electrical delay (RBBB, LV PVC, WPW) or mechanical delay (pulmonary stenosis or subvalvular pulmonary obstruction, large PE, RV dysfunction) of P2, dilated pulmonary artery, ASD; paradoxical splitting may accompany TR, electrical delay (LBBB, RV PVC, RV pacemaker, CAD) of mechanical delay (AS, hypertrophic cardiomyopathy, CAD, PDA, AI) of A2

Table 2.3 Ascultation of Heart Sounds

Finding	Possible Cause
Normal	Physiologic splitting
Normal, P2 > A2	Pulmonary HT
	Aortic stenosis
Narrow, fixed splitting	Pulmonary HT
Wide, fixed split	RBBB
	Pulmonary stenosis
	Partial anomalous pulmonary venous return
	ASD
	MI
Paradoxical (reversed) splitting	PDA with L-to-R shunt
	Tricuspid regurgitation
	LBBB
	Aortic stenosis
	Ischemia
Pseudo-splitting	S2 plus opening snap
	S2 plus S3
	S2 plus pericardial knock
	S2 plus tumor plop

PHYSICAL EXAMINATION

Third Heart Sound (S3): Low-pitched sound occurring in early diastole during rapid ventricular filling; may arise from either ventricle; typically best heard at apex in left lateral decubitus position; may be normal finding in children and young adults; pathological finding in pts > 40 yr; associated with ventricular dysfunction of any cause, increased early diastolic filling (hyperkinetic states, mitral/tricuspid regurgitation, left to right shunts), restrictive/constrictive pericarditis

Fourth Heart Sound (S4): Low-pitched sound occurring just before S1 at/medial to apex; can occur in children as benign finding; in disease is associated with increased resistance to ventricular filling (acute ischemia, LV aneurysm, hypertensive heart disease, dilated or hypertrophic cardiomyopathy, aortic stenosis, systemic or pulmonary HT), increased late diastolic filling (anemia, thyrotoxicosis, AV fistula, acute mitral or tricuspid regurgitation), or delayed AV conduction

Systolic Click: High-pitched sound; early sounds (just after S1) in aortic or pulmonary areas are ejection sounds that may indicate dilation of aorta or main PA, systemic or pulmonary HT, or aortic or pulmonary stenosis (due to opening of stenotic but mobile valve cusps); mid/late systolic clicks heard in mitral valve prolapse syndrome

Opening Snap: Early diastolic high-pitched sound heard in mitral stenosis; valve must be stenotic but mobile; can be confused with widely split S2, but S2-OS interval decreases during inspiration

Heart Murmurs

Characterization and Etiology (Circ 2005;111:e20): See Tables 2.4, 2.5, and 2.6.

Changes with Respiration: During inspiration, right-sided systolic murmurs due to tricuspid regurgitation, pulmonary stenosis, increased flow across normal pulmonary valve, and diastolic

Table 2.4 Systolic Murmurs

Example	Aortic stenosis	Pulmonic stenosis	Mitral regurgitation	Tricuspid regurgitation	VSD
Source	Aortic valve	Pulmonic valve	Mitral valve	Tricuspid valve	VSD
Type	Mid-systolic flow murmur	Mid-systolic flow murmur	Holosystolic regurgitant murmur; late systolic in MVP	Holosystolic regurgitant murmur	Holosystolic regurgitant murmur
Location	2nd RICS; apex	2nd-3rd LICS close to sternum	5th LICS at MCL	4th-5th LICS close to sternum	4th-6th LICS, left sternal border
Radiation	Into carotids; along LSB	Toward left shoulder and neck	Into left axilla	To right of sternum, to LMCL	Across precordium
Intensity	Variable	Variable	Variable; does not increase during inspiration	Variable; increases during inspiration	Frequently loud
Pitch	Medium	Medium	High	High	High
Quality	Often harsh	Often harsh	Blowing	Blowing	Harsh
Possible Associated Findings	Decreased S2 sustained apical impulse, slowed carotid upstroke	Widely split S2, diminished P2, RV lift	Displaced/diffuse PMI, decreased S1, S3 gallop	RV lift, pulsatile liver	

Table 2.5 Diastolic and Continuous Murmurs and Sounds

Typical Lesion	Aortic regurgitation	Mitral stenosis	Pericardial rub	PDA	Venous hum
Source	Aortic valve	Mitral valve	Pericardium	PDA	Jugular veins
Type	Diastolic murmur	Diastolic murmur	Rub with atrial systole, ventricular systole and diastole	Continuous murmur, fades in diastole	Continuous murmur
Location	2nd RICS, LICS	5th LICS at MCL	Usually 3rd LICS but variable	2nd LICS	Above medial portion of clavicles
Radiation	LSB, RSB	Little radiation	Little radiation	Toward left clavicle	1st and 2nd interspaces
Intensity	Variable	Variable; frequently soft	Variable	Loud	Soft/moderate
Pitch	High	Low	High	Medium	Low
Quality	Blowing	Rumbling	Scratchy	Harsh, "machinery-like"	Humming
Possible Associated Findings	Aortic flow murmur, S3 gallop	Increased S1, increased P2, opening snap, RV lift		Loudest in late systole, obscuring S2	Loudest in diastole, may be obliterated by pressure on jugular veins

Table 2.6 Causes of Heart Murmurs

Timing	Source	Examples/Comments
1. Midsystolic (ejection) murmurs	Obstructive aortic lesions	Supra-aortic stenosis, coarctation
		Valvular aortic stenosis/sclerosis
		Obstructive hypertrophic cardiomyopathy
	Increased aortic flow	Hyperkinetic states
		Aortic regurgitation
		Complete heart block
	Dilated ascending aorta	Aortitis
		Ascending aortic aneurysm
	Obstructive pulmonary lesions	Pulmonary artery stenosis
		Pulmonary valve stenosis
		Infundibular pulmonary stenosis
	Increased pulmonary flow	Hyperkinetic states
		L-to-R shunts (ASD, VSD)
	Dilated pulmonary artery	
2. Pansystolic (regurgitant) murmurs	AV valve regurgitation	Mitral regurgitation
		Tricuspid regurgitation
	L-to-R shunt	
3. Early diastolic murmurs	Valvular aortic regurgitation	Rheumatic valvular disease
		Post-endocarditis perforation
		Traumatic
		Post-valvulotomy

continues

Table 2.6 continued

Timing	Source	Examples/Comments
	Dilation of aortic valve ring	Aortic dissection
		Cystic medial necrosis
		HT
	Widening of aortic commissures	Syphilis
	Congenital	Bicuspid valve
	Valvular pulmonary regurgitation	Post-valvulotomy
		Endocarditis
		Rheumatic fever
		Carcinoid
	Dilation of pulmonary valve ring	Pulmonary HT
		Marfan syndrome
	Congenital	Isolated pulmonary regurgitation
		With tetralogy of Fallot
		With VSD
		With congenital pulmonary stenosis

4. Mid-diastolic murmurs	Mitral stenosis	
	Increased flow across anatomically normal mitral valve	Mitral regurgitation VSD PDA High-output states Complete heart block
	Tricuspid stenosis	
	Increased flow across anatomically normal mitral valve	Tricuspid regurgitation ASD Anomalous pulmonary venous return
	Acute rheumatic fever	Carey-Coombs murmur
	Atrial tumors	
5. Continuous murmurs	PDA	
	Ruptured AV fistula	
	ASD	
	Cervical venous hum	
	Anomalous origin of left coronary artery	
	Mammary souffle	
	Bronchial collateral circulation	

murmur of tricuspid stenosis tend to increase. Murmurs rising from left side are typically louder during expiration.

Positional Changes: With standing, most murmurs diminish; murmur of obstructive hypertrophic cardiomyopathy becomes louder, and murmur of MVP becomes longer and often louder. With squatting, most murmurs increase. Exceptions are hypertrophic cardiomyopathy and MVP.

Valsalva Maneuver: Most murmurs decrease in duration and intensity during Valsalva strain. Murmur of obstructive hypertrophic cardiomyopathy becomes louder; murmur of MVP becomes longer and often louder as well.

Exercise: Murmurs due to flow across normal/stenotic valves increase with exercise. Murmurs of aortic and mitral regurgitation and VSD also increase with handgrip exercise, but murmurs of hypertrophic cardiomyopathy often decrease with handgrip exercise.

Effects of Premature Beats: Due to pause following APC or PVC, flow murmurs arising from semilunar valves increase. Murmurs due to regurgitation across AV valve do not change or become shorter (MVP).

Transient Arterial Occlusion: Compression of both arms with cuff inflation (20 mm Hg above systolic BP) produces an increase in murmurs of aortic and mitral regurgitation and VSD.

Amyl Nitrite: Early (hypotensive) response: murmur of aortic stenosis/sclerosis and hypertrophic cardiomyopathy increase, murmurs of aortic and mitral regurgitation and VSD decrease. Late (tachycardia) phase: right-sided murmurs and murmur of MS increase; Austin Flint murmur (mitral diastolic murmur in severe aortic regurgitation) decreases. MVP may produce biphasic response with murmur first diminishing and then increasing; administration of phenylephrine produces opposite responses.

Sensitivity/Specificity: See Table 2.7.

Table 2.7 Differentiation of Murmurs

Maneuver	Murmur	Response	Sensitivity (%)	Specificity (%)
Inspiration	All right-sided	Increase	100	88
Expiration	All right-sided	Decrease	100	88
Valsalva	Hypertrophic cardiomyopathy	Increase	65	96
Stand → squat	Hypertrophic cardiomyopathy	Decrease	95	85
Squat → stand	Hypertrophic cardiomyopathy	Increase	95	84
Leg elevation	Hypertrophic cardiomyopathy	Decrease	85	91
Handgrip	Hypertrophic cardiomyopathy	Decrease	85	75
Handgrip	Mitral regurgitation VSD	Increase	68	92
Transient arterial occlusion	Mitral regurgitation VSD	Increase	78	100
Amyl nitrite	Mitral regurgitation VSD	Decrease	80	90

(Nejm 1988;318:1572)

2.2 Evaluation of Pulses

Jugular Venous Pulses

Examination Technique: Pillow under head, head of exam table at 45°; top of visible vein normally < 4 cm above sternal angle (RA usually 5 cm below sternal angle in this position)

Jugular venous pressure increased in RV failure, tricuspid valve disease, pericardial constriction or tamponade, obstruction of SVC

Normal pulse consists of 4 components: A wave with atrial contraction, X descent with atrial relaxation, V wave in late ventricular systole, Y descent in early ventricular diastole; C wave visible after A wave is reflection of carotid pulse

Jugular pulses can be distinguished from carotid impulses by their several components: Elimination with light pressure, increase with recumbent position, decrease with inspiration

A wave prominent when RA emptying impeded (tricuspid stenosis) or in RVH (pulmonary HT, pulmonic stenosis); A wave absent in Afib; V wave prominent in tricuspid regurgitation; X and Y descents prominent in constrictive pericarditis; X descent prominent in tamponade

Hepatojugular Reflux: Sustained (30-60 sec) pressure applied to RUQ produces > 1 cm increase in JVD indicative of CHF

Kussmaul's Sign: Paradoxical rise in jugular venous pressure during inspiration; can be seen with constrictive pericarditis, tricuspid stenosis (increased venous return not accommodated by right ventricle)

Table 2.8 Assessment of Carotid Arterial Pulse

Finding	Diagnosis
Small weak pulse	Decreased stroke volume (CHF, shock), aortic stenosis
Large bounding pulse	Hyperkinetic states, aortic regurgitation, PDA, increased aortic rigidity (atherosclerosis)
Pulsus alternans	Left-sided heart failure (pulse must be regular)
Bigeminal pulse	Arrhythmia
Pulsus paradoxicus	Constrictive pericarditis, pericardial tamponade, severe COPD
Diagnosis	**Findings**
Anemia, fever, thyrotoxicosis	Increased amplitude and rate
Shock	Reduced amplitude
Aortic stenosis	Slowed upstroke, prolonged duration, pulsus parvus et tardus
Aortic regurgitation	Rapid rise and runoff, may have 2 peaks
Obstructive hypertrophic cardiomyopathy	Bisferiens: rapid rise, abrupt peak and plateau
LV failure	Low amplitude; alternans pulse (strong and weak pulses alternate)
Tamponade or constrictive pericarditis	Pulsus paradoxicus (exaggerated decrease during inspiration)
AV fistula	Rapid rise and runoff

Chapter 3

The EKG

3.1 Abnormal EKG Findings

Table 3.1 P-Wave, QRS-Complex, ST-Segment, and T-Wave Abnormalities

Finding	Diagnostic Criteria
P Wave	
Right atrial enlargement/abnormality (P pulmonale)	P-wave amplitude > 2.5 mm in leads II, III, and aVF with P-wave duration < 0.12 sec; initial positive component of P-wave in lead VI > 1.5 mm; P-wave axis in frontal plane > +75°
Left atrial enlargement/abnormality (P mitrale)	P-wave duration ≥ 0.12 sec and P waves notched in leads I, II, and aVL; abnormal P terminal force in lead V1; P-wave axis in frontal plane is leftward of +15°
Biatrial enlargement/abnormality	Abnormal P terminal force combined with an initial positive P-wave component > 1.5 mm in lead VI; combined wide (> 0.12 sec) and tall (> 2.5 mm) P waves in limb leads
QRS Complex	
Left axis deviation	A frontal plane QRS between −30° and −90°
Right axis deviation (Table 3.3)	A frontal plane QRS between +90° and +270°
Low voltage	Sum of R and S waves in limb leads ≤ 5 mm; sum of R and S waves in precordial leads ≤ 10 mm
Poor R-wave progression	R waves are present in leads V1–V3 but magnitude of R waves in each of the 3 leads ≤ 3.0 mm, and LBBB, pre-excitation (WPW), or criteria for low voltage (above) are not present

continues

Table 3.1 continued

Finding	Diagnostic Criteria
rSR′ V1	rSR′ complex is of normal duration; primary R wave < 8 mm; R′ < 6 mm; R′/S ratio < 1
Electrical alternans	Regular alternation of amplitude of the P, QRS, and/or T waves in complexes originating from a single pacemaker
ST-T Findings/U Waves	
J-point evaluation	1–4 mm upward displacement of ST segment at J junction with upward concavity; T waves are frequently tall, broad, and symmetric
Persistent juvenile T-wave pattern	T-wave inversion in V1 and V2 in an otherwise normal adult
Nonspecific ST-T abnormality	Slight ST depression, ST elevation, or isolated T-wave inversion or other abnormality that cannot be characterized as secondary to a specific abnormality
ST-T abnormalities associated with ventricular hypertrophy	LVH: ST depression with downward concavity and T-wave inversion in left precordial leads; same ST-T changes may be present in leads I, aVL if QRS axis horizontal, or in leads II, III, and aVF with a vertical axis RVH: ST depression with downward concavity and T-wave inversion in right precordial leads
ST-T abnormalities associated with ventricular conduction abnormalities	LBBB: ST depression and T-wave inversion in left precordial leads RBBB: ST depression and T-wave inversion in right precordial leads
Possible myocardial ischemia	Horizontal/downsloping ST depression with or without T-wave inversion in the absence of concomitant ST elevation in additional leads
Possible acute myocardial injury	Horizontal/concave downward ST-segment elevation with or without T-wave inversion; ST depression with upright T wave in leads V1–V2 (posterior wall injury); horizontal/downsloping ST depression with or without T-wave abnormalities in leads opposite those with the ST elevations can reflect ischemia or reciprocal change

Table 3.1 continued

Finding	Diagnostic Criteria
ST-T abnormalities associated with acute pericarditis	Diffuse ST-segment elevation (concave upward) in multiple leads, especially leads I, II, and V5–V6; T wave remains concordant with direction of ST segment in early pericarditis
Digitalis effect	Flattening or inversion of T wave; "sagging" ST segment (down-sloping ST depression, concave upward); slight shortening of QT interval
Peaked T wave	T-wave amplitude $>$ 6 mm in limb leads or $>$ 10 mm in any precordial lead
Post-PVC T-wave abnormality	Nonspecific change in T-wave morphology of sinus beat following PVC
Prolonged QT interval	Corrected QT interval (QTc) = QT interval $\div$ (sq root of R-R interval); upper limit of normal for QTc usually 0.44 sec; approximation formula: QT upper limit 0.40 sec for heart rate of 70, add/subtract 0.02 sec for every 10-beat increase/decrease in heart rate
U Waves	
U waves	U wave usually $\leq$ 1.0 mm; amplitude is proportional to T wave; should be no greater than 25% of height of T wave; U-wave inversion in leads with a normally upright T wave are abnormal

THE EKG

Table 3.2 AV Conduction Abnormalities

Conduction Abnormality	Diagnostic Criteria
1° AV block	Sinus rhythm with PR interval > 0.20 sec
2° AV block, Mobitz type I (Wenckebach block)	Sinus rhythm with progressive decremental lengthening of PR interval (and associated progressive shortening of R-R interval) until a P wave fails to conduct to the ventricles and a beat is dropped; resulting pause is sum of two P-P intervals
2°AV block, Mobitz type II	Sinus rhythm with constant PR interval and intermittent failure of P wave to conduct to the ventricles
3° AV block (complete heart block)	Complete absence of AV conduction; atrial rate > ventricular rate; atria and ventricles depolarize independently of each other
High-grade AV block	Sinus rhythm with conduction of P waves to ventricles in ratio ≥ 3:1; majority (but not all) of P waves fail to conduct to ventricles; identification of occasional conduction to ventricles defines the conduction abnormality as high-grade rather than complete AV block
Accelerated AV conduction	Sinus rhythm with PR interval < 0.12 sec and normal P-wave morphology and QRS duration
Wolff-Parkinson White (pre-excitation) syndrome	Sinus rhythm with PR interval < 0.12 sec, normal P-wave morphology, initial slurring (delta wave) prior to a wide QRS complex ≥ 0.11 sec, and secondary ST-T wave changes
Physiologic AV conduction delay associated with supraventricular tachyarrhythmias	Prolongation of PR interval with 1:1 conduction at atrial rates > 150 beat/min; Wenckebach phenomenon at atrial rates of 130-200 beat/min; 2:1 AV conduction at atrial rates > 200 beat/min in atrial tachycardia; Aflut; Afib with average ventricular response of 100-180 beat/min
Nonphysiologic AV conduction delay associated with supraventricular tachyarrhythmias	PR interval prolongation with 1:1 conduction at atrial rates of 100-150 beat/min; Wenckebach phenomenon at atrial rates of 100-130 beat/min; > 2:1 AV conduction ratio at atrial rates > 200 beat/min in atrial tachycardia and Aflut; Afib with an average ventricular response < 100 beat/min

Table 3.3 Intraventricular Conduction Abnormalities

Finding	Diagnostic Criteria
RBBB	QRS duration ≥ 0.12 sec; rSR′ in right precordial leads with terminal R′ > initial R wave; secondary ST-T abnormalities in right precordial leads; deep S waves in leads I and aVL and in left precordial leads
Incomplete RBBB	Criteria for RBBB, but QRS duration 0.09–0.11 sec
Left anterior fascicular block	Left axis deviation between −30° and −90°; positive terminal deflection in aVL and aVR; QRS < 0.12 sec duration; QR in leads I and aVL; rS in leads II, III, and aVF; S wave in lead III > S in lead II
Left posterior fascicular block	Right axis deviation between +90° and +180°; rS in lead I and aVL; QR in leads II, III, and aVF with Q waves < 0.04 sec; QRS < 0.12 sec; R wave in lead III ≥ R in lead II
LBBB	QRS ≥ 0.12 sec; broad, notched, or slurred R waves in leads I, aVL, and V5-V6 with secondary ST-T wave abnormalities in leads I, aVL, and V5-V6 and absent Q waves in leads I and V5-V6
Nonspecific intraventricular conduction delay	QRS ≥ 0.11 sec in absence of criteria for RBBB or LBBB

Table 3.4 Ventricular Hypertrophy

Finding	Diagnostic Criteria
Left ventricular hypertrophy	Sum of S wave in leads VI or V2 plus R wave in leads VS or V6 $>$ 35 mm **or** R wave in lead aVL $>$ 11 mm **or** Sum of R wave in lead I and S wave in lead III $>$ 25 mm **or** (R lead I − S lead I) + (S lead III − R lead III) $\geq$ 17 *Supporting findings:* T-wave inversions in left precordial leads; prolongation of R peak time (intrinsicoid deflection) $\geq$ 0.05 sec in left precordial leads; left atrial abnormality
Right ventricular hypertrophy	Right axis deviation; R-wave voltage $>$ S wave in lead V1; R wave in lead V1 $\geq$ 7 mm QR pattern in lead V1; rSR′ pattern with normal QRS duration and with R′ $\geq$ 10 mm; R/S ratio in lead V5 or V6 $\leq$ 1 *Supporting findings:* delay in the R peak time (intrinsicoid deflection) in V1; ST depression and T-wave inversion in right precordial leads; S wave in lead V1 $<$ 2 mm
Combined ventricular hypertrophy	Presence of criteria for both RVH and LVH

Table 3.5 Myocardial Infarction

Diagnosis	Diagnostic Criteria
Acute MI	Q waves (or developing Q waves) with horizontal/concave-down ST elevation in the affected leads; ST depression in leads V1-V2 for posterior infarction
Recent or subacute MI	Q waves with resolving ST-segment abnormalities associated with T-wave inversion in affected leads; upright T wave for posterior infarction
Old/indeterminate MI	Diagnostic Q waves (width $\geq$ 0.04 sec, depth $\geq$ 25% of R wave) without associated ST-segment or T-wave abnormalities to suggest acute injury
MI location	
Anteroseptal	Leads V1-V3
Anterior	Leads V1-V5
Lateral	Leads I, aVL
Inferior	Leads II, III, aVF
True posterior	Tall R waves $\geq$ 0.04 sec with R > S leads VI-V2
Possible LV aneurysm	ST elevation in leads containing Q waves that persists for at least 2 wk following MI

Table 3.6 Atrial Arrhythmias

Rhythm	Diagnostic Criteria
Sinus rhythm	Physiologic rhythm initiated in sinus node; rate 50-100 beat/min; P wave upright in leads I, II, aVF but inverted in aVR; P-P interval may vary by 0.16 sec (sinus arrhythmia) Sinus bradycardia: sinus rhythm with rate $<$ 50 beat/min Sinus tachycardia: sinus rhythm with rate $>$100 beat/min
Wandering atrial pacemaker	Sinus rhythm with variable P-wave morphology and PR interval; P wave may become inverted and retrograde as pacemaker wanders to AV junction
Sinus node pause/arrest	Absent P waves/QRS complexes; resulting pause is not a multiple of intrinsic P-P interval
SA node exit block	Abnormal transmission of sinus impulse with progressive shortening of P-P interval leading to dropped P wave (type I block) or pause in P-P cycle that is an exact multiple of the intrinsic sinus rate (type II block)
Ectopic atrial rhythm	Atrial pacemaker with rate $<$ 100 beat/min; P wave morphology different from that of sinus node but PR interval is normal
APC	Atrial premature complex with P-wave morphology different from that of sinus node; PR interval frequently $\geq$ 0.12 sec but can be variable Because of partial refractoriness of conduction system, APC may be abnormally conducted to ventricles, resulting in an alteration in QRS complex (usually RBBB pattern); with complete refractoriness, impulse is not conducted and no QRS follows P wave
Atrial tachycardia	SV rhythm with abnormal P waves, atrial rate 100-250 beat/min; may be paroxysmal or sustained; may not have 1:1 conduction if AV block present
Multifocal atrial tachycardia	Atrial rhythm with rate $>$ 100 beat/min and at least 3 different P-wave morphologies and PR intervals
Atrial fibrillation	SV rhythm characterized by the absence of P waves and presence of irregular atrial fibrillatory waves

Table 3.6 continued

Rhythm	Diagnostic Criteria
Atrial flutter	Atrial rhythm characterized by atrial rate 250-350 beat/min with flutter waves exhibiting sawtooth appearance in leads II, III, aVF, and V1; AV block frequently present
Retrograde atrial activation from a ventricular focus	Retrograde activation of atria from an independent depolarization in ventricles

Table 3.7 Junctional Rhythms

Rhythm	Diagnostic Criteria
AV junctional rhythm	Regular rhythm, rate usually 35-60 beat/min, originating in AV junction; P waves in leads II, III, and aVF usually inverted/ retrograde; P waves may occur prior to, within, or after QRS complex; PR interval usually < 0.12 sec
Accelerated AV junctional rhythm (junctional tachycardia)	More rapid AV junctional rhythm (70-130 beat/min) produced by enhanced automaticity of AV junction; characterized by absence of paroxysmal onset and termination
AV junctional escape rhythm	AV junctional rhythm emerging as a result of conduction failure or slowing of the normally faster sinus node rhythm
AV junctional premature beats	Isolated AV junctional complexes occurring prematurely relative to the basic sinus cycle

Table 3.8 Ventricular Arrhythmias

Rhythm	Diagnostic Criteria
Ventricular premature beats (PVC)	Premature depolarizations relative to intrinsic cycle originating in ventricles and characterized by a wide, abnormal QRST morphology (may see RBBB-type pattern for PVC from LV or LBBB-type morphology for PVC originating in RV) PVC may be unifocal or multifocal, paired, or recurrent (bigeminy, trigeminy, etc)
Interpolated PVC	Ventricular extrasystoles interposed between sinus beats that do not interrupt the sinus rhythm; prolongation of PR interval of second sinus beat may occur secondary to concealed retrograde conduction of PVC to AV junction
Fusion beats	QRS complex representing simultaneous transmission of atrial and ventricular impulses; QRS morphology is intermediate between the 2 depolarization patterns
Ventricular parasystole	Ventricular complexes that are independent of the intrinsic rhythm; characterized by varying coupling intervals and fusion beats; intervals between ventricular beats are constant or are multiples of a common denominator
Accelerated idioventricular rhythm	Three or more ventricular complexes in succession with rate $\leq$ 100 beat/min
Ventricular tachycardia	Three or more ventricular complexes in succession with rate $>$ 100 beat/min
Ventricular fibrillation	Chaotic ventricular rhythm characterized by absence of discernible QRS complexes and by ventricular fibrillatory waves of variable rate and amplitude
Torsades de pointes	Polymorphous ventricular tachycardia with an alternating amplitude and polarity (literally "twisting of the points")

Table 3.9 Electrolyte Disturbances

Abnormality	Diagnostic Findings
Hypokalemia	Concave ST-segment depressions; T-wave flattening; U waves that may fuse with T wave; arrhythmias (especially if the pt is taking digoxin), including worsening AV block, PEA, or asystole
Hyperkalemia	Peaked T waves (tenting); prolonged PR interval; flattening and ultimate disappearance of visible P waves; progressive widening QRS complex with deepened S waves and merging of S and T waves (sine-wave formation); PVC, idioventricular rhythm, VF
Hypomagnesemia	Flattening or inversion of precordial P waves; widening of QRS; prolonged QT and PR intervals; ST-segment depression and T-wave inversion; torsades de pointes; treatment-resistant VF
Hypermagnesemia	Increased PR and QT intervals and QRS duration; variable decrease in P-wave voltage; peaked T waves; complete AV block; asystole
Hypocalcemia	Terminal T-wave inversion; QT prolongation; heart block; VF
Hypercalcemia	Prolonged PR and QRS interval; increased QRS voltage; notching of QRS; T-wave flattening and widening; shortened QT interval ($Ca^{++} > 13$ mg/dL); AV block; cardiac arrest (when serum calcium > 15-20 mg/dL)

Chapter 4

Cardiac Testing

4.1 Exercise Stress Testing

Circ 2002;106:1883; J Am Coll Cardiol 2002;40:1531

Indications

- Pts with intermediate pretest probability of CAD with normal EKG, RBBB, <1 mm resting ST depression but not pre-excitation (Wolff-Parkinson-White) syndrome, paced ventricular rhythm or complete LBBB
- Pts with suspected vasospastic angina
- Risk assessment in pts with CAD undergoing initial evaluation or who have significant change in clinical status
- Asymptomatic low-risk pts with unstable angina 8-12 hr post-presentation
- Asymptomatic intermediate-risk pts with unstable angina 2-3 d post-presentation
- Pts post-MI: submaximal at 4-7 d, symptom-limited at 14-21 d or at 3-6 wk if early exercise test was submaximal
- Pts with multiple risk factors or who are at high risk for CAD due to other diseases; men > 40 yr and women > 50 yr who plan to start vigorous exercise, who are in occupations in which impairment might affect public safety, or who are at high risk for CAD due to other diseases
- Evaluation of asymptomatic adult pts with diabetes mellitus who have additional CAD risk factors or microvascular disease

- Pts with chronic aortic regurgitation who require evaluation of functional capacity
- Pts with recurrent sx suggesting ischemia after revascularization
- Evaluation of exercise-induced arrhythmias and of ablative therapy in such pts
- Evaluation of patients with congenital complete heart block
- Identification of appropriate settings in pts with rate-adaptive pacemakers

Contraindications

Absolute Contraindications

- Acute MI (within 2 d)
- High-risk, unstable angina
- Uncontrolled cardiac arrhythmias causing symptoms or hemodynamic compromise
- Symptomatic severe aortic stenosis
- Uncontrolled symptomatic CHF
- Acute pulmonary embolus or pulmonary infarction
- Acute myocarditis or pericarditis
- Acute aortic dissection

Relative Contraindications

- Left main coronary stenosis
- Moderate stenotic valvular heart disease
- Electrolyte abnormalities
- Systolic BP $>$ 200 mm Hg or diastolic BP $>$ 100 mm Hg
- Tachyarrhythmias or bradyarrhythmias
- Hypertrophic cardiomyopathy and other forms of outflow tract obstruction
- Mental or physical impairment leading to inability to exercise adequately
- High-degree AV block

Procedure

Exercise Protocols: Bruce protocol is the most widely used

Preparation

- Pt assessment; informed consent
- No eating or smoking for 3 hr before test
- Loose clothing; appropriate footwear
- Examine for murmur, gallop, wheezing, rales
- Consider withdrawal of medication such as β-blockers that could interfere with test
- 12-lead EKG prior to exercise; standing EKG and BP

Absolute Indications for Cessation of Stress Test

- Drop in systolic BP (persistently below baseline) despite an increase in workload
- Increasing anginal pain
- CNS symptoms (eg, ataxia, dizziness, or near-syncope)
- Signs of poor perfusion (cyanosis or pallor)
- Serious arrhythmias (ie, high-grade ventricular arrhythmias such as multiform complexes, triplets, and runs of VT)
- Technical difficulties monitoring the EKG or systolic BP
- Subject's request to stop

Relative Indications for Cessation of Stress Test

- ST or QRS changes such as excessive ST displacement, extreme junctional depression, or marked axis shift
- Fatigue, shortness of breath, wheezing, leg cramps, or claudication
- Less serious arrhythmias, including supraventricular tachycardias
- Development of BBB that cannot be distinguished from VT

Interpretation & Findings

Sensitivity/Specificity: Sensitivity of stress testing without imaging reported in meta-analyses to be 67-72%, sensitivity 69-77%, predictive accuracy 68-74%

ST-segment depression: Represents subendocardial ischemia; abnormal response ≥ 1 mm (0.1 mV) horizontal/downsloping ST-segment depression 0.08 sec past J point; exercise-induced ST-segment depression less specific in presence of baseline EKG abnormalities; amount, time of appearance, duration, and number of leads with ST-segment depression all correlate with probability/severity of CAD; ST depression at lower workload or double product worsens prognosis and increases likelihood of multivessel disease

Downsloping ST-segment depression is a stronger predictor of CAD than horizontal depression. Both are more predictive than upsloping depression. Ischemic ST-segment changes developing during recovery from treadmill exercise in apparently healthy individuals have adverse prognostic significance similar to those appearing during exercise (Circ 1998;97:2117).

Lead V5 outperforms the inferior leads or combination of lead V5 with II, because lead II has a high false-positive rate. In pts without prior MI and normal resting EKG, precordial leads alone are a reliable marker for CAD and monitoring of inferior limb leads adds little additional diagnostic information. In pts with normal resting EKG, exercise-induced ST-segment depression confined to inferior leads is of little value for identification of CAD.

ST elevation in leads without Q waves occurs in only 1 of 1000 pts. ST elevation on a normal EKG (other than in aVR or V_1) represents transmural ischemia caused by spasm or a critical lesion, is very rare (0.1% in a clinical lab), and is very arrhythmogenic and localizes ischemia. If resting EKG shows old MI, ST elevation may indicate wall motion abnormalities or residual viability in the infarcted area.

R-Wave Changes: Many factors affect the R-wave amplitude response to exercise; response does not have diagnostic significance.

LBBB: Exercise-induced ST depression usually occurs with LBBB and has no association with ischemia; ~0.5% of pts develop new LBBB during exercise; exercise-induced LBBB associated with adjusted relative risk of 2.78 for death and major cardiac events (Jama 1998;279:153).

RBBB: Exercise-induced ST depression usually occurs with RBBB in leads V1-V3 and is not associated with ischemia; ST depression in lead V5-V6 or in inferior leads has same significance as in normal EKG.

LVH with Repolarization Abnormalities: Associated with decreased specificity of exercise testing, but sensitivity is unaffected

Resting ST-Segment Depression: Identified as marker for adverse cardiac events in pts with and without known CAD; 2-mm additional exercise-induced ST-segment depression or downsloping depression of 1 mm or more in recovery useful markers for dx of CAD

Attenuated heart rate response to exercise is predictive of increased mortality and CAD incidence (Framingham). In pts having a stress test, chronotropic incompetence is an independent predictor of all-cause mortality (Circ 1996;93:1520; Jama 1999;281:524).

PVC: Frequent ventricular ectopy (> 7 PVC/min) during exercise predicted an increased 5-yr risk of death, and frequent ectopy in recovery period was an even stronger predictor (Nejm 2003;348:781).

Women: Exercise-induced ST depression less sensitive in women than men; exercise EKG commonly viewed as less specific in women than men; significant gender differences are modest and do not preclude use of treadmill exercise testing in women; possible explanations offered include greater prevalence of mitral valve prolapse and syndrome X in women, differences in microvascular function (leading perhaps to coronary spasm), and possibly hormonal differences

Digoxin: Produces abnormal exercise-induced ST depression in 25-40% of apparently healthy normal subjects; prevalence of abnormal responses directly related to age; repolarization effects alleviated 2 wk post cessation of administration

β-Blockers: Exercise testing may have reduced diagnostic value due to inadequate heart rate response; β-blockers should not be stopped in pts exhibiting possible sx of ischemia.

Flecainide: Associated with exercise-induced ventricular tachycardia

Scoring of Results: *Pretest likelihood of CAD* can be estimated (Table 4.1) on basis of pt's age, sex, and description of chest pain (*typical* angina: substernal chest discomfort with characteristic quality and duration, provoked by exertion/emotional stress, relieved by rest/TNG; *atypical* angina pain meeting 2 of above characteristics; *noncardiac* chest pain meets ≤ 1 of the typical angina characteristics) (J Am Coll Cardiol 1983;1:574)

Duke treadmill score formula: Exercise time − (5 × ST deviation) − (4 × exercise angina) with 0 = none, 1 = nonlimiting, and 2 = exercise-limiting

Typical score is −25 to +15. Pts can be stratified to low risk (score +5 or above), moderate risk (score −10 to +4), and high risk (score −11 or below) categories. In the Duke study, 60% of low-risk pts had no coronary stenosis > 75%, 16% had only

Table 4.1 Pretest Probability of CAD Based on Age, Sex, and Pain Description

	Non-anginal Chest Pain		Atypical Angina		Typical Angina	
Age	**Men**	**Women**	**Men**	**Women**	**Men**	**Women**
30-39	4	2	34	12	76	26
40-49	13	3	51	22	87	55
50-59	20	7	65	31	93	73
60-69	27	14	72	51	94	86

(Circ 1981;64:360)

single-vessel > 75% stenosis, 74% of high-risk pts had 3-vessel or left main CAD, and 5-yr mortality was 3%, 10%, and 35% for low-, moderate-, and high-risk groups, respectively (Circ 1998; 98:1622). Prognosis can be formulated using the nomogram in Figure 4.2. Score may have reduced prognostic accuracy in subjects > age 65 (Ann IM 2000;132:862).

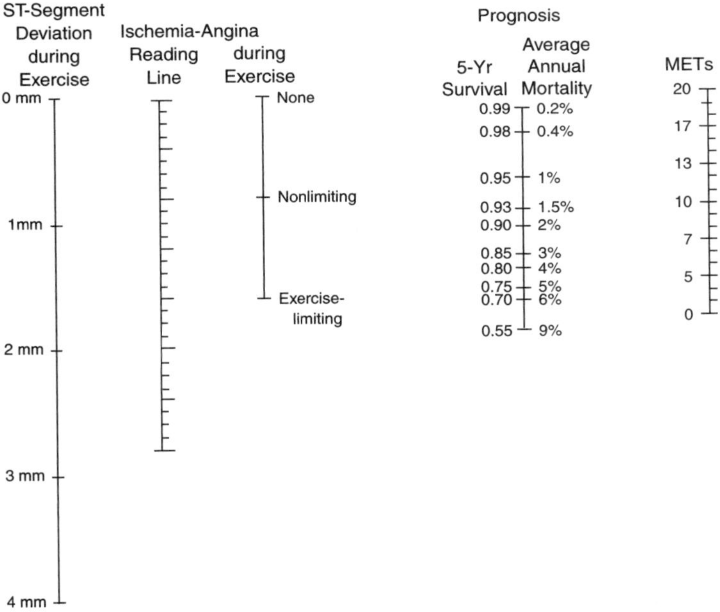

1. Mark observed amount of ST depression on ST-segment deviation line.
2. Mark observed degree of angina on line for angina and connect these two points.
3. Note the point where line intersects ischemia-reading line.
4. Mark observed exercise tolerance on line for duration of exercise.
5. Connect mark on ischemia-reading line and mark on exercise duration line; read estimated 5-yr survival or average annual mortality rate from point at which the line intersects prognosis scale.

Figure 4.1 Duke Treadmill Score Nomogram (J Am Coll Cardiol 1999;33:1756)

4.2 Radionuclide Imaging

Circ 2003;108:1404; J Am Coll Cardiol 2003;42:1318

Indications

Uses of Radionuclide Testing after Acute MI: Assessment of RV/LV function with rest radionuclide angiography; detection of stress-induced ischemia by stress myocardial perfusion imaging, measurement of infarct size by rest myocardial perfusion imaging

Uses of Radionuclide Testing in Pts with Unstable Angina: Identification of ischemia in the distribution of the "culprit" lesion or in remote areas with stress myocardial perfusion imaging; assessment of severity/extent of disease in pts with ischemia with rest and stress myocardial perfusion imaging; measurement of baseline LV function with radionuclide angiography

Uses of Radionuclide Testing in Detection and Assessment of Chronic Ischemic Heart Disease: Dx of ischemia with exercise or with pharmacologic myocardial perfusion imaging (for subjects with pacemakers or those unable to exercise); assessment of ventricular performance (rest or exercise) by radionuclide angiography or gated sestamibi imaging; assessment of myocardial viability in patients with LV dysfunction in planning revascularization [rest-redistribution Tl-201 imaging, stress-redistribution-reinjection Tl-201 imaging (J Am Coll Cardiol 2002;39:1151), or PET F18 fluorodeoxyglucose imaging]; identifying lesions causing myocardial ischemia, if not otherwise known with exercise or pharmacologic myocardial perfusion imaging; risk stratification before noncardiac surgery with pharmacologic or exercise perfusion imaging; assessment of LV performance with rest or exercise radionuclide angiography or gated sestamibi perfusion imaging; assessment of possible restenosis after PTCA or CABG with exercise or pharmacologic perfusion imaging

Uses of Radionuclide Imaging in Myocarditis and Cardiomyopathies:

Determination of initial and serial LV and RV performance in myocarditis or dilated, hypertrophic, and restrictive cardiomyopathy with rest radionuclide angiography; initial and serial evaluation of LV function in pts receiving chemotherapy with doxorubicin with rest radionuclide angiography; differentiation of ischemic and dilated cardiomyopathy with exercise or pharmacologic perfusion imaging; assessment of myocardial ischemia in hypertrophic cardiomyopathy

In general, the pts who benefit most from a stress test with SPECT perfusion scan at the outset are those with an intermediate (15-90%) pretest likelihood of CAD. Exercise EKG stress testing alone is the first test of choice in pts with a likelihood of CAD < 15% (based on age, gender, type of chest pain presentation, number of CAD risk factors, EKG findings at rest). If such pts demonstrate an ischemic ST-segment response that might represent a false-positive test outcome or fail to reach 85% of maximal predicted heart rate, repeat testing with SPECT perfusion imaging indicated (J Am Coll Cardiol 1998;31:1286).

Contraindications

For ischemic disease, same as those under stress testing

Procedure

Nuclear cardiology applications utilize a gamma camera for either planar or SPECT imaging (tomographic reconstructions derived from gamma camera that rotates around pt). Tomographic imaging allows for better separation of myocardial and other nonmyocardial structures and individual coronary artery beds and is inherently quantitative.

Equilibrium or gated blood pool radionuclide angiography most commonly utilizes technetium-99m (Tc-99m) pertechnetate bound to red blood cells. Acquisition of images is synchronized with the EKG QRS complex, with the cardiac cycle divided temporally into frames and corresponding frames from all cycles added together for an acquisition time ranging from 2 to 10 min. This approach generates reliable LV and RV ejection fraction values and offers a means for assessing regional wall motion. Studies can be acquired by both planar and SPECT approaches.

Myocardial perfusion imaging can employ thallium-201 (Tl-201), Tc-99m sestamibi, or Tc-99m tetrofosmin. Tl-201 is very efficiently extracted by viable myocardial cells and distributes in proportion to regional blood flow. Retention is an active process that is a function of cell viability and cell membrane integrity. "Redistribution" of the isotope generally occurs in previously ischemic zones, while defects related to infarcted or scarred myocardium typically do not "redistribute" and remain fixed. Imaging at 24 hr or after reinjection of Tl-201 may show viable but hypoperfused segments not identified by a standard redistribution study at 3-4 hr after isotope injection. Studies can be performed at rest, with exercise or dobutamine stress, or after the myocardial hyperemia induced by iv dipyridamole or adenosine.

Tc-99m sestamibi has a shorter half-life than Tl-201 (6 hr vs 73 hr) and has more favorable imaging characteristics (higher emission energy, less scattered radiation). Like Tl-201, Tc-99m requires intact cell membrane processes for retention.

PET employs radiotracers such as fluorine-18 (F-18, half-life 110 min), nitrogen 13 (N-13, half-life 10 min), or rubidium-82 (Rb-82, half-life 75 sec) coupled to physiologically active molecules to assess myocardial perfusion or metabolism.

Myocardial perfusion imaging is most commonly used in conjunction with exercise stress, with Tl-201 administered iv at peak exercise. The pt then exercises for an additional 30-60 sec. Images are acquired immediately after and again 3-4 hr after Tl administration. Because sestamibi undergoes only a small amount of washout after initial myocardial uptake, distinguishing between transient, stress-induced perfusion defects and fixed perfusion defects requires administration of 2 separate injections, one during stress and one at rest.

CARDIAC TESTING

Adenosine/Dipyridamole Stress Test Protocol

Contraindications: Unstable angina or acute MI; asthma; systolic BP < 100 mm Hg; hemodynamically severe aortic stenosis; high-degree AV block; pregnancy

Pretest Instructions: No aminophylline for 48 hr prior to study; no coffee, tea, cola, chocolate, or other caffeinated beverages for 24 hr prior to study; npo 3 hr prior to study

Protocol: Adenosine, 0.84 mg/kg in 40 mL NS, infused over 6 min; inject radionuclide at 3 min **or** dipyridamole, 0.57 mg/kg (maximum dose 60 mg) in 25-50 mL NS, infused over 4 min; inject radionuclide with 5 min of infusion; monitor vital signs and EKG q 1 min; image 45 min after completion of infusion and preferably after pt has eaten; ambulation (1 mph) during infusion increases image quality (J Nucl Cardiol 2000;7:439)

Side Effects: Headache, nausea/vomiting, dizziness, hypotension, chest pain

Termination Criteria: Same as for exercise stress test

Dobutamine Stress Test Protocol

Contraindications: Unstable angina or acute MI; obstructive hypertrophic cardiomyopathy; hemodynamically severe aortic stenosis; any symptomatic tachyarrhythmia; systolic BP > 180 mm Hg and/or diastolic BP > 110 mm Hg; pregnancy

Pretest Instructions: npo 3 hr prior to study

Protocol: Dobutamine continuous iv infusion at 5 μgm/kg/min for 3 min; increase to 10, 20, 30, 40 μgm/kg/min at 3-min intervals; monitor VS and EKG q 3 min; inject radionuclide after 1 min at maximal infusion rate; continue infusion an additional 2 min; if target heart rate not obtained, administer atropine 0.5-1 mg iv; image 5-10 min after completion of infusion

Side Effects: Palpitations, dizziness, chest pain

Termination Criteria: Same as for exercise stress test

Interpretation & Findings

Comparison with Stress Echo: Advantages of stress radionuclide imaging include higher technical success rate, higher sensitivity (1-vessel CAD), better accuracy in evaluating ischemia if rest wall motion abnormalities are present, and a more extensive published database. Advantages of stress echo include higher specificity, more extensive evaluation of cardiac anatomy, greater convenience/availability, and lower cost (Circ 1999;99:2829). In a meta-analysis, exercise echo had a sensitivity of 85% and specificity of 77%; exercise SPECT had a sensitivity of 87% and specificity of 64-73%; vasodilator SPECT had a sensitivity of 89% and specificity of 75%. Unlike exercise stress testing, ST depression ≥ 2 mm in pts undergoing adenosine SPECT is not specific for CAD (Am Hrt J 2000;140:937). Vasodilator SPECT has better *sensitivity*, especially in pts on β-blockers; echo stress has better *specificity* (Am Hrt J 2001;142:934; Cardiol 2001;95:112). Both echo and SPECT performed significantly better than exercise testing without imaging (Jama 1998;280:913).

Chest pain may occur during adenosine administration in the absence of ischemia (May Clin Proc 1995;70:331).

The diagnostic sensitivity/specificity of SPECT imaging is not diminished in pts with LVH and repolarization abnormalities.

Pts with LBBB have an increased prevalence of false-positive septal perfusion defects. Pharmacologic stress is preferred for such subjects.

Normal-stress SPECT sestamibi images are associated with a 0.6% average annual event rate (death or nonfatal MI). Pts with abnormal images had an annual event rate of 7.4% (J Am Coll Cardiol 1998;32:57).

In a retrospective study, 4649 pts with intermediate-risk Duke treadmill scores and normal/near-normal exercise SPECT perfusion images had cardiovascular survival rates of 99.8% at

1 yr, 99.0% at 5 yr, and 98.5% at 7 yr; cardiac survival free of MI was 96.6% at 7 yr; survival free of MI or revascularization was 87.1% at 7 yr (Circ 1999;100:2140).

Results predicting high risk for adverse outcomes in pts with known or suspected CAD include severe resting or exercise LV dysfunction (LVEF $< 35\%$), high-risk treadmill score (score ≤ -11), stress-induced large perfusion defect (particularly if anterior) or multiple moderate perfusion defects, and large, fixed perfusion defect or moderate stress-induced perfusion defect with LV dilatation or increased lung uptake. Conversely, in men with and without diabetes and in nondiabetic women with no known CAD and a negative test, predicted time to 1% risk was > 1 yr even at age 80 (J Am Coll Cardiol 2003;41:1329).

In pts s/p CABG, the 5-yr survival rate free of cardiac death or MI was 93% for pts without angina and a normal image or small post-exercise perfusion defect vs 71% for patients with angina and a medium or large defect seen on exercise Tl-201 imaging (J Am Coll Cardiol 1998;31:848).

4.3 Echocardiography

J Am Coll Cardiol 2003;42:954; Circ 2003;108:1146

Indications

Two-dimensional echocardiography provides images of the heart, paracardiac structures, and great vessels. Interposition of an air-filled lung between the body surface and heart limits examination in pts with COPD. Pts on ventilators, pts who cannot be rotated into a lateral position, and pts with incisions may not have satisfactory precordial or apical windows. TEE may avoid most of these limitations.

Valvular Heart Disease

Evaluation of Heart Murmurs: Indicated for murmur in pts with cardiorespiratory sx, murmur in asymptomatic pts if clinical features indicate a moderate probability that the murmur is reflective of structural heart disease, murmur in asymptomatic pts in whom dx of heart disease cannot be reasonably excluded

Valvular Stenosis: Dx/assessment of hemodynamic severity; assessment of LV and RV size, function, and/or hemodynamics; reevaluation of pts with known valvular stenosis with changing si/sx or with LV dysfunction or hypertrophy; assessment of changes in hemodynamic severity and ventricular compensation in pts with known valvular stenosis during pregnancy; reevaluation of asymptomatic pts with severe stenosis; assessment of hemodynamic significance of mild/moderate valvular stenosis by stress Doppler echocardiography

Native Valvular Regurgitation: Dx/assessment of hemodynamic severity; initial assessment and reevaluation when indicated of LV and RV size, function, and/or hemodynamics; reevaluation of pts with mild/moderate valvular regurgitation with changing sx; reevaluation of asymptomatic pts with severe regurgitation; assessment of changes in hemodynamic severity and ventricular compensation in pts with known valvular regurgitation during pregnancy; reevaluation of pts with mild/moderate regurgitation with ventricular dilation without clinical sx; assessment of effects of medical therapy on severity of regurgitation and ventricular compensation and function; evaluation of valvular morphology and regurgitation in pts with h/o anorectic drug use

Mitral Valve Prolapse: Dx/assessment of hemodynamic severity, leaflet morphology, and/or ventricular compensation in pts with physical signs of MVP; to exclude MVP in pts who have been diagnosed but without clinical evidence to support the dx; to exclude MVP in pts with first-degree relatives with known myxomatous valve disease; risk stratification in pts with physical signs of MVP or known MVP

Infective Endocarditis of Native Valves: Detection and characterization of valvular lesions, their hemodynamic severity, and/or ventricular compensation; detection of associated abnormalities (eg, abscesses, shunts); evaluation of pts with high clinical suspicion of culture-negative endocarditis; evaluation of bacteremia without known source; risk stratification in established endocarditis (TEE may provide incremental value in all of above); detection of vegetations and characterizations of lesions in pts with congenital heart disease suspected of having infective endocarditis; reevaluation studies in complex endocarditis (eg, virulent organism, severe hemodynamic lesion, aortic valve involvement, persistent fever or bacteremia, clinical change, or symptomatic deterioration)

Infective Endocarditis of Prosthetic Valves: Detection and characterization of valvular lesions, their hemodynamic severity, and/or ventricular compensation; detection of associated abnormalities (eg, abscesses, shunts); reevaluation in complex endocarditis (eg, virulent organism, severe hemodynamic lesion, aortic valve involvement, persistent fever or bacteremia, clinical change, or symptomatic deterioration); evaluation of suspected endocarditis and negative cultures; evaluation of bacteremia without known source; evaluation of persistent fever without evidence of bacteremia or new murmur (TEE may provide incremental value)

Interventions for Valvular Heart Disease and Prosthetic Valves: Assessment of timing of valvular intervention based on ventricular compensation, function, and/or severity of primary and secondary lesions; selection of alternative therapies for mitral valve disease; use of echocardiography (especially TEE) in performing interventional techniques; postintervention baseline studies for valve function early and ventricular remodeling late; reevaluation of pts with valve replacement with changing clinical si/sx; suspected prosthetic dysfunction stenosis, regurgitation, or thrombosis; guiding performance of valve interventions through intraprocedure TEE

ASHD

Pts with Chest Pain: Dx of underlying cardiac disease in pts with chest pain and clinical evidence of valvular, pericardial, or primary myocardial disease; evaluation of chest pain in pts with suspected acute myocardial ischemia, when baseline EKG is nondiagnostic, and when study can be obtained during pain or soon after its abatement; evaluation of chest pain in pts with suspected aortic dissection; chest pain in pts with severe hemodynamic instability

Acute Myocardial Ischemic Syndromes: Dx of suspected acute ischemia or MI not evident by standard means; measurement of baseline LV function; pts with inferior MI and bedside evidence suggesting possible RV infarction; assessment of mechanical complications and mural thrombus; identification of location/severity of disease in pts with ongoing ischemia; assessment of myocardial viability to define potential efficacy of revascularization with low-dose dobutamine infusion

Risk Assessment/Prognosis/Assessment of Therapy in Acute Myocardial Ischemic Syndromes: Assessment of infarct size and/or extent of jeopardized myocardium; in-hospital assessment of ventricular function when the results are used to guide rx; in-hospital or early postdischarge assessment of the presence/extent of inducible ischemia whenever baseline abnormalities are expected to compromise EKG interpretation; in-hospital or early postdischarge exercise or pharmacological stress echo for assessment of the presence/extent of inducible ischemia in the absence of baseline abnormalities expected to compromise EKG interpretation; dobutamine stress echo for assessment of myocardial viability when required to define potential efficacy of revascularization; reevaluation of ventricular function during recovery when results are used to guide therapy; assessment of ventricular function after revascularization

Dx and Prognosis of Chronic Ischemic Heart Disease: Assessment of global ventricular function at rest; exercise or pharmacological stress echo for dx of myocardial ischemia in symptomatic individuals, assessment of functional significance of coronary lesions if not already known in planning PTCA, dx of myocardial ischemia in selected pts with an intermediate or high pretest likelihood of CAD, assessment of asymptomatic pts with positive results from a screening treadmill test; dobutamine stress echo for assessment of myocardial viability hibernating myocardium for planning revascularization

Assessment of Interventions in Chronic Ischemic Heart Disease: Assessment of LV function when needed to guide institution and modification of drug rx in pts with known or suspected LV dysfunction; exercise or pharmacological stress echo for assessment for restenosis after revascularization in pts with recurrent sx; assessment of LV function in pts under consideration for AICD implantation

CHF

Echocardiography in Pts with Dyspnea, Edema, or Cardiomyopathy: Assessment of LV size and function in pts with suspected cardiomyopathy or clinical diagnosis of CHF; edema with clinical signs of elevated CVP when a potential cardiac etiology is suspected or when CVP cannot be estimated with confidence and clinical suspicion of heart disease is high; dyspnea with clinical signs of heart disease; pts with unexplained hypotension, especially in ICU (TEE indicated when TTE studies not diagnostic for above); pts exposed to cardiotoxic agents; reevaluation of LV function in pts with established cardiomyopathy and documented change in clinical status or who are being considered for dual-chamber pacing (see Chapter 9)

Pericardial Disease

Pts with suspected pericardial disease, including effusion, constriction, or effusive-constrictive process; pts with suspected bleeding in the pericardial space (eg, trauma, perforation); follow-up study to evaluate recurrence of effusion or to diagnose early constriction; pericardial friction rub developing in acute MI accompanied by sx such as persistent pain, hypotension, nausea; follow-up studies to detect early signs of tamponade in the presence of large or rapidly accumulating effusions; a goal-directed study may be appropriate; echocardiographic guidance and monitoring of pericardiocentesis

Cardiac Masses and Tumors

Evaluation of pts with clinical syndromes and events suggesting an underlying cardiac mass; evaluation of pts with underlying cardiac disease known to predispose to mass formation for whom a therapeutic decision regarding surgery or anticoagulation will depend on the results of echocardiography; follow-up/surveillance studies after surgical removal of masses known to have a high likelihood of recurrence; pts with known primary malignancies when echocardiographic surveillance for cardiac involvement is part of staging process

Thoracic Aortic Disease

TTE preferred for aneurysm of aortic root, aortic root dilatation in Marfan or other connective tissue syndromes, follow-up of aortic dissection—especially after surgical repair without suspicion of complication or progression, first-degree relative of a pt with Marfan syndrome or other connective tissue disorder; TEE preferred in aortic dissection, aortic rupture, degenerative or traumatic aortic disease with clinical atheroembolism, follow-up of aortic dissection—especially after surgical repair when complication or progression is suspected

Pulmonary Disease

Suspected pulmonary HT, follow-up of PA pressures in pts with pulmonary HT to evaluate response to rx, lung disease with clinical suspicion of cardiac involvement, suspected cor pulmonale, measurement of exercise PA pressure; TEE may be indicated for pts with pulmonary emboli and suspected clots in RA, RV, or main pulmonary artery branches to distinguish cardiac from noncardiac etiology of dyspnea in pts in whom all clinical and laboratory clues are ambiguous, or in pts being considered for lung transplantation or other surgical procedure for advanced lung disease

Hypertension

When assessment of resting LV function, hypertrophy, or concentric remodeling is important in clinical decision making; follow-up assessment of LV size and function in pts with LV dysfunction when there has been documented change in clinical status; identification of LV diastolic filling abnormalities; stress echo for detection and assessment of functional significance of concomitant CAD

Neurological/Other Vascular Occlusive Events

Pts of any age with abrupt occlusion of a major peripheral or visceral artery; pts < 45 yr with cerebrovascular events; pts > 45 yr with neurological events without evidence of cerebrovascular disease or other obvious cause; pts for whom a clinical rx decision will depend on the results of echocardiography; pts with suspicion of embolic disease and with cerebrovascular disease of questionable significance

Arrhythmias/Palpitations

Arrhythmias with clinical suspicion of structural heart disease; arrhythmia in pts with family h/o genetically transmitted cardiac lesion associated with arrhythmia (tuberous sclerosis, rhabdomyoma, hypertrophic cardiomyopathy); evaluation of pts before electrophysiological ablative procedures; TEE guidance of transseptal catheterization and catheter placement during ablative procedures

Cardioversion

Evaluation of pts for whom a decision concerning cardioversion will be affected by knowledge of prognostic factors such as LV function, coexistent mitral valve disease, etc; TEE for pts requiring urgent but not emergent cardioversion for whom extended precardioversion anticoagulation is not desirable, pts who have had prior cardioembolic events thought to be related to intra-atrial thrombus, pts for whom anticoagulation is contraindicated and for whom a decision about cardioversion will be influenced by TEE results, pts for whom intra-atrial thrombus has been demonstrated in previous TEE

Syncope

Syncope in pts with clinically suspected heart disease; periexertional syncope; syncope in pts in high-risk occupations

Screening

Pts with family h/o genetically transmitted cardiovascular disease; potential donors for cardiac transplantation; pts with phenotypic features of Marfan syndrome or related connective tissue diseases; baseline studies and reevaluations of pts undergoing chemotherapy with cardiotoxic agents; first-degree relatives of pts with unexplained dilated cardiomyopathy

Critical Injuries

Serious blunt or penetrating chest trauma with suspected pericardial effusion or tamponade; mechanically ventilated multiple-trauma or chest trauma pts; suspected preexisting valvular or myocardial disease in trauma pts; hemodynamically unstable multiple-injury pts without obvious chest trauma but with a mechanism of injury suggesting potential cardiac or aortic injury deceleration or crush; potential catheter, guidewire, pacer electrode, or pericardiocentesis needle injury with or without signs of tamponade; evaluation of hemodynamics in multiple-trauma or chest trauma pts with pulmonary artery catheter monitoring and data disparate with clinical situation

TEE in Critically Ill and Injured Pts: For hemodynamically unstable pts on a ventilator; major trauma or postoperative pts unable to be positioned for adequate TTE; suspected aortic dissection/injury; post-injury widening of the mediastinum

Congenital Heart Disease

Adults: Pts with clinically suspected congenital heart disease as evidenced by si/sx such as murmur, cyanosis, or unexplained arterial desaturation, and an abnormal EKG or radiograph suggesting congenital heart disease; pts with known congenital heart disease on follow-up when there is a change in clinical findings; pts with known congenital heart disease for whom there is uncertainty as to the original dx or when the precise nature of the structural abnormalities or hemodynamics is unclear; periodic echo in pts with known congenital heart lesions and for whom ventricular function and AV valve regurgitation must be followed (functionally single ventricle after Fontan procedure, transposition of great vessels after Mustard procedure, l-transposition and ventricular inversion, palliative shunts); pts with known congenital heart disease for whom following pulmonary artery pressure is important (VSD, ASD, single ventricle, or any of the above with an additional risk factor for pulmonary HT); periodic echo in pts with surgically repaired or palliated congenital heart disease with the following: change in clinical condition or clinical suspicion of residual defects, LV or RV function that must be followed, or possibility of hemodynamic progression or h/o pulmonary HT; to direct interventional catheter valvotomy, radiofrequency ablation valvotomy interventions in the presence of complex cardiac anatomy; identification of site of origin of coronary arteries

Infants, Children, Adolescents: Atypical or pathological murmur or other abnormal cardiac finding in an infant or older child; cardiomegaly on CXR; dextrocardia, abnormal pulmonary or visceral situs on clinical, EKG, or radiographic examination; pts with a known cardiac defect to assess timing of medical or surgical rx; immediate preoperative evaluation for cardiac surgery of pts with known cardiac defect to guide cardiac surgical management and inform pts and family of risks of surgery; pts with known cardiac lesion and change in physical findings; postoperative congenital or acquired heart disease with clinical suspicion of residual or recurrent abnormality, poor ventricular function, pulmonary artery HT, thrombus, sepsis, or pericardial effusion; presence of a syndrome associated with CVD and dominant inheritance or multiple affected family members; pts with family h/o genetically transmitted myocardial disease, with or without abnormal cardiac findings; phenotypic findings of Marfan syndrome or Ehlers-Danlos syndrome; baseline and follow-up exam of pts with neuromuscular disorders having known myocardial involvement; presence of a syndrome associated with a high incidence of congenital heart disease when there are no abnormal cardiac findings; exercise-induced precordial chest pain or syncope; "atypical," "nonvasodepressor" syncope without other cause

Pediatric Pts with Arrhythmias/Conduction Disturbances: Arrhythmia in the presence of abnormal cardiac findings; arrhythmia in pts with family h/o a genetically transmitted cardiac lesion associated with arrhythmia (tuberous sclerosis, hypertrophic cardiomyopathy); complete AV block or advanced second-degree AV block; complete or high-degree AV block; arrhythmia requiring rx; ventricular arrhythmia in pts referred for evaluation for competitive sports; evidence of pre-excitation on EKG

Pediatric-Acquired Cardiovascular Disease

Baseline studies and reevaluation as clinically indicated on all pediatric pts with suspected or documented Kawasaki disease, myopericarditis, HIV, or rheumatic fever; postcardiac or cardiopulmonary transplant to monitor for signs of acute or chronic rejection, thrombus, and cardiac growth; baseline studies and reevaluation of pts receiving cardiotoxic rx agents; pts with clinical evidence of myocardial disease; pts with severe renal disease and abnormal cardiac findings; donors undergoing evaluation for cardiac transplantation; acutely ill child with suspected bacterial sepsis or rickettsial disease

Contraindications

TTE is associated with little, if any, pt discomfort. No risks have been identified with the procedure. Use of exercise or vasoactive drugs (dipyridamole, dobutamine) is associated with minimal risks of arrhythmia, ischemia, and hypotension.

TEE involves some discomfort and minimal, but definite, risk of pharyngeal and esophageal trauma and even rarely esophageal perforation. TEE is contraindicated in pts with esophageal varices. Rare instances of infective endocarditis have been associated with TEE, and an occasional patient has a reaction to either the sedative or the local anesthesia used.

Contraindications to dobutamine stress echo include critical aortic stenosis, hypertrophic cardiomyopathy, uncontrolled HT, uncontrolled Afib, known severe ventricular arrhythmias, and severe electrolyte abnormalities (mainly hypokalemia). The addition of atropine is contraindicated in pts with narrow-angle glaucoma, myasthenia gravis, obstructive uropathy, or obstructive gi disorders.

Procedure

For a stress echo, a 2-D echo is acquired, the pt is stressed per the usual protocols, and echo images are obtained again immediately after the cessation of exercise.

For a dobutamine echo, rest EKG and 2-D echo are acquired. Dobutamine is administered iv by pump starting at 5 μgm/kg/min for 3 min, 10 μgm/kg/min for 3 min, and then increased by 10 μgm/kg/min every 3 min to maximum of 40-50 μgm/kg/min. In pts not achieving 85% of the predicted maximal heart rate (max HR = 220 − the pt's age—eg, if you are 50, your max HR = 170) and without si/sx of myocardial ischemia, atropine is administered on top of the maximal dose of dobutamine (0.25 mg iv and repeated to max of 1.0 mg within 4 min) with continuation of the dobutamine infusion. BP and EKG are monitored and recorded in each stage. The echo is continuously monitored and recorded at low- and maximum-dose dobutamine and in recovery. The test should be terminated in the event of severe or extensive new wall motion abnormalities, horizontal/downsloping ST-segment depression or ST-segment elevation, severe angina, symptomatic BP reduction > 40 mm Hg from baseline or BP > 240/120 mm Hg, or significant tachyarrhythmias. An iv β-blocker must be available.

Interpretation & Findings

(See also chapters on the disease entities listed earlier.)

TEE-guided cardioversion with short-term anticoagulation therapy may allow cardioversion to be done earlier (Ann IM 1997;26:200).

In high-risk patients with Afib, subsequent rates of thromboembolism are correlated with dense spontaneous echocardiographic contrast, thrombus of atrial appendage, and aortic plaque. Adjusted-dose warfarin reduces the rate of stroke among pts with dense contrast and complex plaque (SPAF study) (Ann IM 1998;128:639).

A *normal stress echocardiogram* is defined by a uniform increase in wall motion and systolic wall thickening. A positive test is denoted by the development of new wall motion dyssynergy or by worsening of regional dyssynergy in one or more segments. In pts with rest wall motion abnormalities, initial improvement of dyssynergy at a low dose followed by worsening of dyssynergy at a high dose represents a positive test (J Am Coll Cardiol 1997;30:595).

Pts with normal stress echo have a cardiac event rate of 0.9%/yr (J Am Coll Cardiol 2003;42:1084).

In pts with CAD, treadmill exercise induces greater ischemic burden than dobutamine–atropine infusion. When adequate exercise can be performed, exercise echo is better than dobutamine echocardiography for diagnosing ischemia (J Am Coll Cardiol 1997;30:1660). ST segment changes have less dx value during dobutamine stress.

Dobutamine echo has sensitivity of 80%, specificity of 84%, and accuracy of 81% for the detection of CAD. Sensitivities for 1-, 2-, and

3-vessel disease were 74%, 86%, and 92%, respectively. Sensitivities for detection of LCx, LAD, and RCA disease were 55%, 72%, and 76%, respectively. Less than 5% of pts have an inadequate acoustic window; 10% have nondiagnostic test results. Vfib or MI occurs in < 1 of every 2000 studies; no deaths have been reported (J Am Coll Cardiol 1997;30:595).

In pts with CAD, the ischemic threshold measured during dobutamine stress echo correlates with the number of stenosed vessels (Circ 1995;92:2095). Results predicting high risk for adverse outcomes in pts with known/suspected CAD include echocardiographic wall motion abnormality involving > 2 segments developing at dobutamine dose ≤ 10 μgm/kg/min or at HR < 120 beat/min.

In multivariate regression analysis, positive results on dobutamine echo were independently predictive of future cardiac death (J Am Coll Cardiol 1997;29:969). Normal dobutamine stress echo was associated with an 1.3% annual event rate (cardiac death or MI) over a 5-yr period (Circ 1999;99:757).

In medically treated pts with severe global LV dysfunction early after acute MI, presence of myocardial viability identified by low-dose dobutamine echo is associated with a higher probability of survival; presence of inducible ischemia is a predictor of cardiac death (Circ 1998;98:1078).

In patients with CAD and severe LV dysfunction who demonstrated myocardial viability during dobutamine echo, revascularization improved survival compared with medical rx (J Am Coll Cardiol 2002;39:1151).

Intravascular ultrasound is an invasive procedure employing a 2.6-3.5 French US catheter with axial resolution ~150 μm. It can be useful in assessment of angiographically indeterminate coronary/vascular lesions, left main CAD, transplant CAD, and unstable plaque/thrombus (Circ 2001;103:604).

4.4 Ambulatory EKG Monitoring

Circ 1999;100:886

Indications

Pts with unexplained syncope, near-syncope, episodic dizziness, or recurrent palpitations; pts with neurological events when transient Afib/Aflut is suspected; pts with sx in whom a probable cause has been identified but in whom sx persist despite rx; assessment of antiarrhythmic drug response; detection of proarrhythmic responses; assessment of rate control in Afib; detection of asymptomatic nonsustained arrhythmias during rx; in pts with pacemakers/ICDs for evaluation of sx to assess device function so as to exclude myopotential inhibition and pacemaker-mediated tachycardia and to assist in programming, evaluation of suspected component failure/malfunction when device interrogation is not definitive, and assessment of response to adjunctive pharmacological rx in pts receiving frequent ICD therapy; ST-segment monitoring of pts with suspected variant angina, with chest pain (if pt cannot exercise), or with known CAD and atypical chest pain syndrome

In pediatric pts for assessment of syncope, near-syncope, or dizziness in conjunction with recognized cardiac disease, previously documented arrhythmia, or pacemaker dependency; assessment of syncope, especially with exertion, when cause is not established; evaluation of pts with hypertrophic or dilated cardiomyopathies; evaluation of possible/documented long QT syndromes; assessment of palpitation in pts with prior surgery for congenital heart disease and significant residual hemodynamic abnormalities; evaluation of antiarrhythmic drug efficacy during rapid somatic growth; evaluation of pts with symptomatic congenital complete AV block (nonpaced); evaluation of cardiac rhythm after initiation of an antiarrhythmic rx, particularly when associated with a significant proarrhythmic potential; evaluation of cardiac rhythm after transient AV block associated with heart surgery or catheter ablation; evaluation of rate-responsive or physiological pacing function in symptomatic pts; evaluation of asymptomatic pts with prior surgery for congenital heart disease, particularly when there are either significant or residual hemodynamic abnormalities, or a significant incidence of late postoperative arrhythmias; evaluation of pts < 3 yr old with prior tachyarrhythmia to determine whether unrecognized episodes of the arrhythmia have recurred; evaluation of pts with suspected incessant atrial tachycardia or with complex ventricular ectopy on EKG/exercise test

Contraindications

Inability of pt to cooperate with monitor requirements

Procedure

Three choices: (1) continuous recorder (Holter monitor); (2) intermittent (event) recorder (stores period of EKG activity when activated by pt) for intermittent/unpredictable events; (3) loop recorder (record EKG continuously but store EKG recording in memory when activated by pt) for intermittent and very brief episodes

Event monitors are usually smaller and have fewer/simpler electrodes than Holter monitors. Newer recorders exist that can be implanted for longer-term monitoring.

Interpretation & Findings

Frequency, duration, and depth of ischemic ST-segment depression are highly variable. Most ischemic episodes during routine daily activities are due to increases in HR. The variability of ischemia between recording sessions may reflect variability of the pt's physical or emotional activities. The optimal duration of recording to detect/quantify ischemia episodes is probably 48 hr.

In one study, 75% of pts with AECG ischemia had multivessel CAD; 50% had complex plaque (J Am Coll Cardiol 1997;29:78).

To ensure that a change in arrhythmia is due to rx effect and not to spontaneous variability, a 65-95% reduction in arrhythmia frequency after intervention is necessary.

4.5 Right Heart Catheterization

J Am Coll Cardiol 1998;32:840

Indications

Conditions in which there is general agreement that RHC is warranted

CHF: Differentiation between hemodynamic and permeability pulmonary edema or dyspnea when a trial of diuretic and/or vasodilator rx has failed or is associated with high risk; differentiation between cardiogenic and noncardiogenic shock when a trial of intravascular volume expansion has failed or is associated with high risk; guidance of therapy in pts with concomitant manifestations of "forward" (hypotension, oliguria, and/or azotemia) and "backward" (dyspnea and/or hypoxemia) heart failure; determination of whether pericardial tamponade is present when clinical assessment is inconclusive and echocardiography is unavailable, technically inadequate, or nondiagnostic; guidance of perioperative management in selected pts with decompensated heart failure undergoing intermediate- or high-risk noncardiac surgery; detection of pulmonary vasoconstriction and determination of its reversibility in pts being considered for heart transplantation

Acute MI: Differentiation between cardiogenic and hypovolemic shock when initial rx with intravascular volume expansion and low doses of inotropic drugs has failed; guidance of management of cardiogenic shock with pharmacologic and/or mechanical support or of acute mitral regurgitation or ventricular septal rupture before surgical correction; guidance of management of RV infarction with hypotension and/or signs of low cardiac output not responding to intravascular volume expansion, low doses of inotropic drugs, and/or restoration of heart rate and AV synchrony; guidance of management of acute pulmonary edema not responding to rx with diuretic drugs, TNG and other vasodilator agents, and low doses of inotropic drugs

Perioperative Use in Cardiac Surgery: Differentiation between causes of low cardiac output (hypovolemia vs ventricular dysfunction) when clinical and/or echo assessment is inconclusive; differentiation between right and left ventricular dysfunction and pericardial tamponade when clinical and/or echo assessment is inconclusive; guidance of management of severe low-cardiac-output syndromes; dx and guidance of management of pulmonary HT in pts with systemic hypotension and evidence of inadequate organ perfusion

Primary Pulmonary HT: Exclusion of postcapillary (elevated PAOP) causes of pulmonary HT; establishment of dx and assessment of severity of precapillary (normal PAOP) pulmonary HT; selection and establishment of safety and efficacy of long-term vasodilator therapy based on acute hemodynamic response; assessment of hemodynamic variables before lung transplantation

Conditions in which reasonable differences of opinion exist

CHF: Differentiation between hemodynamic and permeability pulmonary edema or dyspnea when a trial of diuretic and/or vasodilator therapy is associated with low/intermediate risk; differentiation between cardiogenic and noncardiogenic shock when a trial of intravascular volume expansion is associated with intermediate risk; facilitation of titration of diuretic, vasodilator, and inotropic therapy in patients with severe CHF; guidance of perioperative management in pts with compensated CHF undergoing intermediate- or high-risk noncardiac surgery

Acute MI: Guidance of ongoing management of hypotension responding to initial therapy with intravascular volume expansion and/or low doses of inotropic drugs; short-term guidance of pharmacologic and/or mechanical management of acute mitral regurgitation or ventricular septal rupture if operation is delayed or not contemplated; guidance of management of RV infarction, after correction of hypotension and/or signs of low cardiac output by intravascular volume expansion, low doses of inotropic drugs, and/or restoration of heart rate and AV synchrony; guidance of management of acute pulmonary edema with vasodilator agents and/or inotropic drugs after initial rx with diuretic drugs and TNG has failed; confirmation of the diagnosis of pericardial tamponade associated with subacute myocardial rupture when clinical and echo assessments are inconclusive

Perioperative Use in Cardiac Surgery: Guidance of inotropic and/or vasopressor therapy after pts with significant cardiac dysfunction have achieved hemodynamic stability; guidance of management of hypotension and evidence of inadequate organ perfusion when a therapeutic trial of intravascular volume expansion and/or vasoactive agents is associated with moderate risk

Primary Pulmonary HT: Evaluation of long-term efficacy of vasodilator therapy, particularly prostacyclin; exclusion of significant L-to-R or R-to-L intracardiac shunt

Conditions in which RHC is not warranted

CHF: Routine management of pulmonary edema; differentiation between cardiogenic and non-cardiogenic shock before a trial of intravascular volume expansion, when such a trial is associated with low risk; institution or titration of diuretic and/or vasodilator therapy in pts with mild or moderate CHF; marked hemodynamic instability in pts in whom pericardial tamponade is certain or probable by clinical and/or echo criteria, and RHC would delay rx; guidance of perioperative management in pts with compensated CHF undergoing low-risk noncardiac surgery

Acute MI: Guidance of management of post-infarction angina; guidance of ongoing management of pulmonary edema responding promptly to treatment with diuretics and TNG; pericardial tamponade with marked hemodynamic instability, when the dx is certain or likely by clinical and/or echo criteria, and RHC would delay treatment

Perioperative Use in Cardiac Surgery: Routine management of uncomplicated cardiac surgical pts with good LV function and hemodynamic stability; initial management of postoperative hypotension when a therapeutic trial of volume expansion and/or vasoactive agents is associated with low risk

Contraindications

Absolute Contraindications: Right-sided endocarditis; mechanical tricuspid (or pulmonic) valve prosthesis; presence of thrombus or tumor in right heart chamber; terminal illness for which aggressive management is considered futile

Relative Contraindications: Coagulopathy; anticoagulant therapy that cannot be temporarily discontinued; recent implantation of permanent pacemaker or cardioverter-defibrillator; LBBB; bioprosthetic tricuspid (or pulmonic) valve; thrombolytic therapy

Procedure

Balloon flotation catheters have 4 lumens, including 2 for transmission of pressure signals from the PA and RA, 1 for balloon inflation, and 1 for a thermostat located near the catheter tip. Multipurpose electrode catheters incorporate atrial and ventricular electrodes for recording of intra-atrial and intraventricular EKG, facilitating dx of complex arrhythmias and temporary pacing. Newer catheters have a fifth lumen containing fiber-optic bundles for measurement of mixed venous O_2 saturation.

RHC allows for measurement of CVP or RA pressure; PA systolic, diastolic and mean pressures; PAOP or "wedge" pressure; thermodilution CO; and O_2 saturation. Current practice is to measure right heart pressures relative to zero pressure defined at the midaxillary line. Current ICU practice is to record PAOP and other pressures at end-exhalation.

Sterile technique is essential. Even with a protective sleeve, the catheter should preferably not be advanced after 24 hr. It should be left in place for no more than 3 d (routine replacement of catheters over guidewires has not been demonstrated to reduce the risk of infection). Fluoroscopic guidance should be considered in the presence of a temporary or recently placed permanent pacemaker or implantable cardioverter-defibrillator, RA/RV, severe tricuspid regurgitation, or LBBB (standby transcutaneous pacing allows for RHC in the presence of LBBB).

Adverse events may include arterial puncture, bleeding at insertion site, nerve injury, pneumothorax, air embolism, arrhythmias (usually minor; sustained ventricular arrhythmias requiring rx primarily occur in pts with myocardial ischemia/infarction or preexisting ventricular arrhythmias), RBBB, knotting of catheter, pulmonary artery rupture, thrombophlebitis, venous or intracardiac thrombus formation, pulmonary infarction, endocarditis, and other catheter-related infections. Risk factors for pulmonary artery rupture include pulmonary HT and recent cardiopulmonary bypass. Incidence of pulmonary infarction is reported to range from 0% to 1.3%. The risk of infection increases significantly when catheters remain in place > 3-4 d. Catheter colonization is observed in 18-63% of pts with catheters in place for an average of 3 d; bloodstream infections are documented in up to 5% of such cases.

Interpretation & Findings

The pressure recorded when a pulmonary artery branch is occluded by a balloon (PAOP) reflects pulmonary venous (LA) pressure. In the presence of PEEP, inaccurate estimation of LA pressure is likely when the catheter is above the level of the LA or when the catheter is at the level of the LA but LA pressure is low. (In one study, 43% of catheters placed through the internal jugular approach lodged at or above the level of the LA, yielding inaccurate assessment of LA pressure in the presence of PEEP.) PEEP may also affect measurement of intravascular pressures because positive airway pressure is transmitted to central vessels; this problem is particularly significant when > 10 cm H_2O of PEEP are used.

Pulmonary capillary pressure exceeds PAOP by only a few mm Hg in the normal lung but can exceed PAOP by 10-15 mm Hg in sepsis and other inflammatory disorders. PAOP reflects LA pressure and LV diastolic pressure only in the absence of mitral stenosis or more than mild mitral regurgitation. The relationship between LV pressure and volume in diastole depends on ventricular compliance, which is often abnormal in critically ill pts.

The traditional values for "optimal" PAOP (14-18 mm Hg) are based on early data from pts with acute MI. Effective vasodilator treatment of pts with heart failure results in higher output and lower PAOP, with no "lower limit" or optimal PAOP.

Thermodilution CO may be inaccurate in the presence of arrhythmias, tricuspid regurgitation, or intracardiac shunting.

4.6 Cardiac Catheterization and Coronary Angiography

J Am Coll Cardiol 1999;33:1756

Indications

Pts with known/suspected CAD who are asymptomatic or who have stable angina and have class III/IV angina, high-risk criteria on noninvasive testing, or progressively worsening abnormalities on serial tests

or

- Pts with angina who cannot be adequately risk stratified by other means
- Pts with class I/II angina with failure of medical rx
- Individuals whose occupations affect the safety of others with abnormal stress test results, or multiple clinical features that suggest high risk

Pts with nonspecific chest pain and high-risk findings on noninvasive testing

Pts with unstable coronary syndromes and

- Suspected Prinzmetal-variant angina
- High or intermediate risk for adverse outcome in pts with unstable angina—emergent catheterization if sx refractory to initial adequate medical rx or recurrent after initial stabilization
- Low-short-term-risk unstable angina subsequently reclassified as high risk on noninvasive testing where risk is defined as follows:
    1. *High risk:* Chest pain at presentation that has lasted $\geq$ 20 min; chest pain with associated pulmonary edema, hypotension, S3 gallop, new/worsening rales, or murmur of MR; > 1-mm ST depressions accompanying angina at rest
    2. *Intermediate risk:* No high-risk features but hx of angina at rest > 20 min in pt with moderate/high likelihood of CAD; rest angina relieved by TNG; nocturnal angina; angina with dynamic T-wave changes; new-onset angina in past 2 wk; angina in pt with Q waves or ST depressions $\leq$ 1 mm
    3. *Low risk:* None of the above but angina now occurring at lower workload or of increasing frequency/severity/duration; onset of angina 2 wk to 2 mon before presentation; angina with normal EKG

Pts with ischemia after revascularization and

- Suspected abrupt closure/stent thrombosis
- Recurrent angina or high-risk criteria on noninvasive evaluation
- Recurrent angina inadequately controlled by medical rx

Pts successfully resuscitated from sudden cardiac death or who have sustained (> 30 sec) monomorphic VT or nonsustained (< 30 sec) polymorphic VT

Pts with acute MI

- As an alternative to thrombolytic rx in pts who can undergo PTCA within 12 hr of the onset of sx or in whom ischemic sx persist

- Pts within 36 hr of an acute MI who develop cardiogenic shock, are < 75 yr old, and in whom revascularization can be performed within 18 hr of the onset of shock
- Pts who have a contraindication to fibrinolytic therapy
- Evolving large/anterior MI after thrombolytic rx when it is believed that reperfusion has not occurred (rescue PTCA)
- Suspected acute MI, no ST-segment elevation, with persistent/recurrent (stuttering) episodes of symptomatic ischemia or shock, severe pulmonary congestion, or continuing hypotension
- Recurrent ischemia during recovery, with acute mitral regurgitation, ventricular septal defect, pseudoaneurysm or LV aneurysm, or persistent hemodynamic instability
- Suspected coronary embolism, arteritis, trauma, metabolic or hematologic disease, or coronary spasm
- EF < 0.40, CHF, prior revascularization, or malignant ventricular arrhythmias
- CHF during the acute episode with subsequent EF > 0.40

Pts with recent MI and
- Ischemia at low levels of exercise and > 1-mm ST-segment depression, functional capacity < 5 METs, inadequate BP response (peak systolic BP < 110 mm Hg or < 30 mm Hg increase from resting level), and/or imaging abnormalities
- Clinically significant CHF during the hospital course
- Inability to perform an exercise test and EF < 0.45

Pts with suspected/known CAD scheduled for noncardiac surgery and
- Unstable angina or angina unresponsive to medical rx
- Noninvasive testing indicating significant ischemia
- Equivocal noninvasive tests in pts with recent MI and evidence of important residual ischemic risk, decompensated CHF, high-degree AV block, symptomatic ventricular arrhythmias with known structural heart disease, severe symptomatic valvular heart disease in pts undergoing high-risk operations, or aortic or major vascular or prolonged surgical procedure

- Prior MI, CHF, diabetes, and planned vascular surgery
- Urgent noncardiac surgery while convalescing from acute MI

Pts with valvular heart disease and

- Planned valve procedure, chest discomfort, and/or ischemia by noninvasive imaging or multiple risk factors for CAD
- Infective endocarditis with evidence of coronary embolization

Pts with CHF and

- Angina/regional wall motion abnormalities/scintigraphic evidence of ischemia
- Planned cardiac transplantation
- Ventricular aneurysm or other mechanical complications of MI
- Systolic dysfunction with unexplained cause
- Episodic CHF with suspected ischemia

Other

- Aortic dissection/aneurysm with known CAD
- Hypertrophic cardiomyopathy with angina despite medical rx
- Prospective immediate cardiac transplant donors with risk factors for CAD
- Pts with Kawasaki disease and coronary artery aneurysms on echo
- Blunt chest trauma and suspicion of acute MI without evidence of preexisting CAD

Contraindications

Absolute Contraindications: None

Relative Contraindications: Renal failure (acute or chronic secondary to diabetes), acute gi hemorrhage, untreated infection or unexplained fever, acute CVA, severe anemia, severe uncontrolled HT, severe symptomatic electrolyte imbalance, severe concomitant illness, digitalis toxicity, documented anaphylactoid reaction to contrast, severe peripheral disease that limits vascular access, decompensated CHF or acute pulmonary edema, severe coagulopathy, aortic valve endocarditis, severe lack of pt cooperation

Procedure

Risks of cardiac catheterization and coronary angiography include death (0.11%), MI (0.05%), CVA (0.075%), arrhythmia (0.38%), vascular complications (0.43%), contrast reaction (0.37%), hemodynamic complications (0.26%), and perforation of heart chamber (0.03%).

Predictors of major complications of coronary angiography include shock, acute MI within 24 hr, renal insufficiency, cardiomyopathy, aortic or mitral valve disease, CHF, HT, and unstable angina.

Interpretation & Findings

See Chapter 5 on ASHD and Chapter 16 on valvular disease.

Chapter 5

Atherosclerotic Coronary Artery Disease

5.1 Atherosclerosis

Nejm 2005;352:1685; Circ 2004;109:SupplII; 2001;104:365

Cause: This fatty streak develops by early adulthood. It is caused by oxidation of lipids trapped in the extracellular matrix of the subendothelial space, leading to inflammation. Risk factors include advancing age, dyslipidemia, DM, HT, cigarette smoking, obesity, and some forms of psychological stress (Circ 1998;97:1837; 1999;99:2192). *Chlamydia pneumoniae* and possibly CMV and herpes viruses have been found in atherosclerotic lesions; their role in development of ASHD is still unclear (Circ 1997;96:4095; J Am Coll Cardiol 1998;31:1217; Clin Inf Dis 1998;26:719).

Epidem

- In U.S. pts, fatty streaks increase rapidly in prevalence and extent between ages 15 and 34; by ages 15-19, intimal lesions are present in the RCA in > 50% of subjects (Jama 1999;281:727). Risk factor reduction can account for about 50% of the decline in coronary mortality in the U.S. during 1980-1990, but > 70% of the decline occurred in pts who already had documented CAD.
- Atherosclerosis risk is increased in diabetes, HT, obesity (Circ 1996;93:1372; Arch IM 1998;158:1855), dyslipidemia,

pseudoxanthoma elasticum, myotonic dystrophy, alkaptonuria, and ochronosis. In one study, children of parents with early CAD were overweight from childhood and developed adverse cardiovascular risk factor profiles at an increased rate (Jama 1997;278:1749). Poor fitness in young adults is associated with development of cardiac risk factors (Jama 2003;290:3092).

- There is an association between glycemic control and risk for CAD in middle-aged and elderly pts with NIDDM (Ann IM 1996;124:127). Compared with nondiabetic PTCA pts, diabetic pts have more extensive and diffuse atherosclerotic disease. Diabetic pts without MI have as high a risk of AMI as nondiabetic pts with prior MI (Nejm 1998;339:229). The 9-yr mortality was twice as high in diabetic pts and 9-yr rates of nonfatal MI, CABG, and repeat PTCA were higher in diabetics than in nondiabetics (Circ 1996;94:1818).
- Low HDL with borderline/high triglycerides increases risk (Circ 1995;92:1430). In elderly pts, LDL level is more predictive than total HDL (Circ 1996;94:2381). Increased triglycerides levels, small LDL particle diameter, and decreased HDL levels are all associated with progression of ASHD; debate exists as to whether triglycerides and LDL size are independent risk factors (Jama 1996;276:875,882; Circ 1998;97:1029). Lp(a) may not be an independent risk factor but may increase risk in conjunction with other lipid factors (Circ 1997;96: 1390; J Am Coll Cardiol 1998;31:519; 1998;32:2035).
- Up to 80% of pts with unstable CAD have one or more risk factors (Jama 2003;290:898), as do 87-100% of pts with fatal coronary events (Jama 2003;290:891).
- Elevated homocysteine levels have been associated with increased risk of vascular disease (Arch IM 1997;159:2299; 1999;159:1077; Jama 1997;277:1775). Reduced red cell folate and vitamin B_6 levels are also associated with increased risk (Circ 1998;97:437). In contrast to cross-sectional and

case-control studies, results of prospective studies have indicated less or no predictive ability for plasma homocysteine in ASHD (Arch IM 2000;160:422).

- Estrogens convey a protective effect against ASHD (Nejm 1999;340:1801), although the HERS trial failed to demonstrate reduced CAD mortality with estrogen replacement. In women with ASHD, severity of disease at angiography is associated with polycystic ovary disease (Ann IM 1997;126:32). Subclinical hypothyroidism is a strong indicator of risk for atherosclerosis and MI in elderly women (Ann IM 2000;132:270).
- Moderate alcohol consumption decreases risk (Circ 1996;94:3023; Nejm 1997;337:1705; Ann IM 1997;126:372), as does regular exercise (Circ 1997;96:2534; Arch IM 1998;158:1633). Conversely, low fitness is an important precursor of mortality (Jama 1996;276:205).
- Approximately 33% more deaths due to CAD occur in December-January than in June-September (Circ 1999;100:1630). Compared with the 1950-1969 reference period, the CAD death rate has been lower in subsequent decades, despite the lack of significant temporal changes in risks for recurrent MI or CHF (Framingham) (Circ 1999;100:2054).
- Causal association between peridontal disease and CAD risk has been suggested but was not confirmed by NHANES data (Jama 2000;284:1406).

Pathophys

- NO interferes with monocyte and leukocyte adhesion to the endothelium and with platelet–vessel wall interaction, decreases endothelial permeability, decreases the flux of lipoproteins into the vessel wall, and inhibits vascular smooth muscle cell proliferation. Major risk factors for atherosclerotic vascular disease (hypercholesterolemia, diabetes, HT, and smoking) are associated with impaired NO activity. Reduction in NO synthesis is the primary process involved in endothelial dysfunction and is due to reduced availability of the NOS substrate L-arginine (Circ 1998;97:108).

- Trapped LDL particles undergo progressive oxidation and are internalized by macrophages, facilitating the accumulation of cholesterol esters and resulting in the formation of foam cells. Injury increases the permeability and adhesiveness of the endothelium with respect to leukocytes and platelets. It also induces the endothelium to have procoagulant instead of anticoagulant properties.
- Modified LDL is chemotactic for other monocytes and can upregulate the expression of genes for macrophage colony-stimulating factor and monocyte chemotactic protein. It can also expand the inflammatory response by stimulating replication of monocyte-derived macrophages and entry of new monocytes and specific subtypes of T lymphocytes into lesions.
- Mediators of inflammation (tumor necrosis factor α, interleukin-1, macrophage colony-stimulating factor) increase binding of LDL to endothelium and smooth muscle and, in turn, increase the transcription of the LDL-receptor gene. Modified LDL initiates induction of urokinase and inflammatory cytokines such as interleukin-1. The inflammatory response stimulates migration and proliferation of smooth muscle cells.
- Progression of lesions is also associated with activation of genes that induce arterial calcification, which in turn changes the mechanical characteristics of the artery wall and predisposes it to plaque rupture at sites of monocytic infiltration. Plaque rupture exposes blood to tissue factors in the lesion and induces thrombosis, which is the proximate cause of clinical events. Ruptured plaques may also heal slowly, producing plaque progression (J Am Coll Cardiol 2005;45:652).

- Homocysteine is toxic to endothelium, is prothrombotic, increases collagen production, and decreases the availability of NO.
- Hypertension increases the formation of hydrogen peroxide and free radicals in plasma, which in turn can reduce formation of NO by endothelium, increase leukocyte adhesion, and increase peripheral resistance. Angiotensin II is a potent vasoconstrictor that also stimulates growth of smooth muscle and increases oxidation of LDL (Circ 1995;91:2488; Nejm 1999;340:115).
- Pts with DM have a reduced ability to develop collateral blood vessels in the presence of CAD (Circ 1999;99:2224).
- Multiple metabolic risk factors tend to cluster, resulting in the *metabolic syndrome* (Circ 1997;95:1; 1997;96:3243; Jama 1997; 278:1759).
- Persistent vasospasm may cause progression of atherosclerosis (Circ 1995;92:2446).

Sx: Atherosclerosis typically produces no symptoms until lesions become occlusive; "silent" ischemia can also occur (Cardiologia 1998;43:1159). Plaque rupture may occur with varying clinical presentations (Jama 2002;40:904).

Si: Arcus senilis; tendinous xanthomas in familial hypercholesterolemia; tuberoeruptive and planar xanthomas in familial dysbetalipoproteinemia

Crs: Progressive without intervention (Circ 1998;97:1876); possibly reversible with risk factor modification (Jama 1998;280:2001). Evidence exists for reduction in sequelae with smoking cessation (Nejm 1985;313:1511), hyperlipidemia (Lancet 1994;344:1383; Nejm 1995;333:1301; 1996;335:1001), and HT (Arch IM 1991;151:1277). There may also be an association between cessation of vasospastic activity and regression of atherosclerosis (Circ 1995;92:2446).

Lab: Measure fasting serum cholesterol: Pts with total cholesterol level > 200 mg/dL or who have hx of MI, angina, CABG, PTCA, TIA or known blockage of a carotid artery, abdominal aortic aneurysm, or ischemic peripheral arterial disease should have a complete lipid screen (NHLBI NIH Pub No 95-3045).

Elevated hsCRP level is an independent risk factor for CAD (Circ 2003;107:363; 2002;105:1135). Whether hsCRP contributes directly to the development of plaque remains uncertain (Nejm 2005;352:29).

X-ray: Studies listed under disease entries

Rx

- *Diet:* Moderate restriction of dietary fat (Circ 1997;95:2701; Jama 1997;278:1509). One egg/day has little impact (Jama 1999;281:1387). Extreme restriction of fat intake offers little further advantage and may have potentially undesirable effects in hyperlipidemic subjects.

  A high-fiber diet reduced CAD risk in middle-aged Finnish male smokers (Circ 1996;94:2720). Neither dietary fish consumption nor omega-3 fatty acid intake reduces the risk of MI, nonsudden cardiac death, or total CV mortality. Eating fish did reduce total mortality and risk of sudden cardiac death in men (Jama 1998;279:23); meta-analysis of 11 studies showed an inverse relationship between fish consumption and fatal CAD (Circ 2004;109:2705). The Mediterranean diet provides protection in pts with prior MI (Lancet 1994;343:1454; Circ 1999;99:779).
- *Physical exercise:* There is a dose-response relationship between the amount of exercise performed per week and all-cause mortality and CVD mortality in middle-aged and elderly populations. The greatest potential for reduced mortality is in sedentary individuals who become moderately active (Circ 1996; 94:857). Exercise retards progression of CAD (Circ 1997; 96;2534). Women with ASHD who participate in cardiac

rehab programs showed greater lipid benefits than men (Circ 1995;92;773).

- *Smoking:* The goal is complete cessation. There is a possible increased risk from exposure to second-hand smoke (Circ 1997;95:2374). Smoking cessation programs are cost-effective (Jama 1997;278:1759). For pts with CAD, smoking cessation reduces the crude relative mortality risk by ~36% (Jama 2003;290:86).
- *Lipid management:* Goals as listed above. Statins have proven clinical benefit (Circ 1998;97:946). Fibrates lower triglycerides and usually raise HDL (Circ 1998;98:2088). Gemfibrozil may retard the progression of ASHD in men with low HDL cholesterol as their primary lipid abnormality (Circ 1997;96:2137). Administration of atorvastatin to pts with ACS did not reduce frequence of recurrent events (Lancet 2003;361:809).
- *Diabetes:* In pts with NIDDM and microalbuminuria, multiple risk factor interventions reduce the risk of CAD events by 50% (Nejm 2003;348:383), and statin therapy reduces the risk of the first CAD event independent of LDL level (Lancet 2004;364:685; 2003;361:2005). Treatment with fenofibrate may slow the progression of plaque buildup (Lancet 2001; 357:905).

Antioxidants reduce the susceptibility of LDL to oxidation (J Am Coll Cardiol 1997;30:392). Vitamin E improves vasodilation in pts with coronary artery spasm (J Am Coll Cardiol 1998;32:1672) and improves relaxation in resistance vessels in smokers (J Am Coll Cardiol 1999;33:499), but meta-analysis of clinical trials did not show mortality reduction from vitamin E or β-carotene administration (Lancet 2003;361: 2017). AHA recommends that antioxidant vitamins be derived from foods (Circ 1996;94:1795). Pts with personal or family hx of premature ASHD, malnutrition, malabsorption syndromes, hypothyroidism, renal failure, or SLE and those taking nicotinic acid, theophylline, bile acid–binding resins, methotrexate, and L-dopa might benefit from supplemental vitamins (0.4 mg folic acid, 2 mg vitamin B_6, and 6 μg vitamin B_{12} with appropriate medical evaluation and monitoring (Circ 1999;99:178).

Addressing multiple risk factors provides long-term continuing benefits (Circ 1996;94:946).

5.2 Stable Angina Pectoris

Circ 2003;107:149; 1999;99:2829

Cause: Imbalance between myocardial oxygen supply and perfusion pressure (aortic diastolic pressure), coronary artery tone and resistance, presence of epicardial coronary artery stenoses, and myocardial O_2 demand. "Stable angina" by definition is a state in which this imbalance can be corrected.

In syndrome X, pts have angina and abnormal stress tests in the presence of angiographically normal coronary arteries.

Epidem: Stable angina is the mode of presentation of ~50% of all pts with CAD.

Pathophys

- *Conditions that can increase O_2 demand:* Hyperthermia, hypothyroidism, cocaine use, HT, mental stress, AV fistula, hypertrophic or dilated cardiomyopathy, AS, tachycardia
- *Conditions that can decrease O_2 supply:* Anemia, hypoxemia (COPD, asthma, pneumonia, pulmonary HT, interstitial pulmonary fibrosis, obstructive sleep apnea), sickle cell disease, hyperviscosity (polycythemia, leukemia), AS, hypertrophic cardiomyopathy (J Am Coll Cardiol 1999;33:2092)
- *Mental stress:* In the laboratory, ischemia is associated with peripheral vaoconstriction and increased afterload. During daily life, ischemia is accompanied by increased inotropy (J Am Coll Cardiol 1999;33:1476).

Syndrome X pts may have a decreased coronary vasodilator capacity and microvascular dysfunction (CV Res 1998; 40:410; Am J Cardiol 1999;83:149).

Sx

- *Typical angina:* Substernal chest discomfort with characteristic quality and duration, provoked by exertion/emotional stress, relieved by rest/TNG; *atypical angina:* Pain meeting 2 of preceding characteristics; *noncardiac chest pain;* Meets ≤ 1 of the typical angina characteristics (J Am Coll Cardiol 1983;1:574)
- *Functional status classification:* Class I: Ordinary physical activity does not cause angina. Class II: Slight limitation of ordinary activity (climbing stairs rapidly or after meals or in cold). Class III: Marked limitations of ordinary physical activity (walking 1-2 blocks on level; climbing 1 flight of stairs at a normal pace). Class IV: Inability to carry on any physical activity without discomfort (Circ 1976;54:522).
- *Differential dx:* Aortic dissection, pericarditis, pulmonary embolus, pneumothorax, pleuritis, esophageal spasm and reflux, cholecystitis, peptic ulcer disease, pancreatitis, chest wall pain, herpes zoster, panic disorder

  Only 28% of diabetic pts with abnormal Tl stress tests reported exertional pain during the test; up to 75% of ischemic episodes (measured by AECG) in pts with stable angina are asymptomatic (Circ 1996;93:2089).

Si: During ischemia, may hear paradoxically split S2, transient S3 or S4, or murmur of MR

Crs: Average annual mortality in pts with CAD is 1-4%; about 1.5% for 1- and 2-vessel disease; and about 7% for 3-vessel disease (Circ 1994;90:2645). Risk stratification can also be based on noninvasive testing. Duke treadmill score (DTS) = exercise time − (5 × ST deviation) − (4 × exercise angina), with 0 = none, 1 = nonlimiting, and 2 = exercise-limiting (Circ 1998;98:1622). The 5-yr survival rates range from 95% for pts with 1-vessel disease to 59% for pts with 3-vessel disease and severe proximal LAD stenosis (J Am Coll Cardiol 1996;27:964).

Noninvasive Risk Stratification

High risk (greater than 3% annual mortality rate)

1. Severe resting LV dysfunction (LVEF < 35%)
2. High-risk treadmill score (score ≤ −11)
3. Severe exercise LV dysfunction (exercise LVEF < 35%)
4. Stress-induced large perfusion defect (particularly if anterior)
5. Stress-induced multiple perfusion defects of moderate size
6. Large, fixed perfusion defect with LV dilation or increased lung uptake (Tl-201)
7. Stress-induced moderate perfusion defect with LV dilation or increased lung uptake (Tl-201)
8. Echo wall motion abnormality (involving > 2 segments) developing with low-dose dobutamine (< 10 mg/kg/min) or at a low heart rate (< 120 beat/min)
9. Stress echo evidence of extensive ischemia

Intermediate risk (1-3% annual mortality rate)

1. Mild/moderate resting LV dysfunction (LVEF = 35-49%)
2. Intermediate-risk treadmill score (−11 < score < +5)
3. Stress-induced moderate perfusion defect without LV dilation or increased lung intake (Tl-201)
4. Limited stress echo ischemia with a wall motion abnormality only at higher doses of dobutamine involving ≤ 2 segments

Low risk (less than 1% annual mortality rate)

1. Low-risk treadmill score (score ≥ +5)
2. Normal or small myocardial perfusion defect at rest or with stress
3. Normal stress echo wall motion or no change of limited resting wall motion abnormalities during stress

Although the published data are limited, pts with these findings will probably not be at low risk in the presence of either a high-risk treadmill score or severe resting LV dysfunction (LVEF < 35%) (J Am Coll Cardiol 1999;33:2092).

Lab: AHA recommends EKG, FBS, hgb, and lipid profile.

Exercise EKG without imaging: For pts with an intermediate likelihood of CAD, including those with complete RBBB or < 1-mm resting ST depression, but not WPW, LBBB, digoxin rx, paced rhythm, > 1-mm resting ST depression

- *Absolute contraindications:* Acute MI within 2 d, arrhythmias causing symptoms or hemodynamic compromise, symptomatic and severe AS, symptomatic CHF, acute pulmonary embolus or pulmonary infarction, acute myocarditis or pericarditis and acute aortic dissection
- *Relative contraindications:* Left main coronary stenosis, moderate AS, electrolyte abnormalities, systolic HT > 200 mm Hg, diastolic BP > 110 mm Hg, tachyarrhythmia or bradyarrhythmia, hypertrophic cardiomyopathy and other forms of outflow tract obstruction, mental or physical impairment leading to an inability to exercise adequately, high-degree AV block

Exercise EKG with radionuclide or echo imaging: For pts who have an abnormal rest EKG, who are using digoxin, or for whom PTCA is planned. Dipyridamole or adenosine myocardial perfusion or dobutamine echo are recommended for pts who are unable to exercise. Chemical stress with nuclear scanning is preferred for pts with LBBB or paced rhythm (see Chapter 4 on tests for the relevant protocols). Stress echo provides higher specificity, greater versatility, better convenience/efficacy/availability, and lower cost. Stress perfusion imaging has a higher technical success rate, higher sensitivity (especially for 1-vessel CAD), and better accuracy in evaluating possible ischemia when multiple rest LV wall motion abnormalities are present, and it has a more extensive published database.

Echocardiogram: During chest pain, with murmur suggestive of AS, MR, or hypertrophic cardiomyopathy; echo or RVG for pts with h/o prior MI, pathological Q waves, or si/sx suggestive of CHF or with complex ventricular arrhythmia to assess LV function

Coronary angiography: For pts with disabling (classes III/IV) chronic stable angina despite medical rx, pts with high-risk criteria on noninvasive testing regardless of anginal severity, pts with angina who have survived sudden cardiac death or serious ventricular arrhythmia or who have si/sx of CHF, and pts who have clinical characteristics that indicate a high likelihood of severe CAD; may also be used for pts with significant LV dysfunction (ejection fraction < 45%), class I/II angina, and demonstrable ischemia but less than high-risk criteria on noninvasive testing, and those with inadequate prognostic information after noninvasive testing

X-ray: CXR in pts with si/sx of CHF, valvular heart disease, pericardial disease, or aortic dissection/aneurysm

In a study of 3895 asymptomatic pts undergoing EBCT, no subject with a Ca^{++} score < 10 had an abnormal SPECT compared with 2.6% of those with scores of 11-100, 11.3% of those with scores 101-399, and 46% of those with scores > 400 (Circ 2000;101:244).

Rx: *Medical:* ASA; β-blockers; sl TNG or TNG spray; intermittent transdermal TNG rx increases exercise duration and maintains anti-ischemic effects for 12 hr after patch application without significant evidence of nitrate tolerance (Circ 1995;91:1368); calcium antagonists and/or long-acting nitrates when β-blockers are contraindicated, are not successful, or lead to unacceptable side effects (short-acting dihydropyridine calcium antagonists should be avoided); clopidogrel when ASA is absolutely contraindicated; lipid-lowering therapy in pts with documented or suspected CAD and non-HDL cholesterol > 130 mg/dL with a target LDL < 100 mg/dL; ACEIs in pts with diabetes and/or LV systolic dysfunction; PEACE trial (8290 pts) showed no reduction in CV death rate from ACEIs for pts with normal LV systolic function (Nejm 2004;351:20).

- In low-risk pts with stable CAD, aggressive lipid-lowering rx was reported to be as effective as angioplasty and usual care in reducing the incidence of ischemic events (Nejm 1999;341:70).
- In a meta-analysis, β-blockers provided similar clinical outcomes and were associated with fewer adverse events than Ca^{++} antagonists in randomized trials of pts with stable angina (Jama 1999;281:1927).
- The presence of other medical conditions may influence drug choice.
- Enhanced external counterpulsation (EECP) reduces angina and extends time to exercise-induced ischemia in pts with symptomatic CAD (J Am Coll Cardiol 2003;41:1918; 1999; 33:1833).
- Chelation rx has not been shown to have beneficial effects in pts with stable angina and a positive treadmill test (Jama 2002;287:481).
- Azythromycin did not alter the risk of cardiac events in pts with stable CAD (Nejm 2005;352:1637).

Revascularization: PTCA or other catheter-based techniques, CABG, laser surgical transmyocardial revascularization

- CABG for significant left main CAD or left main equivalent (> 70% stenoses of proximal LAD and LCx), for 3-vessel disease (survival benefit greater in pts with abnormal LV function: ejection fraction < 40%), for 2-vessel disease with significant proximal LAD disease and either abnormal LV function (ejection fraction < 50%) or demonstrable ischemia on noninvasive testing, for 1- or 2-vessel CAD without significant proximal left anterior descending CAD in survivors of sudden cardiac death or sustained VT, and for ongoing ischemia or hemodynamic compromise after failed PTCA

- PTCA or CABG for pts (1) with 1- or 2-vessel CAD without significant proximal LAD disease but with a large area of viable myocardium and high-risk criteria on noninvasive testing; (2) with prior PTCA and recurrent stenosis associated with a large area of viable myocardium and/or high-risk criteria on noninvasive testing; or (3) who have not been successfully treated by medical rx and can undergo revascularization with acceptable risk
- PTCA for pts with 2- or 3-vessel disease with significant proximal LAD disease, who have anatomy suitable for catheter-based rx and normal LV function, and who do not have treated diabetes
- Evidence favors repeat CABG for pts with multiple saphenous vein graft stenoses and PTCA or CABG for pts with 1- or 2-vessel CAD *without* significant proximal LAD disease but with a *moderate* area of viable myocardium and demonstrable ischemia on noninvasive testing or with 1-vessel disease with significant proximal LAD disease.
- Among 1018 pts randomly assigned to PTCA or medical rx, PTCA improved the perceived quality of life compared with continued medical rx (J Am Coll Cardiol 2000;35:907).

Stents: Pts with multivessel CAD who receive stents have 3-yr survival rates without MI or CVA that are identical to the rates for pts who receive CABG (Circ 2004;109:1114), but 1-yr revascularization rates for pts with bare metal stents remain higher than for pts with CABG (Lancet 2002;360:965). In pts with in-stent restenosis, brachytherapy (intra-coronary γ irradiation) reduced the 12-mon recurrence rate in saphenous vein grafts from 57% to 17%; however, restenosis after brachytherapy is common at 3 yr

(Circ 2003;107:2274,2283; Nejm 2002;346:1194). Compared with bare metal stents, stents containing sirolimus (rapamycin), an inhibitor of cytokine- and growth factor–mediated cell proliferation, reduced incidence of stent failure at 270 d from 21% to 8.6% (Jama 2005;293:165; Circ 2005;111:1040; Nejm 2003;349:1315); stents treated with paclitaxel reduced restenosis rates at 9 mon from 26.6% to 7.9% (Nejm 2004;350:221).

Sex: Bypass graft surgery is associated with equally low mortality in women and men (1.4% vs 1.1%) (Circ 1995;92:80).

Age: Long-term results as measured by cumulative survival and cardiac event-free survival in pts who underwent CABG reoperation are good. The perioperative mortality rate for repeat CABG is reported to be 3%, with cumulative survival rates of 90.1%, 74%, and 63.4%. Cardiac event-free survival rates were 91.5%, 83.4%, and 67.8% at the 5-, 10-, and 15-yr follow-ups, respectively. Advanced age, HT, and a decreased LVEF significantly increase surgical risk (Chest 1999;115:1593). Cardiac mortality may be less than that expected in these pts because of a high risk of noncardiac death (J Am Coll Cardiol 1997;30:881). In pts > 80 yr old, survival at 1-5 yr was similar for medical or invasive rx (Circ 2004;110:1213; Jama 2003;289:1117). Pts > age 75 who had recurrent sx despite medical rx benefited from revascularization (Lancet 2001;358:951).

Functional status (BARI): Use of anti-ischemic medication was higher in pts post-PTCA than in those post-CABG. Among pts who were angina-free at 5 yr, 52% of pts who had PTCA required revascularization vs 6% of pts who had CABG, but differences in angina-free rates between pts assigned to PTCA and CABG decreased from 73% vs 95% at 4-14 weeks to 79% vs 85% at 5 yr (Jama 1997;277:715).

CHF: Hx of CHF is associated with increased early and intermediate-term mortality in pts undergoing PTCA (J Am Coll Cardiol 1998;32:936).

Diabetes (BARI): Pts with diabetes have higher rates of revascularization and lower 1-yr survival rates than nondiabetic pts (J Am Coll Cardiol 2004;43:1348). The 5-yr cardiac mortality in pts with multivessel disease was greater after PTCA than CABG. No differences were found for the composite end point of cardiac mortality or MI between groups or for cardiac mortality in nondiabetic pts; a difference was found in diabetic pts on drug therapy (Circ 1997;96:2162). In diabetics, the better survival with CABG vs PTCA (5.8% vs 20.6%) was due to reduced cardiac mortality in pts receiving at least one LIMA graft (Circ 1997;96:1761). Pts with advanced 3-vessel CAD and IDDM should be revascularized by CABG. Diabetic pts (especially those taking oral hypoglycemic agents) with minimal multivessel disease could be considered for PTCA. Those with moderate ASHD, especially pts requiring insulin, should be considered for surgery until the results of future trials are completed (Circ 1999;99:847).

Repeat surgery: In-hospital (11.5% vs 4.4%), 1-yr (19.3% vs 7.9%), and 3-yr mortality rates (28.8% vs 13.1%) after CABG were significantly higher in pts of age 80 yr compared with younger pts. Although their initial surgical risk was high, octogenarians who underwent CABG had a long-term survival rate similar to that for the general U.S. octogenarian population (Circ 1995;92:85). The 10-yr patency for saphenous vein grafts is 61% vs 89% for LIMA grafts (J Am Coll Cardiol 2004;44:2149).

Risk factors: Treatment of HT according to Joint National Conference VI guidelines; smoking cessation therapy; management of diabetes and hyperlipidemia; exercise training programs; weight reduction in obese pts in the presence of HT, hyperlipidemia, or DM

- Gemfibrozil produced a significant reduction in risk of major cardiovascular events in pts with CAD whose primary lipid abnormality was a low HDL cholesterol level (Nejm 1999;341:410).

- Nicotine patches can also reduce the extent of exercise-induced myocardial ischemia as assessed by exercise Tl-201 SPECT (J Am Coll Cardiol 1997;30:125). All currently available nicotine replacement therapies appear to be equally efficacious, approximately doubling the quit rate compared with placebo. Concomitant behavioral rx increases quit rates, and combining the patch with nicotine gum or the patch with bupropion may increase the quit rate compared with any single rx (Jama 1999;81:72).

Under investigation: Folate supplementation, identification and appropriate treatment of clinical depression, and intervention directed at psychosocial stress reduction (J Am Coll Cardiol 1999;33: 2092; 1999;34:1262)

- In pts at high risk for cardiovascular events, rx with vitamin E had no apparent effect on cardiovascular outcomes (Nejm 2000;342:154).
- In patients with angina refractory to medical rx and CAD that precluded CABG/PTCA, transmyocardial revascularization improved cardiac perfusion and clinical status over a 12-mon period (Nejm 1999;341:1021).
- Ramipril reduced rates of death, MI, and CVA in high-risk pts not known to have a low EF or CHF (Nejm 2000;342:145).

5.3 Acute Coronary Syndrome

(In older literature: Ustable angina and non–Q-wave MI)

Circ 2002;106:1893; Nejm 2000;342:101; J Am Coll Cardiol 1999;33:107; CV Res 1999;41:323

Cause: Unstable angina results from an imbalance between myocardial O_2 supply and demand. The most common cause is nonocclusive thrombus on a fissured or eroded nonocclusive plaque, but other causes include dynamic obstruction due to Prinzmetal angina (focal spasm of a segment of an epicardial coronary artery with or without nonobstructive plaque); nonfocal constriction of arteries containing plaque that is caused by adrenergic stimuli, cold immersion, or cocaine; microcirculatory angina with constriction of small intramural coronary resistance vessels; progressive mechanical obstruction; inflammation and possibly infection; or extrinsic causes (eg, tachyarrhythmia, fever, thyrotoxicosis, hyperadrenergic states, HT or hypotension, aortic stenosis, anemia, hypoxemia).

Epidem: Similar to that for stable angina and AMI. In 1991, 570,000 hospitalizations for this principal diagnosis in the U.S. resulted in 3.1 million hospital days (AHCPR Pub 94-0602, 1994).

Elevated total homocysteine levels on admission predict late cardiac events in acute coronary syndromes (Circ 2000;102:605).

Pathophys: Inciting event is the rupture of an atherosclerotic plaque. Enzyme degradation and external mechanical shear forces in the artery rupture the fibrous cap and expose the underlying procoagulant atheromatous material. Macrophage deposition and infiltration ensue, with the release of enzymes resulting in digestion of the fibrous cap's collagen and elastin. Cytokines enhance the plaque destabilization by inhibiting collagen synthesis. Circumferential stresses cause further plaque breakdown. The absence of Q waves is determined by the size of the infarct rather than the transmural extent (J Am Coll Cardiol 2004;44:554).

The ruptured plaque favors thrombus formation. Secretion of thromboxanes, serotonin, and other vasoactive substances promotes further platelet aggregation, and vasospasm contributes to both plaque rupture and thrombus formation.

Increasing severity of UA by Braunwald classification (see below) has been associated with increasing prevalence of thrombus, cellularity, atheroma, and neovasculature in plaque fragments (CV Res 1999;41:369).

Sx: Ischemic chest pain at rest, of new onset, or in a progressive pattern. Key elements: change in frequency, increase in severity or duration of sx, occurrence of episodes lasting > 20 min, progression from effort or stress-related sx to sx at rest, new onset of nocturnal sx, decrease in amount of stress or effort necessary to provoke sx.

- Original Braunwald classification:
  Class I: New onset (< 2 mon duration), severe, or accelerated (increasing frequency or with less exertion)
  Class II: Angina at rest but not within past 48 hr
  Class III: Angina at rest within past 48 hr (Circ 1989;80:410)
  Expanded classification subdivides angina into class A, B, or C, depending on whether pain (A) develops in the presence of an extracardiac condition that intensifies myocardial ischemia, (B) develops in the absence of such a condition, or (C) develops within 2 wk of AMI.
- Braunwald class III: Increased age, DM, or need for iv nitrates indicate a high-risk pt (J Am Coll Cardiol 1999;33:107). The 30-day risk for death and MI is as high as 20% in class IIIB-$_{Tpos}$ but < 2% in class IIIB-$_{Tneg}$. Troponins can effectively guide rx with glycoprotein IIb/IIIa antagonists or LMW heparins (Circ 2000;102:118).

Si: As in stable angina: possible paradoxical splitting of S2, transient S3 or S4, or murmur of MR during ischemic episode. Ddx: AMI , aortic dissection, leaking or ruptured thoracic aneurysm, pericarditis, pneumothorax, and pulmonary embolism.

Crs: Among pts with chest pain anticipated to have a low prevalence of CAD, positive cardiac troponin T identifies a subgroup with high prevalence of extensive CAD and increased risk for long-term adverse outcomes (J Am Coll Cardiol 2000;35:1827).

Cmplc: Pts with CK-MB elevation > 5 times normal after PTCA with stenting had higher late mortality and more unfavorable event-free survival rates than pts with normal or lower CK-MB elevations (J Am Coll Cardiol 2000;35:1134).

In pts with a first non–ST-segment-elevation acute MI, those with lateral ST-segment depression had higher rates of death (14.3% vs 2.6%,), severe CHF (14.3% vs 4.1%), and angina with EKG changes (20.0% vs 11.6%); a lower LVEF; and more frequent left main coronary artery or 3-vessel disease (J Am Coll Cardiol 2000;35:1813).

Pts may be classified in terms of short-term risk of death/nonfatal MI (Circ 2002;106:1905):

- High risk: Pain (> 20 min) at rest, pulmonary edema, new/worsening MR murmur, S3 gallop, hypotension, bradycardia, tachycardia, age > 75 yr, transient ST changes > 0.05 mV, BBB, VT, or elevated TnT or TnI levels
- Intermediate risk: Hx of prior MI, CVA, CABG, ASA use, rest angina relieved by TNG, age > 70 yr, T-wave inversions, or mild TnT or TnI elevations

Lab: TIMI-III: 1-mm ST-segment deviation, 0.5-mm ST-segment deviation, or LBBB-identified high-risk pts. T-wave inversion did not predict outcome (J Am Coll Cardiol 1997;30:133).

Elevation of CK-MB level is strongly related to mortality in pts with acute coronary syndromes without ST-segment elevation, and the increased risk begins with CK-MB levels just above normal (PURSUIT trial) (Jama 2000;283:347).

The combined incidence of death and nonfatal MI in pts with UA without and with elevated troponin-I levels was 5.8% vs 27.3%, respectively. At 1 yr, 68% of pts with elevated cTnI and 90% of pts without elevations were free of cardiac events (Circ 1997;95:2053). (See Table 5.1.)

X-ray: CHF on CXR in UA indicates high likelihood of severe CAD.

Rx: *Initial triage:* Pts should be referred to a facility that allows evaluation by a physician and recording of 12-lead EKG. If resting chest discomfort > 20 min duration, hemodynamic instability, or syncope/presyncope is present, refer to ER.

Table 5.1 Cardiac Markers in Acute Coronary Syndromes

Marker	Advantages	Disadvantages	Point-of-Care Test Available	Comment	Clinical Recommendation
CK-MB	Rapid, cost-efficient accurate assays Ability to detect early reinfarction	Loss of specificity in setting of skeletal muscle disease or injury including surgery Low sensitivity during very early MI (< 6 hr after symptom onset) or later after symptom onset (> 36 hr) and for minor myocardial damage (detectable by troponins)	Yes	Familiar to majority of clinicians	Prior standard and still acceptable diagnostic test in most clinical circumstances
CK-MB isoforms	Early detection of MI	Specificity profile similar to CK-MB Current assays require special expertise	No	Experience to date predominantly in dedicated research centers	Useful for extremely early (3–6 hr after symptom onset) detection of MI in centers with demonstrated familiarity with assay technique.
Myoglobin	High sensitivity Useful in early detection of MI Detection of reperfusion Most useful in ruling out MI	Very low specificity in setting of skeletal muscle injury or disease Rapid return to normal range limits sensitivity for later presentations	Yes	More convenient early marker than CK-MB isoforms because of greater availability of assays for myoglobin	Should not be used as only diagnostic marker because of lack of cardiac specificity

continues

Table 5.1 continued

Marker	Advantages	Disadvantages	Point-of-Care Test Available	Comment	Clinical Recommendation
				Rapid-release kinetics make myoglobin useful for noninvasive monitoring of reperfusion in patients with established MI	
Cardiac troponins	Powerful tool for risk stratification Greater sensitivity and specificity than CK-MB Detection of recent MI up to 2 wk after onset Useful for selection of rx Detection of reperfusion	Low sensitivity in very early phase of MI ($<$ 6 hr after symptom onset) and requires repeat measurement at 8-12 hr, if negative Limited ability to detect late minor reinfarction	Yes	Data on diagnostic performance and potential therapeutic implications increasingly available from clinical trials	Useful as a single test to efficiently diagnose NSTEMI (including minor myocardial damage), with serial measurements; clinicians should familiarize themselves with diagnostic "cutoffs" used in their local hospital laboratory

(Circ 2000;102:1193)

A 12-lead EKG should be obtained within 10 min in pts with ongoing chest discomfort. Biomarkers of cardiac injury should be measured (cardiac-specific troponin preferred; CK-MB also acceptable). In pts with negative cardiac markers within 6 hr of onset of pain, another sample should be drawn in 6-12 hr. CRP may also be useful.

Use hx, exam, 12-lead EKG, and initial cardiac markers to stratify pts as having noncardiac pain, chronic stable angina, possible or definite ACS. Pts with definite or possible ACS and initially normal EKG and cardiac markers should be observed in facility with cardiac monitoring, and repeat EKG and markers should be obtained 6-12 hr after the onset of sx. If follow-up data are normal, a stress test may be performed and low-risk pts with a negative stress test can be managed as outpts.

Pts with definite ACS and ongoing pain, positive cardiac markers, new ST-segment deviations, new deep T-wave inversions, hemodynamic abnormalities, or a positive stress test should be admitted for further management. Pts with definite ACS and ST-segment elevation should be evaluated for immediate reperfusion rx.

Anti-ischemic rx: Bed rest with continuous EKG monitoring for pts with ongoing rest pain; sl TNG followed by iv administration; O_2 for pts with cyanosis or respiratory distress with finger pulse oximetry or ABGs to confirm $SaO_2 > 90\%$; morphine iv when sx not immediately relieved with TNG or when acute CHF and/or severe agitation present; iv β-blocker if ongoing chest pain, followed by po administration in the absence of contraindications; ACEI when HT in pts with LV systolic dysfunction/CHF/diabetes; po long-acting Ca^{++} antagonists for recurrent ischemia if β-blockers and nitrates fully used; intra-aortic balloon pump counterpulsation for severe ischemia despite intensive medical rx or for hemodynamic instability in pts pre- or post-coronary angiography.

Antiplatelet/anticoagulation rx (Chest 2004;126:513S): Administer ASA as soon as possible after presentation and continue indefinitely. Give clopidogrel for pts who are unable to take ASA because of hypersensitivity or major GI intolerance; add clopidogrel to ASA for pts in whom an early noninterventional approach is planned (Jama 2004;292:45,89). Anticoagulation with IV unfractionated heparin or SC LMW heparin should be added to antiplatelet rx. In pts with unstable angina or non–Q-wave MI, a meta-analysis showed a 33% reduction in risk of MI or death in pts with unstable angina treated with ASA plus heparin compared with those teated with ASA alone (Jama 1996;276:811). Enoxaparin was reported to reduce rates of recurrent ischemic events with a sustained benefit at 1 yr (TIMI IIB, ESSENCE trials) (J Am Coll Cardiol 2000;36:693; Circ 1999;100:1602).

A platelet GP IIb/IIIa receptor antagonist should be administered in addition to ASA and heparin in pts with continuing ischemia or with other high-risk features and in pts in whom a PCI is planned; eptifibatide and tirofiban are approved for this use. Abciximab can also be used for 12-24 hr in pts with unstable angina in whom a PCI is planned within the next 24 hr. IIb/IIIa inhibitors have been shown to decrease the incidence of death or MI in pts not scheduled for early revascularization (Lancet 2002;359:189).

The OASIS trial reported that fondaparinux, a synthetic Factor Xa inhibitor, is as effective as enoxaparin (LMWH) in reducing the risk of ischemic events at 9 days and reduced major bleeding by 48%, as well as, short (30 days) and long-term (180 days) mortality; the agent has not yet been approved by the FDA for such use (NEJM 2006;354:1464).

Risk stratification: Noninvasive stress testing is recommended for (1) low-risk pts who are free of ischemia at rest or low-level activity and free of CHF for a minimum of 12-24 hr and (2) intermediate-risk pts who are free of ischemia at rest or low-level activity and free of CHF for a minimum of 2-3 d. An imaging modality is added in pts with > 1 mm resting ST-segment depression, LVH, BBB, intravascular conduction defect, pre-excitation, or digoxin use. Pharmacological stress testing with imaging may be performed when physical limitations (eg, arthritis, amputation, severe peripheral vascular disease, severe COPD, general debility) preclude adequate exercise stress. Prompt angiography without noninvasive risk stratification is appropriate in case of failure of stabilization with intensive medical rx. An echo or radionuclide angiogram may be used to evaluate LV function in pts with definite ACS who are not scheduled for coronary arteriography and left ventriculography.

An early invasive strategy is mandated in pts who experience recurrent angina or ischemia at rest or low-level activities despite intensive medical rx or with recurrent angina or ischemia, elevated TnT/TnI levels, new ST depressions, CHF sx, S_3 gallop, pulmonary edema, worsening rales, or new/worsening mitral regurgitation, high-risk findings on noninvasive stress testing, EF < 0.40, hypotension, sustained VT, PCI within 6 mon or prior CABG; this strategy is optional in all other ACS pts (Jama 2003;290:891). The FRISC-II (7457 pts) and RITA-3 (1810 pts) trials showed reductions in mortality, refractory angina, and late revascularization with early use of an invasive strategy in pts with ACS (J Am Coll Cardiol 2002;40:1902; Lancet 2002;360:743).

CABG is used for pts with significant left main CAD, 3-vessel disease (the survival benefit is greater in pts with EF < 0.50), and 2-vessel disease with significant proximal LAD disease and demonstrable ischemia or EF < 0.50. PCI or CABG is used for pts with 1- or 2-vessel CAD without significant proximal LAD disease but with a large area of viable myocardium and high-risk criteria on noninvasive testing. PCI is used for pts with multivessel disease, suitable coronary anatomy, normal LV function, and no diabetes. An iv platelet GP IIb/IIIa inhibitor is administered in pts undergoing PCI.

Repeat CABG for pts with multiple SVG stenoses, especially when there is significant stenosis of a graft that supplies the LAD. PCI is appropriate for focal SVG lesions or multiple stenoses in pts who are poor candidates for reoperative surgery. PCI or CABG is used for pts with 1- or 2-vessel CAD without significant proximal LAD disease but with a moderate area of viable myocardium and ischemia on noninvasive testing and for pts with single-vessel proximal LAD disease.

CABG with the internal mammary artery is appropriate for pts with multivessel disease and treated DM.

At discharge, all pts should be given sl or spray TNG, ASA 75-325 mg/d in the absence of contraindications, and clopidogrel 75 mg/d (Jama 2002;288:2411). Give β-blockers in the absence of contraindications. Lipid-lowering agents and diet are appropriate strategies in pts with LDL cholesterol > 125 mg/dL. Give ACEIs to pts with CHF, LVEF < 0.40, HT, or diabetes. Low-risk medically treated pts and revascularized pts should return in 2-6 wk; higher-risk pts should return in 1-2 wk. Pts managed initially with a conservative strategy who experience recurrent unstable angina or class III sx despite medical rx should undergo coronary arteriography. Pts who have tolerable stable angina or no sx at follow-up visits should be managed medically.

Risk factor modification: Specific instructions should be given regarding the lifestyle factors—smoking cessation, achievement/maintenance of optimal weight, daily exercise, and diet; BP control with target < 130/85 mm Hg; control of hyperglycemia in diabetes; HMG-COA reductase inhibitors for LDL cholesterol > 130 mg/dL or if LDL cholesterol > 100 mg/dL after dietary modifications (Lancet 2001;357:1063; Jama 2001;285:1711); and fibrates or niacin in pts with HDL cholesterol < 40 mg/dL. Experimental animal models suggest that statins may foster plaque stability through reduction in macrophages and cholesterol ester content, increased volume of collagen and smooth muscle cells, and inhibition of platelet aggregation (Jama 1998;279:1643).

There should be a low threshold for angiography in post-CABG pts. Stress testing should, in general, involve imaging in post-CABG pts.

Pts using cocaine should receive TNG and oral Ca^{++} antagonists if ST-segment elevation or depression accompanies ischemic chest discomfort; immediate coronary arteriography is appropriate for pts whose ST segments remain elevated after TNG and Ca^{++} antagonists. Thrombolysis (with or without PCI) is used if thrombus is detected. Consider using iv Ca^{++} antagonists for pts with ST-segment deviation suggestive of ischemia and β-blockers for pts with systolic BP > 150 mm Hg or pulse > 100 beat/min. Begin thrombolytic rx if ST segments remain elevated despite TNG and Ca^{++} antagonists and coronary arteriography is not possible.

Variant (Prinzmetal) angina: Use coronary arteriography in pts with episodic chest pain and ST-segment elevation that resolves with TNG and/or Ca^{++} antagonists. Rx with nitrates and Ca^{++} antagonists is appropriate in pts whose coronary arteriogram is normal or shows only nonobstructive lesions. Consider provocative testing in pts with a nonobstructive lesion on coronary arteriography, a clinical picture of coronary spasm, and transient ST-segment elevation.

Pts with syndrome X: Provide reassurance and medical rx with nitrates, β-blockers, and Ca^{++} antagonists, and institute risk factor reduction. Order intracoronary US to rule out missed obstructive lesions. If no EKGs are available during chest pain and coronary spasm cannot be ruled out, consider coronary arteriography and provocative testing with methylergonovine, acetylcholine, or methacholine; use estrogen replacement rx in postmenopausal women unless there is a contraindication, or imipramine for continued pain.

The troponin T level may identify members of the high-risk subgroup suitable for PTCA who would benefit from antiplatelet rx with abciximab (CAPTURE) (Nejm 1999;340:1623).

The 10-yr survival and event-free survival rates are similar in pts with stable and unstable angina rx with PTCA. No evidence of an increased rate of recurrent cardiovascular events has been found in the unstable group (J Am Coll Cardiol 998;32:1603). Abciximab and stent implantation confer complementary long-term clinical benefits (EPISTENT trial) (Nejm 1999;341:319).

Off-pump CABG is as safe as the on-pump procedure in low-risk populations (Lancet 2002;360:327). Off-pump pts had improved cognitive outcomes at 3 mon but no difference from on-pump pts at 1 yr (Jama 2002;287:1405).

Use of antibiotics that are effective against C. *pneumoniae* did not reduce the rate of cardiac events after hospitalization for acute coronary syndrome (Nejm 2005;352:1646).

5.4 Acute Myocardial Infarction

Circ 2005;111:940; 2004;110:e82; CV Res 1999;41:323; Ann IM 1999;131:47; Chest 1998;114:634S

Cause: Atherosclerotic plaque rupture and resulting intracoronary thrombosis account for most acute coronary syndromes (unstable angina, non–Q-wave MI and Q-wave MI).

Epidem: Risk factors are the same as for other forms of ASHD: HT, DM, hyperlipidemia, cigarette use, and increased homocysteine levels.

- There is a seasonal pattern in the occurrence of AMIs characterized by a marked peak of cases in the winter and a nadir in the summer months (J Am Coll Cardiol 1998;31:226).
- Exertion-related MI tends to occur in habitually inactive people with multiple cardiac risk factors (Jama 1999;282:1731).

- The risk of AMI is elevated by 23.7 times over baseline in the 60 min after cocaine use (Circ 1999;99:2737).
- The 30-d mortality in AMI rx with thrombolysis was 12.5% for pts with IDDM, 9.7% for pts with NIIDDM, and 6.2% for pts without diabetes. The incidence of CVA, cardiac failure, shock, AV block, and Aflut/Afib was greater in diabetic pts. Diabetes remained an independent predictor for mortality at 1-yr follow-up (14.5% vs 8.9%) (J Am Coll Cardiol 1997;30:171).
- Sexual activity can trigger AMI, but the absolute risk increase caused by sexual activity is 1 chance in 1 million for a healthy individual. The relative risk is not increased in pts with prior h/o CAD. Regular exercise appears to prevent triggering (Jama 1996;275:1405).

Pathophys: Acute nonfatal cardiac events result predominantly from development of significant new coronary lesions, not initially severe enough to cause ischemia (Jama 1997;277:318), with rupture of atheromatous plaque. Non–Q-wave MI often occurs after rapid progression of atherosclerotic lesions at a recently minimally diseased site or as transient occlusion at the site of severe stenosis in the presence of extensive collateral circulation. In non–Q-wave MI, complex-appearing lesions actually resolve over the course of 2-3 mon (CV Res 1999;41:323).

The duration of occlusion > 20 min, resulting in CPK leakage from the myocardium. Reperfusion usually occurs within 2 hr, preventing Q-wave MI. In 75% of pts with non–Q-wave MI, the infarct-related artery is patent with an extensive collateral circulation.

Q-wave MI results from persistent complete occlusion of the artery without adequate compensatory collateral circulation post-MI. Healing of the infarct-related lesion requires > 1 mon, and unstable yellow plaque with adherent thrombus is common during that period (Circ 1998;97:26).

Acute MI slows flow globally. Relief of the culprit artery stenosis by PTCA restores culprit artery flow to that in the non-culprit artery but both are 45% slower than normal flow (J Am Coll Cardiol 2005;45:652).

The mechanism of MI in smokers is more often thrombosis of a less critical atherosclerotic lesion compared with nonsmokers (Circ 1995;91:298).

Sx: Chest discomfort radiating to left arm, neck, jaw; diaphoresis; dyspnea; nausea/vomiting; sx may be less in pts with DM; 25-30% of pts with MI by EKG cannot recall obvious symptoms (Ann IM 1995;122:96).

Si: Pallor; diaphoresis; hypotension; rales; arrhythmias or sinus tachycardia; S_3 or S_4 gallop; transient systolic murmur

Crs: Pts with AMI and LBBB or RBBB had higher 30-d mortality rates (18% vs 11%), more cardiogenic shock (19% vs 11%), AV block/asystole (30% vs 19%), and higher incidence of pacing (18% vs 11%) than controls. BBB also carried an independent 53% higher risk for 30-d mortality (J Am Coll Cardiol 1998; 31:105). In GUSTO-1, persistent BBB was predictive of a higher mortality rate (19.4%) than either transient (5.6%) or no BBB (3.5%) (Circ 1996;94:2424).

Pts who receive AMI rx with thrombolysis and develop a new ST shift after the first 6 hr, but within 24 hr, represent a high-risk group. They may benefit from more aggressive intervention (J Am Coll Cardiol 1998;31:783).

Refractory ischemia doubles the mortality rate in AMI pts with ST-segment elevation and triples the risk among those without ST elevation (GUSTO-IIb) (Circ 1998;98:1860).

Post-infarction angina following thrombolysis greatly increases the risk of reinfarction, especially when accompanied by transient EKG changes. Mortality is markedly increased only in the presence of concomitant hemodynamic abnormalities (J Am Coll Cardiol 1998;31:94).

The benefits of thrombolytic rx in prolonging survival of pts with AMI is sustained up to 10 yr (GISSI-I) (Circ 1998;98: 2659).

Studies comparing first Q-wave and non–Q-wave MIs found no difference in their post-MI course (J Am Coll Cardiol 1999; 33:576).

Cmplc: RV infarction complicates up to half of IWMI; it exhibits spectrum of disease ranging from mild, asymptomatic RV dysfunction to cardiogenic shock, and is associated with increased mortality in elderly. Survivors generally have restoration of normal RV function with resolution of hemodynamic abnormalities (Nejm 1994;330:1211; Circ 1998;98:1714).

Cardiogenic shock occurs in 10% of pts with AMI; it is due to extensive MI, ventricular septal rupture, and papillary muscle rupture (Circ 1995;91:873). An aggressive rx strategy (early angiography and revascularization when appropriate) is associated with reduced mortality in pts with AMI and cardiogenic shock who receive thrombolytic rx (GUSTO-I) (Circ 1997;96:122). Early PCI or CABG also improves survival (J Am Coll Cardiol 2003;42:1380); 88% of pts with AMI complicated by cardiogenic shock alive at 30 days survived at least 1 yr (Circ 1999;99:873).

Cardiac rupture most often occurs 2-5 d post-AMI. Risk factors include first transmural AMI, absence of overt CHF, advanced age, delayed hospital admission, and undue in-hospital physical activity. Recurrence of ischemia or infarction can be potential trigger (J Am Coll Cardiol 1998;32:135).

Intraocular hemorrhage after thrombolytic rx for AMI is extremely uncommon. The incidence of intraocular hemorrhage in pts with diabetes in GUSTO-1 was 0.05% (J Am Coll Cardiol 1997;30:1606).

Cardiovascular death and/or LV dilatation occurs in > 50% of survivors of AMI with LV dysfunction. Pts with h/o prior MI, low EF, early CHF, or older age are at high risk for dilatation and adverse cardiovascular events (Circ 1997;96:3294).

Pseudoaneurysm may be asymptomatic. Surgical repair is the rx of choice, but conservative management in selected pts with increased surgical risk is also reasonable (Ann IM 1998;128:299).

Pericarditis occurs in 20% of pts 1-42 d post-AMI.

Mild MR is an independent predictor of post-MI mortality. Pts with MR have higher rates of cardiovascular mortality (29% vs 12%) and severe CHF (24% vs 16%) pts without MR (Circ 1997;96:827).

Abnormal renal function increases the risk for cardiovascular complications post-MI (Nejm 2004;351:1285).

Lab: Elevated serum CK, CK-MB, troponin-I, troponin-T

- In pts with acute coronary syndromes, troponin I levels identify pts with increased risk. Each increase of 1 ng/mL is associated with a significant increase in the risk ratio for death (Nejm 1996;335:1342).
- Right-sided precordial lead should be used in IWMI; 1-mm ST elevations suggest RV infarct (J Am Coll Cardiol 1998;32:882; Nejm 1998;338:978).
- See Chapter 3 for EKG diagnostic criteria for acute MI.

X-ray: CXR may show CHF. Portable echo is useful in risk stratification.

Rx (AHA Guidelines)

General measures: EKG monitoring based on infarct location and rhythm; bed rest with bedside commode privileges for initial 12 hr in hemodynamically stable pts free of ischemic-type chest discomfort; avoidance of Valsalva; careful attention to maximum pain relief; O_2 for pts with overt pulmonary congestion or SaO_2 < 90%; may also be justifiable for all pts with uncomplicated MI during the first 6 hr

Iv TNG: For first 24-48 hr in pts with acute MI and CHF, large anterior infarction, persistent ischemia, or HT; continued use in pts with recurrent angina or persistent pulmonary congestion or complicated MI; contraindicated in pts with systolic BP < 90 mm Hg or suspected RV infarct

ASA: 160-325 mg administered pre-hospital or on d 1 of acute MI and continued indefinitely qd thereafter. Clopidogrel may be substituted if true ASA allergy is present or if pt is unresponsive to ASA. ASA use is associated with absolute risk reduction in AMI of 137 events/10,000 persons (Jama 1998;280:1930).

Morphine sulfate: 2-8 mg iv q 15 min for pain management

Oral β-blockers: For pts without contraindications

Thrombolysis: ST elevation > 0.1 mV, 2 or more contiguous leads; time to rx < 12 hr; EKG findings of true posterior MI; BBB obscuring ST-segment analysis and hx suggesting acute MI for pts < age 75. Among pts age 76-86, thrombolytic rx has not been shown to offer survival benefits in any clinical subgroup and may carry a significant survival disadvantage (Chest 2004;126:549S; Circ 2000;101:2239).

Contraindications to fibrinolysis

- Absolute: Prior intracranial hemorrhage, known structural cerebral vascular lesion, malignant intracranial neoplasm, ischemic stroke within 3 mon *except* acute ischemic stroke within 3 hr, suspected aortic dissection, significant closed head/facial trauma within 3 mon, active bleeding
- Relative: Hx of poorly controlled HT or BP > 180 systole or > 110 mm Hg diastolic on presentation, h/o ischemic stroke > 3 mon, traumatic or prolonged (> 10 min) CPR, major surgery in last 3 wk, internal bleeding in last 2-4 wk, noncompressible vascular puncture, pregnancy, active peptic ulcer, current use of anticoagulants

Fibrinolytic rx is preferred for pts presenting within 3 hr of symptom onset if access to primary PCI within 90 min is not available. Each 30-min increase in sx duration before thrombolytic rx begins is associated with an increase in infarct size of 1% of the myocardium; prolonged sx-to-rx time is associated with adverse outcomes (J Am Coll Cardiol 2004;44:980). The final infarct size in pts treated 4-6 hr after sx onset is indistinguishable from that in pts who did not receive thrombolytic rx (Circ 1996;93:48). Survival benefits of streptokinase persist for 12 yr after MI (J Am Coll Cardiol 1999;34:62).

Primary PTCA: Utilize PTCA if able to be performed within 12 hr of onset of sx by individuals skilled in the procedure; as a reperfusion strategy in pts who are candidates for reperfusion but who are ineligible for fibrinolytic rx; in pts < 75 yr old in cardiogenic shock (within 18 hr of onset); in pts with acute CHF; and in pts with recurrent ischemia or MI (Lancet 2004;363:1045; Jama 2004;291:736). A review of 23 trials with 7739 pts concluded that primary PTCA produced better results than thrombolysis (Lancet 2003;361:13). Time to rx with direct PTCA is a critical determinant of mortality (GUSTO IIB) (Circ 1999; 100:14). Anemia is associated with increased mortality in pts undergoing primary PTCA for AMI (J Am Coll Cardiol 2004;44:547).

In pts with acute MI, implantation of a stent has clinical benefits beyond those of primary coronary angioplasty alone (Nejm 1999;341:1949), including lower rates of angiographic restenosis (J Am Coll Cardiol 2000;35:1729). Results of primary angioplasty are similar in diabetics and nondiabetics, and it appears to be more effective than thrombolytic rx among diabetics with AMI (GUSTO IIb) (J Am Coll Cardiol 2000; 35:1502). Compared with stenting in nondiabetic pts, however, stenting of coronary arteries in diabetic pts is associated with significantly increased lumen renarrowing (J Am Coll Cardiol 2000; 35:1554). There are no data on the use of drug-eluting stents in AMI (Jama 2005;293:1501).

In a retrospective analysis, rescue PTCA early after failed thrombolysis seemed to be as effective and safe as primary PTCA (J Am Coll Cardiol 2000;36:51).

Pts ≥ 65 yr old who received thrombolytic therapy or primary PTCA had lower mortality at 1 yr compared with those who did not receive a reperfusion strategy. Primary PTCA was also associated with better survival at 30 d (J Am Coll Cardiol 2000;36:366).

Sulfonylurea drug use is associated with increased mortality among pts with DM undergoing PTCA for AMI (J Am Coll Cardiol 1999;33:119).

Thrombolysis or primary PTCA in first 6 hr after AMI may improve short-term survival in pts with associated RV infarction (J Am Coll Cardiol 1998;32:882).

Emergency/urgent CABG: For pts with failed angioplasty with persistent pain or hemodynamic instability and with coronary anatomy suitable for surgery; acute MI with persistent or recurrent ischemia refractory to medical rx in pts with coronary anatomy suitable for surgery who are not candidates for catheter intervention; at the time of surgical repair of post-infarction VSD or mitral valve insufficiency; cardiogenic shock with coronary anatomy suitable for surgery; pts with life-threatening arrhythmias; pts with left main or triple-vessel CAD

Emergency revascularization did not significantly reduce overall mortality at 30 d in pts with cardiogenic shock, but a significant survival benefit was apparent after 6 mon (Nejm 1999;341:625) and 1 yr (Lancet 2002;359:1805; Jama 2002;287:210,1943).

Management of recurrent chest discomfort: ASA for pericarditis; β-blockers iv and po for ischemic-type chest discomfort; (re)administration of thrombolytic rx for pts with recurrent ST elevation; coronary arteriography for ischemic-type chest discomfort recurring after hours to days of initial rx and associated with objective evidence of ischemia in pts who are candidates for revascularization; TNG iv for 24 hr, then topically or po for ischemic-type chest discomfort

Balloon flotation right-heart catheter monitoring: Severe/ progressive CHF or pulmonary edema; cardiogenic shock or progressive hypotension; suspected mechanical complications of acute infarction such as acute VSD, papillary muscle rupture, or pericardial tamponade; hypotension that does not respond promptly to fluid administration in a pt without pulmonary congestion

Intra-arterial pressure monitoring: Pts with severe systolic arterial pressure < 80 mm Hg and/or cardiogenic shock; pts receiving vasopressor agents, iv sodium nitroprusside, or other potent vasodilators

Intra-aortic balloon counterpulsation: Progressive hypotension or cardiogenic shock not quickly reversed with pharmacological rx as a stabilizing measure for angiography and prompt revascularization; acute mitral regurgitation or VSD complicating MI as a stabilizing rx for angiography and repair/revascularization; recurrent intractable ventricular arrhythmias; refractory post-MI angina as a bridge to angiography and revascularization; signs of hemodynamic instability, poor LV function, or persistent ischemia in pts with large areas of myocardium at risk

Rx of Afib: Electrical cardioversion for pts with severe hemodynamic compromise or intractable ischemia; rapid digitalization to slow a rapid ventricular response and improve LV function; iv β-blockers to slow a rapid ventricular response in pts without clinical LV dysfunction, bronchospastic disease, or AV block; iv amiodarone; heparinization; diltiazem or verapamil iv to slow a rapid ventricular response if β-blockers are contraindicated or ineffective

Rx of ventricular tachycardia/ventricular fibrillation: VF and sustained (> 30 sec or causing hemodynamic collapse) polymorphic VT should be treated with unsynchronized electric shock with initial energy of 200 J. If unsuccessful, a second shock of 200-300 J should be given and, if necessary, a third shock of 360 J. Episodes of sustained monomorphic VT associated with angina, pulmonary edema, or hypotension (systolic BP < 90 mm Hg) should be treated with synchronized electric shock of 100-J initial energy; increasing energies should be used if the initial rx not successful. Sustained monomorphic VT *not* associated with angina, pulmonary edema, or hypotension should be treated with one of the following regimens:

- Amiodarone: 150 mg infused over 10 min followed by a constant infusion of 1.0 mg/min for 6 hr and then a maintenance infusion of 0.5 mg/min
- Procainamide: 20-30 mg/min loading infusion, up to 12-17 mg/kg; may be followed by an infusion of 1-4 mg/min
- Synchronized electrical cardioversion starting at 50 J (brief anesthesia necessary)
- AICD for pts with VT/VF more than 48 hr post acute MI

Infusions of antiarrhythmic drugs may be used after an episode of VT/VF but should be discontinued after 6-24 hr and the need for further arrhythmia management assessed. Electrolyte and acid-base disturbances should be corrected to prevent recurrent episodes of VF when an initial episode of VF has been treated.

Prophylactic AICD insertion did not reduce mortality in high-risk MI pts who did not have VT/VF (Nejm 2004; 351:2481).

Atropine: For sinus bradycardia with evidence of low CO and peripheral hypoperfusion or frequent PVC at onset of sx of acute MI; acute inferior MI with type I second- or third-degree AV block associated with sx of hypotension, ischemic discomfort, or ventricular arrhythmias; sustained bradycardia and hypotension after administration of TNG; nausea and vomiting associated with administration of morphine; ventricular asystole; second- or third-degree AV block of uncertain mechanism when pacing is not available

Placement of transcutaneous patches and active (demand) transcutaneous pacing: Sinus bradycardia (rate < 50 beat/min) with systolic BP < 80 mm Hg unresponsive to drug rx; Mobitz type II second-degree AV block; third-degree heart block; bilateral BBB (alternating BBB, or RBBB and alternating left anterior fascicular block and left posterior fascicular block, irrespective of time of onset); newly acquired or age-indeterminate LBBB, LBBB and LAFB, RBBB, and LPFB; RBBB or LBBB and first-degree AV block, or newly acquired or age-indeterminate RBBB

Temporary transvenous pacing: Indicated for asystole; symptomatic bradycardia; bilateral BBB, any age; new or indeterminate-age bifascicular block with first-degree AV block; Mobitz type II second-degree AV block; RBBB and LAFB or LPFB, new or indeterminate age; RBBB with first-degree AV block; LBBB, new or indeterminate age; incessant VT (for atrial or ventricular overdrive pacing); recurrent sinus pauses (> 3 sec) not responsive to atropine

Permanent pacing after acute MI: Persistent second-degree AV block in the His-Purkinje system with bilateral BBB or complete heart block; transient advanced (second- or third-degree) AV block and associated BBB; symptomatic AV block at any level

Emergency/urgent cardiac repair of mechanical defects: Papillary muscle rupture with severe acute mitral insufficiency; post-infarction VSD or free wall rupture; post-infarction ventricular aneurysm associated with intractable ventricular tachyarrhythmias and/or pump failure

Heparin: For pts undergoing percutaneous or surgical revascularization; pts undergoing reperfusion rx with alteplase, reteplase, tenecteplase [PTT > 70 sec associated with higher likelihood of mortality, stroke, bleeding, and reinfarction; aPTT range of 50-70 sec is optimal (GUSTO-I) (Circ 1996;93:870)]. The recommended regimen of unfractionated heparin is 60 U/kg as a bolus at initiation of TPA infusion with initial maintenance dose of ~12 U/kg/hr (maximum 4000 U bolus and 1000 U/hr infusion for pts weighing > 70 kg), adjusted to maintain PTT at 1.5-2.0 times control (50-70 sec) for 48 hr.

For pts treated with nonselective thrombolytic agents (streptokinase, anistreplase, urokinase) who are at high risk for systemic emboli (large or anterior MI, Afib, previous embolus, or known LV thrombus), heparin should be withheld for 6 hr and started when PTT returns to < 2 times control, then infused to keep PTT 1.5-2.0 times control (initial infusion rate ~1000 U/hr). After 48 hr, a change to sc heparin, warfarin, or ASA alone should be considered.

Heparin alone is not associated with an improved 30-d mortality rate in pts > age 65 (J Am Coll Cardiol 1998;31:973).

LMW heparin (eg, enoxaparin 1 mg/kg bid) is recommended for all pts not treated with thrombolytic therapy who do not have a contraindication to heparin or pts < 75 yr old with significant renal dysfunction.

Clopidogrel is appropriate for pts with PCI; 1 mon for bare metal stents, 3-6 mon for drug-eluting stents.

β-Blocking agents: Early rx for pts without contraindications who can be treated within 12 hr of onset of MI, irrespective of administration of concomitant thrombolytic rx; pts with continuing or recurrent ischemic pain; pts with tachyarrhythmias such as Afib with a rapid ventricular response

ACEIs: Orally for pts within first 24 hr of suspected acute MI with ST-segment elevation in 2 or more anterior precordial leads or with clinical CHF in the absence of hypotension (systolic BP < 100 mm Hg) or known contraindications; pts with MI and LV ejection fraction < 40%; pts with clinical CHF on the basis of systolic pump dysfunction during and after convalescence from acute MI. ACEIs are possibly also of value for all pts within the first 24 hr of a suspected or established acute MI, provided significant hypotension or other clear-cut contraindications are absent, and for pts with mildly impaired LV function and hx of old MI. ARBs are preferred for pts who are intolerant of ACEIs.

In high-risk pts, ACEI rx reduced overall mortality by 7-20%. Early treatment with lisinopril in pts with DM and AMI was associated with decreased 6-wk and 6-mon mortality (8.7% vs 12.4%; 37 ± 12 lives saved per 1000 treated pts) (Circ 1997;96:4239; 1998;97:2192).

Ca^{++}-channel blockers: Verapamil or diltiazem may be given to pts in whom β-blockers are ineffective or contraindicated (ie, bronchospastic disease) for relief of ongoing ischemia or control of a rapid ventricular response with Afib after acute MI in the absence of CHF, LV dysfunction, or AV block.

Magnesium: This rx is used for correction of documented magnesium (and/or potassium) deficits, especially in pts receiving diuretics before onset of infarction. Pts with episodes of torsades de pointes-type VT associated with a prolonged QT interval should be treated with 1-2 gm magnesium administered as a bolus over 5 min.

Glycoprotein IIb/IIIa inhibitors: For pts with MI without ST-segment elevation who have high-risk features and/or refractory ischemia and no major contraindications due to bleeding risk

Stress EKG: Indicated before discharge for prognostic assessment or functional capacity (submaximal at 4-6 d or symptom limited at 10-14 d) or soon after discharge for prognostic assessment and functional capacity (14-21 d); late after discharge (3-6 wk) for functional capacity and prognosis if early stress was submaximal. Exercise or vasodilator stress nuclear scintigraphy or exercise stress echo is indicated when baseline abnormalities of the EKG compromise interpretation of results. Dipyridamole or adenosine stress perfusion nuclear scintigraphy or dobutamine echo may be used before discharge for prognostic assessment in pts judged to be unable to exercise. Exercise 2-D echo or nuclear scintigraphy (before or soon after discharge for prognostic assessment) may also be of value. An exercise test may be useful after catheterization to evaluate function or identify ischemia in the distribution of a coronary lesion of borderline severity. The majority of exercise tests after an MI can be done using the Bruce protocol within 3 d of admission with a very low incidence of complications (J Am Coll Cardiol 2000;35:1212).

Coronary angiography and possible PTCA: For pts with spontaneous episodes of myocardial ischemia or episodes of myocardial ischemia provoked by minimal exertion during recovery from infarction; before definitive rx of a mechanical complication of infarction such as acute mitral regurgitation, VSD, pseudoaneurysm, or LV aneurysm; in pts with persistent hemodynamic instability; when MI is suspected to have occurred by a mechanism other than thrombotic occlusion at an atherosclerotic plaque; for survivors of acute MI with LV ejection fraction ≤ 40%, CHF, prior revascularization, or malignant ventricular arrhythmias or who had clinical CHF during the acute episode but subsequently demonstrated well-preserved LV function

DANAMI study: Invasive rx in post-AMI pts with inducible ischemia following thrombolysis reduced the incidence of reinfarction (5.6% vs 10.5%), admissions for unstable angina (17.9% vs 29.5%), and prevalence of stable angina (21% vs 43%) (Circ 1997;96:748).

Lipid management: AHA Step II diet (< 7% of total calories as saturated fat and < 200 mg/d cholesterol) for all pts. Pts with LDL cholesterol levels > 125 mg/dL despite the AHA Step II diet should be placed on drug rx with the goal of reducing LDL cholesterol to < 100 mg/dL. Pts with normal plasma cholesterol levels who have HDL cholesterol levels < 35 mg/dL should receive nonpharmacological rx (eg, exercise) designed to raise it. Drug rx may be added to diet modifications in pts with LDL cholesterol levels < 130 mg/dL but > 100 mg/dL after an appropriate trial of the AHA Step II diet. Pts with normal total cholesterol levels but HDL cholesterol levels < 35 mg/dL despite diet and other nonpharmacological rx may be started on drugs such as niacin to raise their HDL cholesterol levels.

Pts who received statin rx demonstrated a 20-30% reduction in death and major cardiovascular events compared with pts who

Table 5.2 Secondary Prevention in Patients with ST-Elevation MI

Goals	Intervention Recommendations
Smoking: *Goal* complete cessation	Assess tobacco use. Strongly encourage pt and family to stop smoking and to avoid secondhand smoke. Provide counseling, pharmacological rx (including nicotine replacement and bupropion), and formal smoking cessation programs as appropriate.
Blood pressure control: *Goal* < 140/90 mm Hg or < 130/80 mg Hg if chronic kidney disease or diabetes	If blood pressure ≥ 120/80 mm Hg: • Initiate lifestyle modification (weight control, physical activity, alcohol moderation, moderate sodium restriction, and emphasis on fruits, vegetables, and low-fat dairy products) in all patients. If blood pressure ≥ 140/90 mm Hg or ≥ 130/80 mm Hg for pts with chronic kidney disease or diabetes: • Add blood pressure medications, emphasizing the use of β-blockers and inhibition of the renin-angiotensin-aldosterone system.
Lipid management: (TG < 200 mg/dL) *Primary goal* LDL-C *substantially* < 100 mg/dL	Start dietary therapy in all pts (< 7% of total calories as saturated fat and < 200 mg/d cholesterol). Promote physical activity and weight management. Encourage increased consumption of omega-3 fatty acids. Assess fasting lipid profile in all pts, preferably within 24 hr of STEMI. Add drug therapy according to the following guide: LDL-C *substantially* < 100 mg/dL (baseline or on-treatment): • Statins should be used to lower LDL-C. LDL-C ≤ 100 mg/dL (baseline or on-treatment): • Intensify LDL-C–lowering rx with drug rx, giving preference to statins.
Lipid management: (TG ≥ 200 mg/dL) *Primary goal* Non–HDl-C[1] *substantially* < 130 mg/dL	If TG ≥ 150 mg/dL or HDL-C is < 40 mg/dL: • Emphasize weight management and physical activity. Advise smoking cessation.

	If TG is 200-499 mg/dL: • After LDL-C–lowering therapy,[2] consider adding fibrate or niacin.[3] If TG ≥ 500 mg/dL: • Consider fibrate or niacin[3] before LDL-C–lowering therapy.[2] • Consider omega-3 fatty acids as adjunct for high TG.
Physical activity: *Minimum goal* 30 min 3-4 d per wk; optimal daily	Assess risk, preferably with exercise test, to guide prescription. Encourage minimum of 30-60 min of activity, preferably daily, or at least 3-4 times weekly (walking, jogging, cycling, or other aerobic activity) supplemented by an increase in daily lifestyle activities (eg, walking breaks at work, gardening, household work). Cardiac rehabilitation/secondary prevention programs, when available, are recommended for pts with STEMI, particularly those with multiple modifiable risk factors and/or those moderate- to high-risk pts in whom supervised exercise training is warranted.
Weight management: *Goal* BMI 18.5-24.9 kg/m^2 Waist circumference: Women: < 35 in Men: < 40 in	Calculate BMI and measure waist circumference as part of evaluation. Monitor response of BMI and waist circumference to therapy. Start weight management and physical activity as appropriate. Desirable BMI range is 18.5-24.9 kg/m^2. If waist circumference ≥ 35 in in women or ≥ 40 in in men, initiate lifestyle changes and treatment strategies for metabolic syndrome.
Diabetes management: *Goal* HbA1c < 7%	Appropriate hypoglycemic therapy to achieve near-normal fasting plasma glucose, as indicated by HbA1c. Treatment of other risks (eg, physical activity, weight management, blood pressure, and cholesterol management).

continues

Table 5.2 continued

Goals	Intervention Recommendations
Antiplatelet agents/ anticoagulants	Start and continue indefinitely ASA 75-162 mg/d if not contraindicated. Consider clopidogrel 75 mg/d or warfarin if ASA is contraindicated. Manage warfarin to INR of 2.5-3.5 in post-STEMI pts when clinically indicated or for those not able to take ASA or clopidogrel.
Renin-angiotensin-aldosterone system blockers	ACEIs in all pts indefinitely; start, early in stable high-risk pts (anterior MI, previous MI, Killip class ≥ 11 [S_3 gallop, rales, radiographic CHF], LVEF < 0.40). ARBs in pts who are intolerant of ACEIs and who have either clinical or radiological signs of heart failure or LVEF < 0.40. Aldosterone blockade in pts without significant renal dysfunction[4] or hyperkalemia who are already receiving therapeutic doses of an ACEI, have an LVEF ≤ 0.40, and have either diabetes or heart failure.
β-Blockers	Start in all patients. Continue indefinitely. Observe usual contraindications.

BMI, body mass index; in, inches; LDL-C, low-density lipoprotein cholesterol; HDL-C, high-density lipoprotein cholesterol; INR, international normalization ratio; ACE, angiotensin-converting enzyme; CHF, congestive heart failure; LVEF, left ventricular ejection fraction; ARB, angiotensin-receptor blocker and TG, triglycerides.

1. Non–HDL cholesterol equals total cholesterol minus HDL cholesterol.
2. Treat to a goal of non–HDL-C *substantially* less than 130 mg/dL.
3. Dietary-supplement niacin must not be used as a substitute for prescription niacin, and OTC niacin should be used only if approved and monitored by a physician.
4. Creatinine should be ≤ 2.5 mg/dL in men or ≤ 2.0 mg/dL in women.
5. Potassium should be ≤ 5.0 mEq/L.

(Circ 2004;110:626)

received placebo (Arch IM 1999;159:1793). Pravastatin reduced clinical events in revascularized post-MI pts with average cholesterol levels (J Am Coll Cardiol 1999;34:106). In pts > 65 yr old with MI, coronary events occurred in 28.1% of placebo recipients and 19.7% of pravastatin recipients, and coronary death in 10.3% of placebo recipients and 5.8% of the pravastatin group. CVA incidence was 7.3% for placebo recipients and 4.5% for the pravastatin group (CARE study) (Ann IM 1998;129:681).

Pts who continued to smoke after CABG had a greater risk of death than pts who stopped smoking. The former pts also underwent repeat revascularization procedures more frequently (J Am Coll Cardiol 2000;36:878).

Long-term β-blocker rx in survivors of AMI: All pts without a clear contraindication to β-blocker rx should begin this rx within a few days of the event, if not initiated acutely, and continue it indefinitely (Nejm 2003;348:878). β-Blockers are associated with a lower 1-yr mortality rate for elderly diabetic pts to a similar extent as for nondiabetics, without increased risk of readmission for diabetic complications. In pts > 75 yr old, the mortality rate among β-blocker recipients was 43% less than that for nonrecipients, and β-blocker recipients were rehospitalized 22% less often than nonrecipients (Jama 1997;277:115).

With thrombolytic rx, atenolol improves outcomes but early administration is of limited value (J Am Coll Cardiol 1998; 32:634). Benefits extend to pts > 65 yr old (Jama 1998;280:623) and are additive with the use of ACEIs for pts with EF < 40% (J Am Coll Cardiol 1997;29:229).

Long-term anticoagulation after AMI: For secondary prevention of MI in post-MI pts unable to take daily ASA; for post-MI pts with paroxysmal or persistent Afib or pts with LV thrombus or extensive wall motion abnormalities.

Estrogen replacement: Estrogen plus progestin for secondary prevention of coronary events should not be given de novo to postmenopausal women after AMI. Postmenopausal women who are already taking estrogen/progestin at the time of AMI can continue this rx.

Depression is an independent predictor of death after CABG (Lancet 2003;362:392; 2001;358:1766), but rx with SSRIs may not improve survival (Jama 2003;289:3106).

Chapter 6

Congestive Heart Failure

6.1 Acute Pulmonary Edema

Nejm 2003;348:20; Circ 2001;104:2996

Cause: Acute MI; mitral stenosis; rupture of chordae, papillary muscle, or intraventricular septum; myocarditis; LV diastolic dysfunction; hypoalbuminemia; infectious or aspiration pneumonia; radiation pneumonitis; ARDS; phosgene, chlorine or smoke inhalation; septic shock; massive pulmonary embolus; hemorrhagic pancreatitis; DIC; snake venom

Pathophys: Imbalance of Starling forces (pulmonary edema develops when mean PCWP exceeds 20-25 mm Hg), increased negative interstitial pressure (edema post-rx of pneumothorax) or primary alveolar-capillary membrane damage. Noncardiogenic causes of pulmonary edema of uncertain mechanism include high-altitude pulmonary edema, neurogenic pulmonary edema, heroin overdose, eclampsia, and pulmonary edema post-cardioversion.

Sx: Acute severe dyspnea, air hunger, anxiety, terror

Si: Cough, pink sputum, diaphoresis, pallor, cyanosis, tachycardia, HT, rales, rhonchi, wheezing

Crs: Course may vary depending on etiology. Potentially reversible conditions include HT, ischemia, valvular disease, pulmonary embolus, alcohol use, and noncompliance with a diet or drug regimen.

Lab: CBC, electrolytes, BUN, creatinine and cardiac enzymes, B-type naturetic peptide (Arch IM 2004;164:1978; Nejm 2002;347;161; Jama 2002;287:1531), oximetry or ABG, echocardiogram, cardiac catheterization if ASHD is clinically likely and if an acute intervention is planned

Right heart catheterization is indicated for cardiogenic shock not improved by the administration of iv fluid, for CHF that is complicated by hypotension/shock, and for pulmonary edema suspected to be of noncardiogenic origin; see also the section in Chapter 4.

X-ray: For frank pulmonary edema. Cardiomegaly may not be present in acute cardiac disease (eg, acute MI or acute mitral regurgitation).

Rx: Acute pulmonary edema: O_2 to maintain saturation > 90%; MS 2-6 mg iv q 5-10 min initially; iv loop diuretics (initial dose: furosemide 40-160 mg; bumetanide 1-2 mg; torsemide 10-20 mg iv); TNG (0.4 mg sl, 1-2 in 2% paste topically, 10-500 μgm/min iv) for angina or pre- and afterload reduction, but recall that nitrate tolerance develops rapidly with continuous administration; iv dobutamine (0.5-20 μgm/kg/min) if CO is low; dopamine (1-3 μgm/kg/min) to improve/maintain renal perfusion; iv nitroprusside (0.5-8 μgm/kg/min) for severe HT and refractory CHF (titrate dose to maintain systolic BP > 100 mm Hg); digoxin (0.25-1 mg iv loading dose) requires > 3 hr to take effect; for enalaprilat 1.25 mg iv, data on use in acute CHF are limited; thrombolytic rx or primary PTCA for acute MI; neseritide for pts unresponsive to diuretics (Lancet 2003;362:316)

Intubation/mechanical ventilation for severe hypoxia and/or respiratory acidosis; intra-aortic balloon counterpulsation for CHF and cardiogenic shock not responding to above rx, for pts with severe MR or ruptured ventricular septum, for support before/during catheterization/PTCA/CABG, or for pts with CHF awaiting heart transplantation

6.2 Chronic Congestive Heart Failure

Circ 2000;101:558; Nejm 2000;342:1120; 1999;341:1276

Cause: See preceding section. In addition, *high output failure* can be seen with anemia, systemic AV fistula, hyperthyroidism, beriberi heart disease (severe thiamine deficiency), Paget's disease, and multiple myeloma.

Afib can cause severe but reversible LV dysfunction (Circ 2004;109:2839).

In pts with severe lung disease, RV dysfunction is present in 66%, most of whom had pulmonary vascular disease. LV dysfunction (EF < 45%) is present in only 6% (Chest 1998;113:576).

LV diastolic dysfunction is seen in hypertrophic/constrictive cardiomyopathy, constrictive pericarditis, and HT. As many as 40% of pts with diastolic dysfunction also have systolic EF > 35% (Circ 2002;105:1387; 2002;105:1505).

Epidem: Over the past 50 yr, the incidence of CHF has declined among women but not among men (Nejm 2002;347:1397). Approximately 50% of pts with chronic CHF are older than 70 yr. More than 50% of cases are due to ASHD. Diastolic dysfunction is also more common in elderly pts. An elevated homocysteine level is an independent predictor of development of CHF in adults without h/o prior MI (Jama 2003;289:1251).

Pathophys: Salt/water retention; constriction of peripheral resistance vessels; increased sympathetic activity and circulating catecholamines; reduction in cardiac norepinephrine stores and reduced myocardial β-adrenergic receptors; activation of renin-angiotensin-aldosterone system; redistribution of cardiac output; in diastolic dysfunction, abnormal ventricular relaxation and altered ventricular pressure/volume relationships and ventricular filling (Circ 2003;107:659; Nejm 2003;348:2007)

Sx: Fatigue, orthopnea, PND, nocturnal cough, dyspnea on exertion

New York Heart functional classification:

Class I	No limitation
Class II	Mild limitation of physical activity
Class III	Marked limitation of physical activity
Class IV	Unable to carry out any physical activity without distress

Note that these are *different* stages from those in the AHA/ACC Practice Guidelines, in which Stage A represent pts at risk for development of CHF, Stage B pts have structural heart disease without CHF, Stage C pts have heart disease with current/prior sx of CHF, and Stage D pts have severe rest sx (Circ 2001; 104:2996).

Exertional sx correlate with maximal exercise capacity but frequently underestimate functional disability (J Am Coll Cardiol 1999;33:1943).

Si: Weight gain, decreased exercise capacity; JVD (> 4 cm above sternal angle at 45°), rales, cardiac asthma; hepatojugular reflux (gradual continuous compression of right upper quadrant for 1 min), hepatosplenomegaly; cardiomegaly, tachycardia, quiet S_1 and S_2, S_3 gallop, murmur of MR or TR, arrhythmias; edema, ascites, pleural effusion; S_4 in diastolic dysfunction

Crs: *Framingham study:* During 1948-1988, the median survival after dx was 3.2 yr for men and 5.4 yr for women (Circ 1993;88:107). Average annual mortality was 5-10% for class I-II, 20% for class II, and > 50% for class IV.

SOLVD trial: 3-yr mortality was 25% for pts with EF of 30-35% and 50% for pts with EF < 20% (Nejm 1992;327:685; 1991;325:293).

Pts with peripartum cardiomyopathy have a better prognosis than those with other forms of cardiomyopathy. Pts with cardiomyopathy due to infiltrative myocardial disease, HIV infection, or doxorubicin therapy have an especially poor prognosis (Nejm 2000;342:1077).

Sudden cardiac death (SCD) may occur in up to 40% of pts. Digoxin or diuretic use does not decrease incidence of SCD; β-blockers and amiodarone decreased risk in some, but not all, studies (J Am Coll Cardiol 1997;30:1589).

Pts with late-onset CHF following MI have a 10-fold greater risk of death compared with other MI survivors (J Am Coll Cardiol 2003;42:1446). Pts wth EF < 35% and severe ventricular ectopy after exercise also have increased mortality (J Am Coll Cardiol 2004;44:820).

Cmplc: The incidence of pulmonary and systemic embolism in chronic CHF is 2-5%. A retrospective case-control study demonstrated that pts with ischemic cardiomyopathy and LV diastolic diameter > 60 mm have an increased risk of LV thrombi. Peripheral embolic events are related to poor long-term survival in these pts (Chest 2000;117:314).

Use of NSAIDs in elderly pts taking diuretics is associated with doubling of the risk of hospitalization for CHF (Arch IM 1998;158:1108).

Nonsustained VT occurs frequently in pts with CHF but is not an independent predictor of all-cause mortality or sudden death. Suppression of arrhythmias does not improve survival (J Am Coll Cardiol 1998;32:942).

Pancreaticobiliary disease occurs 17.4 times more frequently in pts receiving a heart transplant than in the general population (Ann IM 1996;124:980).

Anemia is common in CHF. Correction of this anemia is associated with improvement in cardiac function, functional class, renal function, and need for diuretics and hospitalization (J Am Coll Cardiol 2000;35:1737). Anemia is associated with greater disease severity (Circ 2004;110:149).

Lab: CBC, UA (pyelonephritis, nephrotic syndrome), electrolytes, BUN/creatinine, glucose, phosphorus, magnesium, calcium, albumin, TSH (hypo- or hyperthyroidism).

EKG: To assess possible MI, ischemia, Afib, LVH (diastolic dysfunction)

Echocardiogram: To assess possible MI, cardiomyopathy, valvular disease, pericardial effusion/tamponade; in evaluation of first-degree relatives of pts with idiopathic dilated cardiomyopathy; Doppler assessment to assess diastolic dysfunction

Stress testing: For pts with high probability of CAD or prior MI

Cardiac catheterization: For pts with angina, suspected CAD, or large areas of ischemic or hibernating myocardium

X-ray: CXR: cardiomegaly; pulmonary vascular redistribution; Kerley B lines; pulmonary edema; pleural effusion

Rx:

Stage A and B pts: Risk reduction, possible ACEI and/or β-blocker rx

For Stage C and D pts: Na^+ restriction (2 gm/d)

Long-term moderate exercise produces an improvement in functional capacity and quality of life (Circ 1999;99:1173).

ACEIs are prescribed unless contraindicated (symptomatic hypotension, hyperkalemia, known intolerance) for all symptomatic pts and for class I pts with significantly reduced LVEF, with h/o diabetes, with HT, or with vascular disease at doses used in clinical trials and continued indefinitely. Reduced doses and careful monitoring are required for pts with serum creatinine > 3 mg/dL. In pts > age 85, ACEIs may demonstrate a benefit but digoxin may have detrimental effects (Arch IM 2000;160:53). Pts treated with high-dose lisinopril had 24% fewer hospitalizations for CHF than those treated with 2.5-5 mg qd, but dizziness and renal insufficiency were also observed more frequently (Circ 1999;100:2312). ARBs are used for pts who are intolerant of ACEIs (Lancet 2003;362:759).

Among 464 pts with ASHD and CHF, 5-yr mortality was 24% for pts on ACEIs plus ASA vs 34% for pts on ACEIs without ASA (J Am Coll Cardiol 1999;33:1920).

Diuretics are used for symptomatic pts with volume overload (in conjunction with ACEIs) and are generally needed indefinitely. Spironolactone added to standard rx reduces morbidity and risk of death among pts with severe CHF (Circ 2003;108: 1790; Nejm 1999;341:709).

Hydralazine and nitrates are used for pts who cannot take or do not respond to ACEIs. They may be added to ACEIs and diuretics if the pt remains symptomatic.

Digoxin (Circ 2004;109:2942) is used in patients with CHF and LV systolic dysfunction not controlled by ACEIs and diuretics and in pts with Afib and rapid ventricular response. Anticoagulation is necessary in case of Afib, prior h/o systemic or pulmonary embolus, intracardiac thrombus, or low EF and chamber dilation. The optimal serum level is 0.7-1.1 ng/mL (Circ 2004;109:2942) and may be as low as 0.5-0.8 ng/mL in men (Jama 2003;289:712). Digoxin reduces the rate of hospitalization but does not reduce overall mortality (Nejm 1997;336:525).

Carvedilol can retard progression of heart failure (Circ 2003;107:1100; Jama 2002;287:883,890) and may partially reverse systolic dysfunction and ventricular remodeling in pts with idiopathic dilated or ischemic cardiomyopathy (Circ 1996;94:2285; Nejm 1996;334:1349; 1996;335:490). Metoprolol may also be of value at a starting dose of 6.25 mg. These pts require close monitoring, as their CHF may worsen initially; the benefit appears over 2-3 mon. In a meta-analysis of studies on 3023 pts, β-blockers were reported to increase EF by 29% and reduce the combined risk of death or hospitalization for CHF by 37%; their effect on NYHA functional class was of borderline significance (Circ 1998;98:1184). Carvedilol may be more effective than metoprolol in extending survival (Lancet 2003;362:7). Carvedilol lowers BP more than metoprolol in pts with CHF, and it may prevent nitrate tolerance in pts with CHF during continuous rx with TNG (J Am Coll Cardiol 1998;32:1194). Pts with class IV sx are more likely to develop adverse events during initiation and dose titration of carvedilol as compared with less symptomatic pts but are more likely to show symptomatic improvement in the long term (J Am Coll Cardiol 1999;33:924). Carvedilol is well tolerated in pts with COPD who have no reversible airway obstruction (J Am Coll Cardiol 2004;44:497).

Low-dose dobutamine infusion is appropriate for pts with stunned/hibernating myocardium that has been revascularized (J Am Coll Cardiol 1999;33:572). It may also relieve symptoms (but be associated with a small increase in the risk of death) of refractory CHF (Nejm 1998;339:1848); it may be administered as outpatient rx.

Amrinone (0.5-0.75 mg/kg bolus, 2-20 μgm/kg/min infusion) and milrinone (50 μgm/kg bolus, 0.25-1 μgm/kg/min infusion) are approved for short-term support in severe CHF but data supporting their efficacy are equivocal (Jama 2002;287:1541). 10% of pts on amrinone develop thrombocytopenia.

Ca^{++}-channel blockers are not of proven benefit in CHF and may be harmful (amlodipine and felodipine may be exceptions).

In the PROMISE study, occurrence of nonsustained asymptomatic VT on ambulatory EKG did not specifically predict sudden death in pts with moderate/severe CHF or identify candidates for antiarrhythmic or AICD rx (Circ 2000;101:40). In a double-blind study, EF increased in 8% of pts started on amiodarone (Circ 1996;93:2128). Amiodarone suppressed ventricular arrhythmias but did not reduce the incidence of sudden death or prolong survival in pts with CHF (Nejm 1995;333:77). It also reduces clearance of digoxin and warfarin.

Implantation of an AICD in pts with non-ischemic dilated cardiomyopathy who were already treated with β-blockers and ACEIs reduced the risk of sudden death from arrhythmia (Nejm 2004;350:2151).

In the SOLVD study, ASA or dipyridamole improved survival and reduced morbidity in pts with CHF. Warfarin was associated with a significant reduction in all-cause mortality risk of death or admission for CHF (J Am Coll Cardiol 1998;31:749).

CABG in pts with CHF and poor LV function is indicated for left main CAD or the equivalent, proximal LAD stenosis with 2- to 3-vessel disease, or significant viable noncontracting revascularizable (hibernating) myocardium (J Am Coll Cardiol 1999;34:1262).

Little is known about long-term survival or LV performance following surgical LV reduction of dilated cardiomyopathy (Circ 2004;110:3734; 2004;110:3858; J Am Coll Cardiol 1998;32: 1809). However, 5-yr outcomes after surgery are good in pts with ischemic LV dilation (J Am Coll Cardiol 2004;44:1439).

Cardiac transplantation is used for pts with severe CHF and refractory ischemia. Contraindications include advanced age; severe diabetes with end-organ damage; active peptic ulcer disease; active infection; severe peripheral vascular or cerebrovascular disease; pulmonary HT; and irreversible pulmonary, renal, or hepatic disease. A total artificial heart may serve as a bridge to transplantation (Nejm 2004;351:859).

For diastolic dysfunction, the goal is reduction of LV ventricular filling pressure while maintaining CO. Diuretics, nitrates, anticoagulation and rate control in Afib, Ca^{++}-channel blockers, β-blockers, and ACEIs may also be of benefit. Avoid use of positive inotropes if systolic function is normal.

In pts with CHF and cardiac dyssynchrony, biventricular pacing may improve sx and lower risk of death (Nejm 2005;352:in press). Pts with QRS duration > 130 ms who remain symptomatic despite medical rx are most likely to benefit from this approach. Pacing appears to improve myocardial O_2 consumption, mitral and/or tricuspid regurgitation, incidence of Afib and other arrhythmias, but improvement in sx is not uniformly seen in all eligible pts (Circ 2004;109:296,300,357; 2003;108:1004,2596; Jama 2003;289:2041). LV tissue Doppler may be useful in identifying responders (J Am Coll Cardiol 2004;44:1834). Intracardiac dyssonchrony is a marker of increased risk for adverse events (J Am Coll Cardiol 2004; 43:248).

Chapter 7

Arrhythmias

7.1 Supraventricular Arrhythmias

Nejm 2004;338:1369; 2001;344:1067; J Am Coll Cardiol 2003;42: 1493; Circ 2003;107:1096; 2002;106:649

Cause: Mechanisms include increased automaticity of ectopic atrial focus (APC), triggered activity associated with disorders of repolarization, and reentrant arrhythmias involving accessory pathways between atria and ventricles (35-40%), within the AV node (60-65%), or within the SA node for SVT or in RA for Aflut, and macro-reentrant circuits within the atria. Afib may also be due to single, rapidly discharging focus, in which case elimination of the focus by radio-frequency ablation also eliminates the arrhythmia (Circ 1997;95:562).

Multifocal atrial tachycardia is typically seen in elderly pts with severe illnesses, most commonly COPD. The mechanism may be delayed after depolarization, leading to triggered activity (Chest 1998;113:203).

Epidem: Prevalence of PSVT is 225/1000 persons; incidence is 35/100,000 person-yr. Other CVD is present in 90% of male pts and 48% of female pts. 90% of pts have AV or AV node reentrant tachycardia (J Am Coll Cardiol 1998;31:150).

The lifetime risk of Afib is 1 in 4 for subjects > 40 yr old (Circ 2004;110:1042). In pts > 65 yr, overall incidence of Afib is 192/1000 person-years (age 65-74: men, 176 and women, 101; age 75-84: men, 427 and women, 216). Use of diuretics, h/o valvular heart disease, CAD, advancing age, higher systolic BP, glucose, and LA size are all associated with increased risk of Afib (Jama 2001;285:2370; Circ 1997;96:2455).

SV arrhythmias occur in 76% of pts undergoing noncardiac surgery. Correlates include male sex, age > 70 yr, significant valvular disease, h/o asthma, CHF, APC on pre-op EKG, and abdominal, vascular, and intrathoracic surgery (Ann IM 1998;129:279). Up to 33% of pts will develop Afib after CABG. Predictors include age > 70 yr, male sex, HT, need for IABP, post-op pneumonia, mechanical ventilation > 24 hr, and h/o Afib or CHF (Circ 1996;94:390; Jama 1996;276:300). Post-op atrial pacing in conjunction with β-blockade reduces the incidence of Afib following CV surgery (J Am Coll Cardiol 2000;35:1411).

Up to 25% of pts with ablation of Aflut develop Afib over 2 yr. The risk is 10% for pts with neither h/o Afib nor EF < 50%; 20% with either of these; and 74% with both (Circ 1998; 98:315).

Pathophys:

PSVT: In 90% of pts with AV node reentrant tachycardia, anterograde conduction occurs over the slow atrioventricular nodal pathway and retrograde conduction over the fast pathway. In most pts, posterior atrionodal input to the AV node serves as the anterograde limb of the reentry circuit, and anterior atrionodal inputs serve as the retrograde limb (Nejm 1995;332:162; 1999;340:534).

Aflut: Due to macro-reentry involving counterclockwise reentrant activation of RA. The critical element of the reentrant circuit is the isthmus between the IVC and tricuspid valve annulus.

Afib: Pts with AMI are prone to Afib. Predictors are 3-vessel CAD, advanced age, higher peak CK levels, worse Killip class (IV vs I), and increased heart rate. The unadjusted mortality rate is higher at 30 d (14.3% vs 6.2%) and at 1 yr

(21.5% vs 8.6%) in patients with Afib (GUSTO-I; J Am Coll Cardiol 1997;30:406).

After cardioversion of chronic Afib to NSR, there is a gradual increase of 56% in CO over 4 wk, due to return and increasing strength of LA mechanical activity. CO decreases transiently after cardioversion of Afib in > 1/3 of pts; the decrease may last 1 wk (Arch IM 1997;157:1070).

Sx: Palpitations; may be associated with lightheadedness, dyspnea, and nausea. Pts treated with radio-frequency ablation report an improvement in sx (Circ 1996;94:1585).

Si: Irregular heartbeat; tachycardia

Crs: In the Framingham Heart Study, Afib was associated with a 15- to 19-fold higher mortality risk after adjustment for preexisting CV conditions (Circ 1998;98:946).

In pts with CHF and Afib, amiodarone produced conversion to NSR in 31% and reduced incidence of recurrent Afib. Pts who converted to NSR had a lower mortality rate than those who did not (Circ 1998;98:257).

Cmplc: 15% of pts presenting with Afib will have atrial thrombi identified by TEE. Pts with Afib have an annual stroke rate of 45%; the rate is 14% for anticoagulated pts. The risk of stroke in Afib pts is 15% for age 50-59 vs 23.5% for age 80-89 (Framingham). Pts with previous TIA, CVA, or systemic embolism; age > 75 yr; HT; poor LV function; prosthetic heart valve (mechanical or tissue valve); or rheumatic mitral valvular disease have an increased risk. Diabetes, CAD, age 65-75 yr, or thyrotoxicosis may also increase this risk (Chest 1998;114:S579).

For pts with Afib clinically estimated to have lasted < 48 hr, the likelihood of cardioversion-related clinical thromboembolism is 0.1%. Approximately 67% will convert spontaneously (Ann IM 1997;126:615).

In pts with Afib for < 2 wk before cardioversion, normal atrial mechanical function returns within 24 hr of cardioversion.

Pts with Afib present for 2-6 wk require up to 1 wk, and those with Afib for < 6 wk require up to 3 wk for full recovery of atrial mechanical function (Circ 1998;98:479). Overall, effective mechanical atrial function is recovered by 68% of pts by 3 and by 76% by 7 after cardioversion. Electrical cardioversion produces a greater degree and longer duration of mechanical atrial dysfunction than those who convert pharmacologically or spontaneously (J Am Coll Cardiol 1997;30:481).

Pts with Aflut are also at risk for thromboembolus post-cardioversion (J Am Coll Cardiol 1997;29:582). In one series, TEE showed LA thrombus in 11% of pts with Aflut for 4 ± 9 wk (Circ 1997; 95:962).

Lab: Thyroid function, electrolytes

EKG: (See Chapter 3 for EKG diagnostic criteria.) Wolff-Parkinson-White syndrome—ventricular depolarization through AV node and accessory pathways, with reentrant tachyarrhythmias and characteristic short PR interval and delta wave

TEE: Features independently associated with increased thromboembolic risk in Afib include LA appendage thrombi, dense spontaneous echo contrast, LA appendage peak flow velocity < 220 cm/sec, and complex aortic plaque. Pts with h/o HT have an increased incidence of atrial appendage thrombi on TEE. The presence of complex aortic plaque also distinguishes pts with Afib at high risk from those at moderate risk of thromboembolism (J Am Coll Cardiol 1998;31:1622; Ann IM 1998;128:639).

Rx: See Tables 7.2 through 7.10.

PSVT: More than 90% of tachycardias due to AV or AV nodal reentry are terminated by a 12-mg dose of adenosine. Adenosine also frequently terminates sinus-node reentrant tachycardia and occasionally terminates unifocal atrial tachycardia (Nejm 1995;332:162).

Table 7.1 Acute Management of Stable Regulator Tachycardias

EKG Finding	First Choice	Second Choice
Narrow complex SVT	Vagal maneuvers, adenosine, verapamil, diltiazem	β-Blockers, amiodarone, digoxin
Wide Complex Tachycardias		
SVT with BBB	Vagal maneuvers, adenosine, verapamil, diltiazem	β-Blockers, amiodarone, digoxin
Pre-excitation	Flecanide, ibutilide, procainamide, DC cardioversion	
Wide complex tachycardia of unknown origin	Procainamide, sotalol, amiodarone, DC cardioversion	Lidocaine, adenosine

Table 7.2 Management of Focal Atrial Tachycardias

Clinical Situation	First Choice	Second Choice
Acute Conversion	DC cardioversion	Adenosine, β-blockers, verapamil, diltiazem, procainamide, flecanide, propafenone
Acute Rate Control	β-Blockers, verapamil, diltiazem	Digoxin
Prophylaxis		
Recurrent symptomatic AT	Catheter ablation, β-blockers, verapamil, diltiazem	Disopyramide, flecanide, propafenone, sotalol, amiodarone
Incessant AT	Catheter ablation	

Table 7.3 Long-Term Rx of Recurrent AVNRT

Clinical Situation	First Choice	Second Choice
Hemodynamically unstable AV node reentrant tachycardia	Catheter ablation	β-Blockers, verapamil, diltiazem, sotalol, amiodarone
Recurrent symptomatic AVNRT	Catheter ablation, β-blockers, verapamil, diltiazem	Digoxin
Recurrent AVNRT unresponsive to β- or Ca^{++}-channel blockers	Flecanide, propafenone, sotalol	Amiodarone
PSVT with only dual AV node pathways	β-Blockers, verapamil, diltiazem, flecanide, propafenone	
Infrequent well-tolerated AVNRT	Nothing, vagal maneuvers, "pill in pocket," β-blockers, verapamil, diltiazem, catheter ablation	

Table 7.4 Rx of Junctional Tachycardia

Arrhythmia	First Choice	Second Choice
Focal junctional tachycardia	β-Blockers, flecanide, propafenone, sotalol, amiodarone, catheter ablation	
Nonparoxysmal junctional tachycardia	Correct hypokalemia or digitalis toxicity, treat ischemia	β- or Ca^{++}-channel blockers

Table 7.5 Acute Rx of Atrial Flutter

Clinical Status/Aim	First Choice	Second Choice
Poorly Tolerated		
Conversion	DC cardioversion	
Rate control	β-Blockers, verapamil, diltiazem	Digoxin, amiodarone
Stable		
Conversion	Atrial/transesophageal pacing, DC cardioversion	Ibutilide, flecanide, propafenone, sotalol, procainamide, amiodarone
Rate control	β-Blockers, verapamil, diltiazem	Digoxin, amiodarone

Table 7.6 Long-Term Management of Afib

Clinical Status/Aim	First Choice	Second Choice
Well tolerated, first episode	DC cardioversion	Catheter ablation
Well tolerated, recurrent	Catheter ablation, dofetilide	Amiodarone, sotalol, flecanide, propafenone, procainamide, disopyramide, quinidine
Poorly tolerated	Catheter ablation	
Aflut after use of amiodarone or IC agents	Catheter ablation	

Table 7.7 Drugs for Conversion of Afib and Maintenance of NSR[1]

Drug	Conversion Dose	Maintenance Dose	Comments
Flecainide	300 mg orally (2 mg/kg of body weight iv)	50-150 mg bid	Iv formulation not available in U.S. Approved only for paroxysmal Afib with structurally normal heart.
Propafenone	600 mg orally (2 mg/kg iv)	150-300 mg bid	Same limitations as flecainide.
Procainamide	100 mg iv every 5 min to maximum of 1000 mg	Slow-release formulation, 1000-2000 mg bid	Long-term use associated with lupus. Not FDA approved for Afib.
Quinidine	200 mg sulfate orally, followed 1-2 hr later by 400 mg	200-400 mg sulfate qid, or 324-648 mg gluconate tid	Approved for Afib but risk of death increased during long-term therapy.
Disopyramide	200 mg orally every 4 hr to maximum of 800 mg	100-150 mg qid or 200-300 mg controlled-release formulation bid	Not FDA approved for Afib. Strong negative inotropic effect.
Sotalol	Not recommended (conversion rate is low)	120-160 mg bid	Poor conversion efficacy. Approved for maintenance of sinus rhythm. Hospitalization for initiation is mandatory.

Dofetilide	0.5 mg bid orally (adjust dose downward for patients with renal disease)	0.5 mg bid (adjust dose downward for patients with renal disease)	FDA approved for conversion and maintenance. Hospitalization for initiation is mandatory.
Amiodarone	1200 mg iv in 24 hr	600 mg/day for 2 wk, then 200-400 mg qd (lower dose is preferable)	iv amiodarone moderately effective for conversion, but onset is slow. Good rate slowing in Afib. Not FDA approved for this indication.
Ibutilide	1 mg iv over 10 min in patients weighing $\geq$ 60 kg, or 0.01 mg/kg over 10 min in patients weighing $<$ 60 kg; may be repeated once if arrhythmia does not end within 10 min after end of initial infusion	Not available for maintenance (iv formulation only)	Do not use in patients with hypokalemia, a prolonged QT interval, or torsades de pointes.

1. Iv flecainide and propafenone (the doses of which are given in parentheses) are not available in the United States.

Source: Reprinted with permission, Falk, Medical Progress. Atrial Fibrillation 2001;344:1067–1078, *New England Journal of Medicine.*

Table 7.8 Drugs for Rate Control in Afib

Drug	Control of Acute Episode	Control of Sustained Afib	Comments
Ca^{++}-Channel Blockers			
Diltiazem	20 mg bolus followed, if necessary, by 25 mg given 15 min later. Maintenance infusion of 5-15 mg/hr.	Oral controlled-release formulation, 180-300 mg qd	Long-term control may be better with the addition of digoxin.
Verapamil	5-10 mg iv over 2–3 min, repeated once, 30 min later. Maintenance infusion rate is not reliably documented.	Slow-release formulation, 120-240 mg qd or bid	Causes elevation in digoxin level. May be more negatively inotropic than diltiazem.
β-Blockers[1]			
Esmolol	0.5 mg/kg of body weight iv, repeated if necessary. Follow with infusion at 0.05 mg/kg/min, increasing as needed to 0.2 mg/kg/min.	Not available in oral forms	Hypotension may be troublesome but responds to drug discontinuation.

Metoprolol	5 mg bolus iv, repeated twice at intervals of 2 min. No data on maintenance infusion.	50-400 mg qd in divided doses	Useful if there is concomitant coronary disease.
Propranolol	1-5 mg iv, given over 10 min.	30-360 mg in divided doses or in long-acting form	Noncardioselective: Use cautiously in patients with a history of bronchospasm.
Digoxin	1.0-1.5 mg iv or orally over 24 hr in doses of 0.25–0.5 mg.	0.125-0.5 mg qd	Renally excreted. Slow onset even if given iv, with less effective control than other agents, although may be synergistic with them. Poor efficacy for exertional heart-rate control.

1. The β-blockers listed are representative of agents in this category. Other iv or po β-blockers may be equally acceptable.

Reprinted with permission, Falk, Medical Progress. Atrial Fibrillation 2001;344:1067–1078, *New England Journal of Medicine.*

Table 7.9 Rx of Accessory Pathway-Mediated Arrhythmias

Arrhythmia	First Choice	Second Choice
WPW, well-tolerated	Catheter ablation	Flecanide, propafenone, sotalol, amiodarone, β-blockers
WPW, poorly tolerated	Catheter ablation	
AV reentrant tachycardia without pre-excitation, poorly tolerated	Catheter ablation	Flecanide, propafenone, sotalol, amiodarone, β-blockers
AV reentrant tachycardia without pre-excitation, infrequent	Nothing, vagal maneuvers, "pill in pocket"	β-Blockers, verapamil, diltiazem, catheter ablation
Pre-excitation, asymptomatic	Nothing	Catheter ablation

Table 7.10 Treatment of PSVT during Pregnancy

Strategy	First Choice	Second Choice
Acute conversion	Vagal maneuvers, adenosine, DC cardioversion	Metoprolol, propranolol
Prophylaxis	Digoxin, metoprolol	Propranolol, sotalol, flecanide

Single episodes of well-tolerated tachycardia can be treated conservatively (observation without drugs or ablation therapy). Radio-frequency ablation is first-line rx in symptomatic pts and has a success rate of 85-100%. Complication prevalence: death, 0.08%; cardiac tamponade, 0.5%; AV block, 0.5% (Nejm 1999; 340:534).

Symptomatic recurrent SVT that is reproducibly terminated by pacing after drugs and catheter ablation fail to control the arrhythmia or produce intolerable side effects and recurrent SVT or Aflut that is reproducibly terminated by pacing as an alternative to drug rx or ablation are indications for permanent pacemakers that automatically detect and pace to terminate tachycardias (Circ 1998;97:1325). Third generation ICDs can detect SVT/Afib. Discrimination of SVT from Afib permits successful pacing therapy for a significant fraction of SVTs (Circ 2000; 101:878).

MAT: Metoprolol, Mg^{++}, and verapamil have been evaluated in few rx studies (Chest 1998;113:203).

Aflut: Ibutilide is effective for terminating Aflut. Close monitoring is required during its administration because of the potential for torsades de pointes (Circ 1998;97:493).

The radio-frequency ablation success rate is > 90%, and the recurrence rate is < 10% (J Am Coll Cardiol 2000;35:1898).

Afib: In one study, spontaneous conversion to NSR occurred in 68% of pts with Afib < 72 hr duration; among pts with spontaneous conversion, 66% had Afib < 24 hr duration, 17% had Afib for 24-48 hr, and 17% had Afib > 48 hr (J Am Coll Cardiol 1998;31:588).

Pts with infrequent episodes of stable Afib not associated with pre-excitation may respond to diltiazem 120 mg plus propranol 80 mg (J Am Coll Cardiol 2001;37:548)—the "pill in the pocket" approach. Pts who respond to flecanide or propafenone may use prn rx with flecanide 200-300 mg or propafenone 450-600 mg po (Nejm 2004;351:2384).

For acute rate control, use iv verapamil, diltiazem, or β-blockers. β-blockers are especially effective in thyrotoxicosis and increased sympathetic tone. For long-term rx, verapamil, diltiazem, and β-blockers are more effective than digoxin, but digoxin remains first-line rx in patients with CHF secondary to impaired systolic LV function. Digoxin plus atenolol has produced the most effective rate control during daily activity and programmed exercise (J Am Coll Cardiol 1999;33:304).

Iv procainamide is the rx of choice for pts with WPW syndrome who have a pre-excited ventricular response during Afib if they are stable. Unstable pts require immediate cardioversion (Circ 1996;93:1262).

Quinidine is not effective in pts with permanent Afib. In PAF, quinidine is more effective than placebo and as effective as most other drugs in maintaining NSR for 6-12 mon. No controlled studies have examined the efficacy of quinidine as compared with low-dose amiodarone (< 200 mg/d) or the long-term efficacy of quinidine as prophylaxis against Afib (Nejm 1998; 338:35).

The incidence of Afib induced by 12 mg of iv adenosine is 12%. A relative contraindication may exist if Wolff-Parkinson-White syndrome is a possibility (Ann IM 1997;127:417).

Propafenone or amiodarone converts Afib in 40-50% of pts; LA diameter and arrhythmia duration are independent predictors of conversion (J Am Coll Cardiol 1999;33:966). Amiodarone is more effective than sotalol and class I agents for maintenance of NSR (Chest 2004;125:377; J Am Coll Cardiol 2003;42:20).

Ibutilide (1 mg iv over 10 min) may produce conversion to NSR from Afib and may increase success rates with DC cardioversion (Nejm 1999;340:1849).

Proarrhythmia (bradyarrhythmia or ventricular tachyarrhythmia, especially torsades de pointes) is the most important risk associated with antiarrhythmic drug rx. It often occurs during initiation of drug rx but is rare in pts with no heart disease and with a normal baseline QT interval. The highest incidence is in pts with CHF.

Digoxin reduces the frequency of symptomatic Afib episodes, but the effect is small and may be due to a reduction in the ventricular rate or irregularity rather than any antiarrhythmic action (Circ 1999;99:2765).

Cardioversion restores NSR in > 80% of pts; the most effective electrode placement for cardioversion is anterior-posterior

(Lancet 2002;360:1275). In Afib of recent onset, pharmacologic rx has a success rate of 40-90%. NSR at 1 yr is maintained in 30% of pts without antiarrhythmic rx vs 50% of pts with rx. Long-term rx is warranted only if recurrences or initial clinical instability is seen (Ann IM 1996;125:311).

Preliminary reports indicate that pts with Afib who receive rate control and anticoagulation have survival rates similar to those treated with rhythm control (Nejm 2002;347:1825, 1834).

Rx of Afib with radio-frequency ablation and pacemaker improves sx, although cardiac performance may not change (Circ 1997;96:2617; 1998;98:953). A meta-analysis of 21 studies with 1181 pts reported that ablation and pacing improve clinical outcomes for pts with medically refractory Afib (Circ 2000;101:1138). Survival after ablation is similar to that for the general population (Nejm 2001;344:1043).

Catheter ablation techniques used for abolition of Afib have included right atrial compartmentalization, ablation of triggering focus, and electrical disconnection of multiple pulmonary veins. Approximately 14.5-76.5% of pts are rendered asymptomatic without drugs after these techniques and 8.8-50.3% of pts are asymptomatic with ablation and previously ineffective drug rx; the rate of major complications is 6% (Circ 2005;111:1100).

Low-energy internal cardioversion can convert Afib to NSR. Indications for implantable atrial defibrillators include recurrent symptomatic, drug-refractory Afib in pts requiring cardioversion q 1-2 mon (Circ 1998;98:1594).

Prevention of thromboembolic events: Pts with Afib of unknown or long duration require anticoagulation with warfarin for 3 wk before elective cardioversion (target INR, 2.5; range, 2.0-3.0) with continuation of anticoagulation for a minimum of 4 wk after successful cardioversion (Jama 2002;228:2441; Mayo Clin Proc 2002;77:897).

AHA recommendations (Nejm 2004;351:2408):

ASA 325 mg

- Pts with Afib and no structural heart disease who are < age 60
- Pts < age 60 with heart disease but no CAD risk factors
- Pts age 61-75 with no CAD risk factors
- Pts with contraindications to warfarin

Warfarin with INR 2.0-3.0

- Pts > age 60 with Afib and CAD or diabetes
- Pts > age 75 (especially women)
- Pts with thyrotoxicosis, HT, or EF < 35%

Warfarin with INR 2.5-3.5

- Pts with rheumatic heart disease
- Pts with h/o prior thromboembolism
- Pts with persistent atrial thrombus on TEE
- Pts with prosthetic heart valves

In pts with nonrheumatic Afib, 89% of thrombi identified on initial TEE study resolved after 4 wk of warfarin. No new thrombi were identified on follow-up study and no pt had a clinical thromboembolic event between studies (Circ 1995;92:160).

In the SPAF trial, among Afib pts given ASA, those with intermittent Afib had stroke rates similar to those of pts with sustained Afib (J Am Coll Cardiol 2000;35:183).

Elderly pts' propensity to fall is not an important factor in the decision to prescribe warfarin (Arch IM 1999;159:677). The intensity of anticoagulation rx and the deviation in INR, but not age, are predictors of risk for bleeding in pts < 80 yr (Ann IM 1996;124:970).

ASA has shown a small effect in preventing stroke in pts with Afib (Arch IM 1997;157:1237).

Ximelagatran is an investigational direct thrombin inhibitor initially reported to be as effective as warfarin for stroke/embolism prevention in Afib (Lancet 2003;362:1691).

7.2 Ventricular Arrhythmias

Nejm 2003;349:1836; Circ 2002;106:2145; 1998;97:1325

Cause: ASHD; hypertrophic, restrictive, dilated cardiomyopathy; valvular heart disease; corrected VSD, tetralogy of Fallot, RV dysplasia; anomalous-origin LCA

Long QT syndrome: Polymorphic VT associated with use of class IA or III antiarrhythmics, TCAs, phenothiazines, lithium, erythromycin, pentamadine, long-acting antihistamines, cocaine, hypokalemia, hypocalcemia, hypomagnesemia

Epidem: Structural CAD causes 80% of fatal arrhythmias; cardiomyopathy is the second leading cause (Nejm 2001;345:1473). In pts with AMI receiving thrombolytic rx, 10.2% had sustained VT, VF, or both. Older age, systemic HT, previous MI, Killip class, anterior infarct, and depressed ejection fraction were associated with a higher risk of sustained VT and VF (Circ 1998;98:2567).

Pathophys: Arrhythmogenic right ventricular cardiomyopathy (ARVD): histological evidence of inflammation with isolated RV displasia, Naxos disease, Venetian cardiomyopathy, syndrome of noncoronary RV precordial ST-segment elevation, RV outflow tract tachycardia, and Uhl's anomaly (Circ 1998;97:1532)

Long QT syndrome: Autosomal dominant; autosomal recessive with congenital hearing loss; sporadic (Nejm 1997; 336:1562)

Sx: Palpitations; lightheadedness; syncope; sudden death

Si: PVCs produce an irregular heartbeat with compensatory pause; VT produces a rapid, mildly irregular heartbeat.

Crs: Among pts with AMI who survived hospitalization, no significant difference was found in 30-d mortality between VT/VF and no VT/VF groups; after 1 yr, however, the mortality rate was significantly higher in the VT and VT/VF groups (Circ 1998; 98:2567).

Of 421 pts with AICD, 54% had recurrent VT/VF and 15% had syncope. Once VT/VF had occurred, 76%, 68%, and 62% of pts remained free of syncope during the following 12, 24, and 36 mon, respectively, and 68%, 64%, and 56% remained free of future syncope. If LVEF > 40%, fast VT had not been induced, and pts had no chronic AF, 96%, 92%, and 92% of pts remained free of syncope after 12, 24, and 36 mon, respectively (J Am Coll Cardiol 1998;31:608).

Sudden death in pts with AICD was associated with VT or VF events in 2/3 of pts. Death occurred despite successful device therapies. The suggested cause is acute cardiac mechanical dysfunction (J Am Coll Cardiol 1999;33:24).

Pts with CAD, LV dysfunction, and asymptomatic, unsustained VT in whom sustained ventricular tachyarrhythmias cannot be induced have a lower risk of sudden death/cardiac arrest and lower overall mortality than pts with inducible sustained tachyarrhythmias (MUSTT) (Nejm 2000;342:1937).

Cmplc: Sudden death

Lab: EKG (see Chapter 3 for diagnostic criteria); ambulatory monitoring; echocardiogram (for cardiomyopathy, valve disease); stress test if CAD clinically suspected; electrolytes, serum Mg^{++}, Ca^{++}

X-ray: CXR may reveal cardiomegaly in pts with cardiomyopathy.

Rx: *PVC:* PVC or nonsustained VT in pts without organic heart disease has a benign prognosis and generally requires no rx (Nejm 1985;312:193).

Rx of PVC following AMI with antiarrhythmics conveys no benefit and may increase mortality (Nejm 1992;327:227). β-Blockers are safe in these pts (Eur Hrt J 1993;14 (Suppl F):18).

Accelerated idioventricular rhythm (AIR): Occurs in 10-20% of pts with AMI; rx is required only if hemodynamic compromise results.

VT/VF: Rx should be initiated in pts with cardiac arrest due to VF or VT not due to a transient or reversible cause; spontaneous sustained VT; syncope of undetermined origin with clinically relevant, hemodynamically significant sustained VT or VF induced at electrophysiological study when drug rx is ineffective, not tolerated, or not preferred; and nonsustained VT with coronary disease, prior MI, LV dysfunction, and inducible VF or sustained VT at electrophysiological study that is not suppressible by a class I antiarrhythmic drug. Rx can also be considered for pts with cardiac arrest presumed to be due to VF when electrophysiological testing is precluded by other medical conditions; severe sx attributable to sustained ventricular tachyarrhythmias while awaiting cardiac transplantation; familial/inherited conditions (long QT syndrome, hypertrophic cardiomyopathy) with high risk for life-threatening ventricular tachyarrhythmias; nonsustained VT in pts with CAD, prior MI, LV dysfunction, and inducible sustained VT or VF at electrophysiological study; and recurrent syncope of undetermined etiology in the presence of ventricular dysfunction and inducible ventricular arrhythmias at electrophysiological study when other causes of syncope have been excluded (Circ 1998;97:1325).

Amiodarone reduced total mortality by 10-19% in pts at risk of sudden cardiac death; it also reduced risk in pts after MI who had CHF or clinically evident arrhythmia (Circ 1997;96:2823). The risks of cardiac death and arrhythmic death or resuscitated cardiac arrest were lower for pts receiving β-blockers and amiodarone than for those not receiving β-blockers, with or without amiodarone (Circ 1999;99:2268). In contrast, β-blocker use was associated with improved survival in patients with VF/symptomatic VT, but a protective effect was not prominent if the pt was already receiving amiodarone or had a defibrillator (J Am Coll Cardiol 1999;34:325).

Iv amiodarone is effective rx for VT/VF. Its suppression rates were in the range of 63-91% in uncontrolled trials. Hypotension is the most frequent side effect (J Am Coll Cardiol 1997;

29:1190). No increase in mortality was observed with a 1000 mg/24 hr dose (Circ 1995;92:3154).

Among survivors of VF or sustained VT causing severe sx, overall survival was greater with AICD than with class III antiarrhythmic drugs. The unadjusted survival rate estimates were 89.3% vs 82.3% at 1 yr, 81.6% vs 74.7% at 2 yr, and 75.4% vs 64.1% at 3 yr (Nejm 1997;337:1576). In pts with prior MI, EF $\leq$ 0.35, nonsustained VT, and inducible, nonsuppressible VT, AICD improved survival compared with amiodarone, β-blockers, or other antiarrhythmic rx (Nejm 1996;335:1933). Electrophysiologically guided rx with AICD, but not with antiarrhythmic drugs, reduced the risk of sudden death in high-risk pts with CAD (Nejm 1999;341:1882). AICDs were more effective than drug rx in reducing arrhythmic cardiac death but rates of nonarrhythmic cardiac death were unchanged; apparent arrhythmic death may constitute 38% of all cardiac deaths despite treatment with an AICD (AVID trial) (J Am Coll Cardiol 1999;34:1552). In a Canadian study, pts at the highest risk of death benefited most from AICD rx (Circ 2000;101:1660).

Major early AICD prevention trials (MADIT, MADIT-II, MUSTT) suffered from design problems (Circ 2004;109:2685). Nonetheless, current major indications for AICD implantation are

- Cardiac arrest due to VT/VF
- Sustained VT with structural heart disease
- Unexplained syncope with inducible VT/VF
- CAD with LV dysfunction and inducible VT
- Chronic CAD with EF < 30%
- High-risk inherited cardiac conditions

Contraindications include

- Unexplained syncope in the absence of structural heart disease or inducible VT/VF
- Irreversible NYHA class 4 CHF
- Terminal illness

Complications include

- Those for pacemaker implantation
- Frequent and/or inappropriate shocks
- Acceleration of VT (J Am Coll Cardiol 2004;44:2166; Nejm 2003;349:1836)

In high-risk pts with hypertrophic cardiomyopathy, AICD is effective in terminating VT/VF (Nejm 2000;342:365).

It is safe for a pt with an ICD to walk through electronic article surveillance systems, but lingering in the surveillance system may result in an ICD shock (Circ 1999;100:387).

When there is only one site of origin of VT, radio-frequency ablation is often curative. Its long-term success rate is 85-100% (Nejm 1999;340:534).

Regular participation in moderate-intensity activities is associated with a reduced risk of pulseless cardiac arrest (Arch IM 1999;159:686).

7.3 Bradycardia and AV Block

Lancet 2004;364:1701; Nejm 2000;342:703; 1996;334:90; Circ 1998; 97:1325

Cause: See Table 7.11.

Epidem: Genetic approaches have defined the molecular basis for long QT syndrome, arrhythmogenic right ventricular dysplasia, idiopathic VF and Brugada syndrome (Circ 2002;106:2514), Afib, progressive familial heart block, and familial WPW syndrome (Circ 1999;99:518; Nejm 1998;339:960).

Pathophys: Lyme disease can be a cause of conduction disturbances.

Sx: Lightheadedness; syncope

Si: Sick sinus syndrome: Sinus bradycardia, sinus pause, arrest, or SA node exit block; Afib with unexplained slow ventricular response

Table 7.11 Causes of Bradycardia

Intrinsic Causes	Extrinsic Causes
Idiopathic degeneration (aging)	Autonomically mediated syndromes
Infarction[1] or ischemia	Neurocardiac syncope
Infiltrative diseases	Carotid-sinus hypersensitivity
Sarcoidosis	Situational disturbances
Amyloidosis	Coughing
Hemochromatosis	Micturition
Collagen vascular diseases	Defecation
Systemic lupus erythematosus	Vomiting
Rheumatoid arthritis	Drugs
Scleroderma	β-Blockers
Myotonic muscular dystrophy	Ca^{++}-channel blockers
Surgical trauma	Clonidine
Valve replacement	Digoxin
Correction of congenital heart disease	Antiarrhythmic agents
Heart transplantation	Hypothyroidism
Familial diseases	Hypothermia
Infectious diseases[1]	Neurologic disorders
Chagas's disease	Electrolyte imbalances
Endocarditis	Hypokalemia
	Hyperkalemia

1. This condition causes AV conduction disturbances only. (Nejm 2000;342:703)

First-degree AV block: PR > 0.20 sec. Second-degree block: Not all P waves are followed by QRS complexes. Third-degree block: No relationship between P waves and QRS complexes.

Crs: Frequently intermittent and unpredictable

Cmplc: Syncope

Lab: (See Chapter 3 for diagnostic EKG criteria.) Holter monitoring is less effective than event (loop) monitoring in documenting arrhythmias (Ann IM 1998;128:890).

Rx: Indications for a permanent pacemaker: Third-degree or advanced second-degree AV block at any anatomic level associated with bradycardia with sx (including those of CHF) presumed to be due to AV block; arrhythmias/other medical conditions that require drugs that result in symptomatic bradycardia; documented periods of asystole > 3.0 sec or any escape rate < 40 beat/min in awake, symptom-free pts; pts s/p catheter ablation of AV junction or with postoperative AV block that is not expected to resolve; pts with neuromuscular diseases (myotonic muscular dystrophy, Kearns-Sayre syndrome, Erb's dystrophy, peroneal muscular atrophy) with AV block with or without sx; second-degree AV block regardless of type or site of block, with associated symptomatic bradycardia; asymptomatic type II second-degree AV block; asymptomatic type I second-degree AV block at intra- or infra-His levels found at electrophysiological study for other indications; and first-degree AV block with sx similar to those of pacemaker syndrome

In pts with chronic bifascicular and trifascicular block and intermittent third-degree AV block, type II second-degree AV block, or alternating BBB with syncope not demonstrated to be due to AV block when other likely causes have been excluded (specifically VT), or who have as an incidental finding at electrophysiological study a markedly prolonged HV interval or pacing-induced infra-His block that is not physiological

Pts with an acute MI who have persistent second-degree AV block in the His-Purkinje system with bilateral BBB or third-degree AV block within or below the His-Purkinje system, transient second- or third-degree infranodal AV block and associated BBB (electrophysiological study may be necessary), or persistent and symptomatic second- or third-degree AV block

Sinus node dysfunction: Pts with documented symptomatic bradycardia, including frequent sinus pauses that produce sx or symptomatic chronotropic incompetence, sinus node dysfunction occurring spontaneously or as a result of necessary drug rx with heart rate < 40 beat/min when a clear association between significant sx consistent with bradycardia and the actual presence of bradycardia has not been documented, or minimally symptomatic patients with chronic heart rate < 30 beat/min while awake

For prevention of tachycardia: In pts with sustained pause-dependent VT, with or without prolonged QT, in which the efficacy of pacing is thoroughly documented, or in high-risk pts with congenital long QT syndrome; can also be considered for pts with AV reentrant or AV node reentrant SVT not responsive to medical or ablative rx and for prevention of symptomatic, drug-refractory, recurrent Afib

Permanent pacing in hypersensitive carotid sinus syndrome and neurally mediated syncope: For pts with recurrent syncope when minimal carotid sinus pressure induces ventricular asystole of > 3 sec duration in the absence of any medication that depresses the sinus node or AV conduction; recurrent syncope without clear, provocative events and with a hypersensitive cardioinhibitory response; syncope of unexplained origin when major abnormalities of sinus node function or AV conduction are discovered or provoked in electrophysiological studies; symptomatic recurrent neurocardiogenic syncope with bradycardia; neurally mediated syncope with significant bradycardia reproduced by a head-up tilt with or without isoproterenol or other provocative maneuvers

Children and adolescents: For pts with advanced second- or third-degree AV block associated with symptomatic bradycardia, LV dysfunction, or low CO; sinus node dysfunction with correlation of sx during age-inappropriate bradycardia; post-op advanced second- or third-degree AV block that is not expected to resolve or persists at least 7 d after cardiac surgery; congenital third-degree AV block with a wide QRS escape rhythm or ventricular dysfunction or congenital third-degree AV block in the infant with a ventricular rate < 50-55 beat/min or with congenital heart disease and a ventricular rate < 70 beat/min; sustained pause-dependent VT, with or without prolonged QT, in which the efficacy of pacing is thoroughly documented; bradycardia-tachycardia syndrome with the need for long-term antiar-

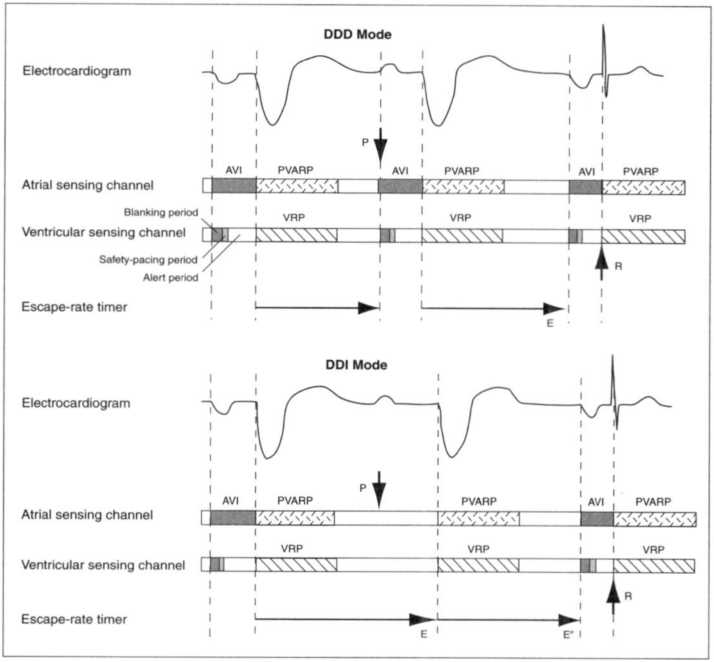

Comparison of the DDD Mode with the DDI Mode in a Dual-Chamber Pacemaker

The upper panel shows timing cycles and refractory periods for a dual-chamber pacemaker in DDD mode. After an atrial stimulus (the first beat), the AV-interval (AVI) timer starts. The atrial sensing channel is refractory throughout the AVI (hatched areas). In the ventricular sensing channel, the AVI is usually divided into the blanking period, the safety-pacing period, and the alert period. During the blanking period (designed to prevent the ventricular channel from sensing the atrial pacing output), the ventricular channel is refractory. During the safety-pacing period (designed to prevent inappropriate inhibition of ventricular output and resulting ventricular asystole), any activity sensed in the ventricular channel is interpreted as noise and triggers a ventricular output at the end of the peiod. In this figure, no activity is sensed during the safety-pacing period, so the alert period begins. Any activity sensed during this period inhibits the ventricular output. If the AVI ends and the ventricular channel has sensed no activity, a ventricular output is delivered (the first paced QRS complex). After an event (sensed or paced) in the ventricular channel, the post-ventricular atrial refractory period (PVARP), the ventricular refractory period (VRP), and the escape-rate timer begin. In the second beat, a spontaneous P wave is sensed (arrow P) and the AVI begins again. This AVI ends without any activity sensed in the ventricular channel, so a ventricular output is delivered, starting the PVARP, the VRP, and the escape-rate timer. In the third beat, the escape-rate timer expires (E) without sensing any atrial activity, so an atrial pacing stimulus is delivered. The AVI timer is interrupted by a spontaneous QRS complex (arrow R) caused by the conducted paced P wave. When the R wave is sensed, the PVARP, the VRP, and the escape-rate timer begin again.

The lower panel shows timing cycles and refractory periods for a dual-chamber pacemaker in DDI mode. Only after an atrial output does the AVI timer start. After the first paced QRS complex, atrial activity is sensed (arrow P); since in this mode the only response to a sensed event is inhibition, the AVI timer does not start, and a ventricular output is delivered only when the escape interval expires (E). After the second paced QRS complex, no atrial activity is sensed, so that when the difference between the escape interval and the AV interval is reached (E"), an atrial output is delivered. In this case, however, intrinsic ventricular activation is sensed before the expiration of the AVI (arrow R), and the ventricular channel is inhibited from delivering a ventricular output. However, the PVARP and VRP do start. Althrough the DDI mode prevents unwanted tracking of atrial activity, it may be associated with less than optimal timing of atrial and ventricular contractions.

Figure 7.1 Programmable Features of Pacemakers *Source:* Reprinted with permission from Kusumoto, Goldschlager, Medical Progress: Cardiac Pacing 1996;334:89–98, *New England Journal of Medicine.*

rhythmic treatment other than digitalis; congenital third-degree AV block beyond the first year of life with an average heart rate $<$ 50 beat/min or abrupt pauses in ventricular rate that are 2 or 3 times the basic cycle length; long QT syndrome with 2:1 AV or third-degree AV block; asymptomatic sinus bradycardia in the child with complex congenital heart disease with resting heart rate $<$ 35 beat/min or pauses in ventricular rate $>$ 3 sec

Meta-analysis suggests that systemic antibiotic prophylaxis reduces the incidence of infective complications after permanent pacemaker implantation (Circ 1998;97:1796).

Dual-chamber and rate-modulating pacing are recommended over ventricular pacing for prevention of Afib, for prevention of pacemaker syndrome, and for preservation of normal QRS duration (Circ 2004;109:443), but are not clearly superior to ventricular pacing for the prevention of stroke or CV death (Nejm 2000;342:1385).

Chapter 8

Valvular Heart Disease

8.1 Aortic Valve Disease

J Am Coll Cardiol 1998;32:1486

Cause: *AS:* Congenital—unicuspid (severe stenosis in infancy), bicuspid (AS in adulthood; AI if infectious endocarditis develops), or tricuspid with commissural fusion; rheumatic; degenerative

AI: Rheumatic fever; infectious endocarditis; diseases of aortic root; VSD; RA; SLE; ankylosing spondylitis; Takayusu's disease; Whipple's disease; Crohn's disease

Epidem: Rheumatic fever and rheumatic AS are decreasing in frequency in the industrialized countries. Degenerative disease remains the most common and most frequent cause of aortic valve replacement (AVR).

Bicuspid valves occur in 1-2% of the population and are associated with dilation of the ascending aorta (Circ 2002; 106:900).

At surgery, 54% of adults with isolated AS are found to have a congenitally malformed valve (Circ 2005;111:920).

In AS, the annual reduction in the aortic valve area is greater in those with milder degrees of stenosis and is accelerated in presence of smoking, hypercholesterolemia, and elevated serum creatinine and Ca^{++} levels (Circ 2000;101:2497).

Pathophys: *AS:* Gradual progression with development of progressive concentric LVH; sarcomeres replicate in parallel and wall thickness/cavity radius ratio increases; critical obstruction develops at valve area/index of 0.8/0.5 cm^2 and transvalvular gradient ≥ 50 mm Hg; CO is then normal at rest but falls with exercise

AI: Volume overload; sarcomeres elongate and replicate in series; chambers dilate but wall thickness/cavity radius ratio remains unchanged; in chronic AI, increased preload produces hemodynamic compensation (Frank Starling law), and EF and CO remain normal until late in disease; with acute AI (endocarditis, trauma, aortic dissection), CHF develops rapidly

In ankylosing spondylitis, development of AI is unrelated to other clinical features and can resolve or progress over time (J Am Coll Cardiol 1998;32:1397).

Sx: *AS:* Angina (⅔ of pts with critical AS; half of these also have significant CAD) (Am Hrt J 1980;100:441); syncope; dyspnea; orthopnea/PND; decreased exercise capacity

AI: Exertional dyspnea; orthopnea/PND; palpitations; syncope is rare

Si: *AS:* Pulsus parvus et tardus; prominent jugular venous A wave; sustained PMI; decreased A2 (in acquired AS); S4; late-peaking harsh systolic murmur at upper-right sternal border and apex that may radiate to carotids—more severe stenosis produces a longer murmur, but murmur may diminish with LV failure; murmur increases with squatting or with administration of amyl nitrite; murmur decreases with standing, moderate exercise, Valsalva maneuver (during strain); murmur is louder after extrasystole and varies in Afib; AI murmur may also be present

AI: Collapsing (water hammer, Corrigan's) pulse; capillary pulsations in lips or fingertips (Quincke's sign); booming femoral pulses (pistol-shot sounds, Traube's sign); widened pulse pressure; PMI laterally displaced or diffuse; systolic thrill; decreased A_2; S_3 gallop; blowing diastolic murmur at left sternal border, 3rd-4th intercostal space; short mid-systolic mumur at base; diastolic rumble at apex (Austin Flint murmur); AI murmur increases when pt is sitting forward or squatting; murmur decreases with administration of amyl nitrite or Valsalva maneuver (strain)

Crs: *AS:* Myocardial ischemia can occur without CAD in severe AS; it is due to inadequate LVH with high systolic and diastolic wall stresses and reduced coronary flow reserve (Circ 1997;95:892). Overall survival with medical rx after dx is 40-65% at 5 yr and 20% at 10 yr (Am J Cardiol 1975;35:221). Asymptomatic pts do well (J Am Coll Cardiol 1990;15:1012; Cardiol Rev 1993;1:344), but the average time to death is 2 yr from onset of CHF, 3 yr from onset of syncope, and 5 yr from onset of angina (Circ 1968;37 suppl V:61; Brit Hrt J 1973;35:41). Statin rx appears to slow the progression of AS; its mechanism of action may not be related to cholesterol lowering (Circ 2004;110:1291).

AI: Asymptomatic pts with nl LV systolic function have mortality < 0.2%/yr, but once pts develop LV dysfunction, 25%/yr develop sx. The mortality rate of symptomatic pts > 10%/yr. Predictors of survival include age, functional class, comorbid conditions, Afib, and LV end-systolic diameter. EF is an independent predictor of overall survival. Surgery for class II sx reduces cardiac mortality rates (J Am Coll Cardiol 1997;30: 746; Circ 1999;99:1851).

Fen-phen: Initial reports indicated that 8% of pts who have taken fenfluramine and phentermine (fen-phen) had moderate or severe AI. The prevalence of valvular regurgitation was 1-2 orders of magnitude lower in a study based on clinical records, and the incidence of clinically overt valvular disease after < 3 mon was < 1 case/1000 pt-yr after 4-yr follow-up (Nejm 1998;339:765). In 1163 pts who had taken fen-phen, mild or greater AI was present in 8.8% of treated pts and 3.6% of controls and moderate or greater MR in 2.6% of treated pts and 1.5% of controls, suggesting that the predominant abnormality is mild AI not accompanied by significant cardiovascular sx (Circ 2000;

101:2071). Spontaneous improvement in AI has been documented in follow-up echocardiograms (Mayo Clin Proc 1999; 74:1191; Circ 1999;100:2161).

Cmplc: Infectious endocarditis; embolic events and angiodysplasia with gi bleeding in calcific AS. Acquired type 2A von Willebrand's disease is common in pts with severe AS (Nejm 2003;349:343).

Lab: *EKG:* LAE; LVH may develop; EKG recommended q 2 yr in adolescents/young adults with AS; q 1 yr if Doppler peak velocity > 3 m/sec because the correlation between EKG findings and severity of AS is better in congenital than acquired AS

Echocardiogram: AS: In all pts for initial evaluation to assess LVH, LV systolic function, severity of AS, valve morphology, presence and severity of other valvular disease; q 2 yr in adolescents/young adults with AS; q 1 yr if Doppler peak velocity > 3 m/sec; Doppler velocity > 4 m/sec indicates > 95% likelihood that AS is severe and pt will require AVR

If pt has vague sx, Doppler echocardiogram; if peak velocity > 3m/sec, exercise test (see below)

If pt is asymptomatic, repeat test annually, advise re sx for Doppler velocity < 3 m/sec, q 6 mon if velocity 3-4 m/sec (pt is unlikely to be asymptomatic if Doppler velocity > 4 m/sec) (Circ 1997;95:2241)

AI: In all pts, to confirm presence and severity of acute AI or chronic AI, assess etiology of regurgitation, valve morphology and aortic root size and morphology, LVH, LV systolic function; if EF abnormal or LV end-diastolic dimension 60-70 mm or end-systolic dimension > 55 mm, pt requires AVR; if LV end-diastolic dimension > 75 mm or end-systolic dimension 45-50 mm, echo q 3 mon if unstable; all others: echo q 12 mon

Fen-phen: Pts should be examined clinically; echocardiography for pts who have a heart murmur or evidence of valvular disease or who received drugs for > 3 mon

Stress test: AS: Contraindicated in pts with severe AS; for pts with vague sx and Doppler echocardiogram peak velocity 3-4 m/sec, consider AVR if pt develops sx, VT, or hypotension during/after exercise test; otherwise follow medically

AI: Assess functional capacity and symptomatic responses, especially in athletes and pts with possible LV dysfunction; pts with normal EF and LV end-diastolic dimension 70-75 mm or end-systolic dimension 50-55 mm on echo will need AVR if sx or EF falls during exercise (measured by echocardiogram or radionuclide imaging)

Consider stress test for adolescents/young adults with AS if Doppler velocity > 3 m/sec and pt plans athletic participation or if clinical findings and echo-Doppler are disparate

See also the recommendations for follow-up in Section 8.4 on prosthetic heart valves.

X-ray: *CXR:* Cardiomegaly in AI; absence of calcium (fluoroscopy) in adults rules out severe AS

Radionuclide ventriculogram: For assessment of LV volume and function in pts with suboptimal echocardiograms or in asymptomatic pts with echocardiogram evidence of significant/progressive LV dysfunction but discordant clinical picture

Cardiac catheterization: In **AS** if other findings indicate severe disease requiring AVR, if noninvasive tests are inconclusive or the clinical picture and test results are inconsistent, or if angiography is required to assess possible concomitant CAD

Up to 22% of pts who undergo retrograde catheterizaton of the aortic valve have MRI evidence of acute cerebral embolic events, though only 3% have clinically apparent neurological deficits (Lancet 2003;361:1241).

In **AI** for pts at risk for CAD or if noninvasive tests are inconclusive or discordant with clinical findings regarding the severity of AI, degree of LV dysfunction, or need for surgery (J Am Coll Cardiol 1998;32:1486)

Rx: *AS:* Symptomatic pts (CHF, syncope, chest pain): valve area < 0.8 cm^2 requires aortic valve replacement; area 0.8-1 cm^2 is "gray area"; if area > 1 cm^2, seek other causes of sx. Pts with moderate or severe AS who are scheduled for CABG or surgery of aorta of other valves also should have AVR; see also the recommendations under stress testing. In asymptomatic pts with AS, surgery may be delayed until sx develop; however, pts with moderate or severe valvular calcification and a rapid increase in aortic-jet velocity are candidates for early valve replacement (Nejm 2000;343:611).

Pts with AS and LV dysfunction (EF $< 35\%$): Operative mortality is 9%. Approximately 58% are alive at 7 yr. Of those surviving, 80% had symptomatic improvement and 76% had improved EF (Circ 1997;95:2395). These pts should be considered for AVR independent of their sx.

Balloon valvotomy is reserved for those pts with severe AS requiring urgent noncardiac surgery or for those pts who are too sick or unstable to undergo AVR immediately but who are likely to be candidates for AVR in future, and for adolescents/young adults with normal CO and catheterization peak gradient > 60 mm Hg **or** peak gradient ≥ 50 mm Hg **and** who are symptomatic (angina, syncope, DOE), have new-onset EKG changes (ST depression, T-wave inversions at rest or during exercise), or want to play competitive sports or become pregnant.

It appears to be relatively safe to delay surgery until sx develop in asymptomatic pts with AS, but the presence of moderate or severe valvular calcification plus a rapid increase in aortic-jet velocity identifies pts with a very poor prognosis who should be considered for early valve replacement independent of their sx (Nejm 2000;343:611).

In pts with severe AS and decompensated CHF, iv nitroprusside may improve LV function acutely; it is safe if the pt is not in cardiogenic shock (Nejm 2003;348:1756).

AI: Fen-phen: Pts should receive endocarditis prophylaxis if they have a heart murmur, "silent" moderate or severe AI on Doppler echocardiography, or mild AI associated and structural valvular lesions (Nejm 1998;339:ed).

Vasodilator rx: For pts with AI and CHF prior to surgery; for pts with severe AI who are symptomatic and/or have LV dysfunction and for whom surgery is not an option; for pts with persistent LV dysfunction after AVR (ACEIs); for asymptomatic pts with severe AI and LV dilatation with normal LV systolic function or who have any degree of AI and HT

AVR: In chronic severe AI, for pts with functional class III or IV sx and preserved LV systolic function; usually for pts with class II sx and preserved LV systolic function and definitely if progressive LV dilatation is present; for pts with declining EF, decreasing exercise capacity, or angina; for pts with only LV dysfunction, especially those receiving nifedipine (J Am Coll Cardiol 2005;45:1025); for pts undergoing CABG, aortic or other valve surgery; and for asymptomatic pts with LV end-diastolic dimension > 75 mm or end-systolic dimension > 55 mm, or pts whose EF falls during exercise (Circ 2003;108:2432). Operative mortality is 2-8% and depends on sx and EF (Nejm 2004;351: 1539). Pts with severe AS but low transvalvular gradient due to poor LV function may have their survival rate improved by AVR (J Am Coll Cardiol 2002;40:410).

In adolescents/young adults, AVR is definitely recommended for symptomatic pts or in asymptomatic pts with LV with EF < 0.50 on serial studies 1-3 mon apart or with progressive LV enlargement. The presence of moderate AS or the appearance of ST depressions or T-wave inversions on EKG may also be indications for AVR.

Pts with severe AI due to disease of the aortic root may require surgical repair/graft of aorta (J Cardiovasc Surg 1994;9 suppl:182).

Percutaneous aortic valvuloplasty does not change the natural course of AI and is not recommended (Circ 2004;109:1572).

See also the recommendations for antithrombotic rx in Section 8.4 on prosthetic heart valves.

8.2 Mitral Valve Disease

J Am Coll Cardiol 1998;32:1486; Ann IM 1989;111:305

Cause: *MS:* Rheumatic fever (Lutembacher syndrome: MS with ASD); congenital very uncommon, seen in infancy

MR: Rheumatic fever, infectious endocarditis, mitral valve prolapse, calcification of mitral annulus, collagen vascular disease (SLE, scleroderma), Marfan syndrome, Ehlers-Danlos syndrome, amyloidosis, sarcoidosis, LA myxoma, trauma, ischemia, congenital abnormalities

Mitral prolapse: Most frequently occurs as a primary condition; also seen in collagen-vascular disease, Marfan syndrome, von Willebrand's disease, myotonic dystrophy

Epidem: Rheumatic: ⅔ of pts are women; 25% of pts with rheumatic fever develop pure MS; another 40% have MS and MR (Eur Hrt J 1991;12 suppl B:77)

In a community-based sample, the prevalence of mitral valve prolapse (MVP) was 2.4% (incidence was previously reported as 3-5%) (Nejm 1999;341:1). Women with this condition outnumber men 2:1.

Pathophys: *MS:* Normal mitral orifice is 5-6 cm^2; orifice is reduced in MS due to fusion of commissures and thickening of cusps and/or chordae. A gradient develops when valve area is reduced to 2 cm^2. LA pressure $\geq$ 25 mm Hg when valves $\leq$ 1 cm^2 (critical MS).

MR: Disorders of mitral leaflets, chordae, or papillary muscles produce a leak. Impedance to LV emptying in systole is reduced and EF remains normal or increased until LV pump failure develops.

Mitral prolapse: Myxomatous proliferation of mitral leaflets and chordae cause billowing of mitral leaflets.

Sx: Exertional dyspnea; orthopnea; palpitations. Sx are usually less in chronic MR than in MS but are acute and severe in acute MR. 15% of pts with MS have angina-like chest pain (Prog Cardiovasc Dis 1973;15:491).

The frequencies of chest pain and dyspnea are similar among subjects with and without prolapse (Nejm 1999;341:1).

Si: *MS:* Prominent jugular A wave; RV heave (if RV enlarged); increased S_1 and P_2; opening snap; diastolic rumble at apex; longer murmur = more severe MS

MR: S_1 normal or decreased; S_2 widely split; P_2 increased in pulmonary HT; S_3 gallop; late/holosystolic murmur radiating to axilla that varies little with cycle length or inspiration

Mitral prolapse: Mid-systolic click, late systolic murmur that decreases with squatting, increases with administration of amyl nitrite and Valsalva maneuver (strain)

Hemoptysis is more common in MS than in MR.

Crs: *MS:* Sx manifest 15-20 yr after an episode of rheumatic fever and progress over 3-4 yr (Am J Cardiol 1975;35:221).

Reported 7-yr survival for pts treated with balloon commissurotomy was 83%. The 1-, 3-, 5-, and 7-yr event-free survival rates (survival without MVR or repeat CBC) were 80%, 77%, 65%, and 65%, respectively. Pts with MVA of 1.5 cm^2 could be subdivided into high- and low-risk subgroups based on mean PCW pressure > 18 mm Hg and cardiac index $<2.5\ L \cdot min^{-1} \cdot m^{-2}$ (Circ 1997;95:382; 1999;99:1580).

MR: LV contractile impairment is reversible in many pts with long-term MR, and surgery can preserve LV contractility (Circ 1995;92:811).

If CHF develops after surgical correction of MR, survival is poor: 44% at 5 yr (Circ 1995;92:2496).

Mitral prolapse: The Framingham study reported the incidence of severe MR in pts with MVP to be 6.5% (J Am Coll Cardiol 2002;40:1298). 15% of pts develop worsening MR over 10-15 yr. Men > 50 yr are at greatest risk (Circ 1988;78:10).

Cmplc: Infectious endocarditis; chordal rupture and flail leaflet in MR; embolic events also reported with mitral prolapse. MR increases the mortality risk in pts receiving thrombolysis or PTCA for acute MI (J Am Coll Cardiol 2004;43:1368).

Lab: *EKG:* LAE, coarse Afib, incomplete RBBB in MS. Only 15% of pts with MR show LAE.

Echocardiogram: MS: For all pts to confirm dx; determine mean gradient, mitral valve area, PA pressure, and RV dimensions; evaluate valve (see below); identify other valve lesions; or for pts with worsening sx

Echocardiographic mitral morphology score: Leaflet rigidity, leaflet thickening, valvular calcification, and subvalvular disease are each graded from 1+ to 4+. Lower scores are correlated with post-balloon valvulotomy valve area of 1.5 cm^2, without 2-grade increase in the severity of MR and without L-to-R shunt of 1.5:1 across the intra-atrial septum. The complication rate is low if score > 8 (Circ 2004;109:1572; 1998;97:223).

MR: In all pts for initial assessment of MR and LV function and to identify cause; subsequently for periodic measure of LV function and dimensions in asymptomatic pts, for changing sx, and after valve repair/replacement

Recommended frequency in pts with chronic MR:

- Mild MR with nl EF, nl end-systolic LV diameter (ESD), echo every 5 yr
- Moderate MR with nl EF, nl ESD, echo every 1-2 yr
- Moderate MR, EF < 0.65 or EDV > 40 mm, echo every yr
- Severe MR with nl EF and EDV, echo every yr
- Severe MR, EF < 0.65 or EDV > 40 mm, echo every 6 mon (Nejm 2001;345:740)

In asymptomatic pts, echo quantification of MR (regurgitant volume, effective regurgitant orifice) predicts clinical outcome (Nejm 2005;352:875).

Mitral prolapse: In all pts, to demonstrate systolic billowing of leaflets and to assess severity of MR; repeat study for changing sx and/or to follow degree of prolapse and MR and chamber dimensions; for suspected infectious endocarditis

TEE: For pts with mitral valve disease and inadequate transthoracic echocardiogram or suspected LA thrombus or endocarditis; also used intraoperatively

X-ray: *MS:* Enlargement of LA, RV, or RA, pulmonary arteries; pulmonary edema

MR: Enlargement of LV or LA; CHF

Cardiac catheterization: MS: Indicated to assess MR severity in candidates for balloon valvotomy if clinical and echocardiographic data are discordant; to measure PA, LA, and LV diastolic pressures if clinical and echo/Doppler data are discordant with the severity of MS by 2-D and Doppler echocardiography; or to gauge hemodynamic response of PA and LA pressures during exercise if clinical symptoms and resting hemodynamics are discordant

MR: For pts with angina, prior MI, or suspected ischemia; for pts with CAD risk factors who are scheduled for mitral valve surgery; or for pts with inconclusive/discrepant noninvasive studies

Rx: *MS:* Endocarditis prophylaxis; anticoagulation for pts with Afib or embolic events

Balloon valvuloplasty: For pts with class II-IV sx **and** valve area ≤ 1.5 cm^2 or valve area > 1.5 cm^2 and pulmonary HT (PA systolic pressure 50 mm Hg at rest or 60 mm Hg with exercise) **and** mild or no MR, no LA thrombus, and reasonable valve morphology, **or** for asymptomatic pts with the same characteristics and pulmonary HT, Afib, or pregnancy (Circ 2004;109:1572)

VALVULAR HEART DISEASE

Mitral valve replacement: For pts with class III-IV sx and valve area ≤ 1.5 cm^2 **or** pts with class I-II sx, valve area ≤ 1.5 cm^2, and PA systolic pressure > 60-80 mm Hg who are not candidates for balloon valvotomy

MR: Endocarditis prophylaxis; medical rx of HT and CHF (qv)

Follow up q 3-6 mon and yearly echo if pt is assessed as functional class I and EF > 60%

Mitral valve surgery: For mitral valve repair in acute symptomatic MR, for class II-IV sx, and for asymptomatic pts if MR is severe (mitral valve repair of flail leaflet improves long-term survival rate and decreases cardiac mortality and morbidity), if ventricle enlarges with exercise, if there is progressive end-systolic LV dilation (end-systolic diameter > 40-45 mm), if LV systolic function is abnormal (EF < 60%; fractional shortening < 30-32%), or if pt develops Afib or pulmonary HT (PA systolic pressure 50 mm Hg at rest or 60 mm Hg with exercise). The exception is the pt with class III-IV sx and EF < 30% for whom no improvement or deterioration results from surgery (Circ 1997; 95:548; 1997;96:1819; 1999;99:338; J Am Coll Cardiol 1998; 32:1486). Mitral valve repair has a lower operative mortality than replacement, but it may not be optimal for rheumatic or severely myxomatous valves (Circ 2003;108:2432). The rate of recurrence of MR after repair is 35-40% at 5 yr (Circ 2003; 107:1609).

MV repair vs replacement: Overall survival at 10 yr 68% vs 52%, overall operative mortality 2.6% vs 10.3% (in pts < 75 yr, 1.3% vs 5.7%), late survival at 10 yr 69% vs 58% , and EF higher after valve repair (Circ 1995;91:1022)

MVP: Endocarditis prophylaxis for pts with mid-systolic click and late systolic murmur or with click and echocardiographic evidence of MVP with MR; ASA for pts with TIA, CVA when anticoagulants are contraindicated, or age < 65 yr with Afib; warfarin for pts with CVA, TIA despite ASA rx, or with

Afib and age > 65 yr. Mitral valve repair for MVP is associated with survival rates of 80-94% at 5-10 yr (Nejm 2001;345:740).

8.3 Rheumatic Fever

Circ 1999;100:1576; Peds 1995;96:758; Jama 1992;268:2069

Cause: Inflammatory process involving heart, joints, CNS, following group A streptococcal infection

Epidem: Current incidence < 2 cases/100,000 population in U.S. The risk of developing rheumatic fever after untreated strep pharyngitis is 3%; 33% of pts with acute rheumatic fever have mild/asymptomatic pharyngitis. Up to 50% of pts with a prior episode of rheumatic fever will have a recurrence after untreated strep pharyngitis.

Pathophys: Exudative and proliferative inflammatory reaction with fibrinoid degeneration of collagen

Sx: Arthralgia, antecedent sore throat

Si: Major: Carditis, polyarthritis, chorea, erythema marginatum, subcutaneous nodules. Minor: Fever, pharyngitis.

Cmplc: Rheumatic valvular heart disease. Up to 1/3 of pts with valve disease cannot provide h/o prior rheumatic fever.

Lab: Elevated ESR, CRP (minor criteria); also leukocytosis

EKG: Prolonged PR interval (minor diagnostic criterion); also sinus tachycardia, AV block, ST-T abnormalities

Echocardiogram: LV dysfunction; mitral or aortic regurgitation; pericardial effusion

X-ray: CXR: Pulmonary edema

Rx: Prevention of rheumatic fever

Primary: Benzathine penicillin G 600,000 U im (1.2 million U im for pts > 60 lb) **or** penicillin G 250 mg po tid × 10 d for children, 500 mg po bid-tid × 10 d for adults. For individuals allergic to penicillin: Erythromycin estolate 20-40 mg/kg/d po bid-qid (maximum 1 gm qd) × 10 d **or** erythromycin ethylsuccinate 40 mg/kg/day po bid-qid (maximum 1 gm qd) × 10 d **or** azithromycin 500 mg po on d 1 and 250 mg po qd × 4 d thereafter

Secondary: Benzathine penicillin G 1.2 million U im q 4 wk (q 3 wk for high-risk pt) **or** penicillin G 250 mg po bid **or** sulfadiazine 0.5 mg po qd (1 gm po qd for pts > 60 lb). For individuals allergic to penicillin: Erythromycin 250 mg po bid. Duration: 10 yr since last episode of RF or into adulthood if pt has no valvular disease; 10 yr or at least to age 40 with valvular disease (Peds 1995;96:758).

Acute rheumatic fever: Bed rest; ASA for 1-3 mon; prednisone 1-2 mg/kg/min for pts not responsive to ASA; diuretics for CHF. There is no evidence that anti-inflammatory rx reduces the incidence of subsequent valvular disease.

8.4 Prosthetic Heart Valves

Chest 2004;126:457S; J Am Coll Cardiol 1998;32:1486

Sx: Progressive dyspnea may be a sx of valve thrombosis.

Si: Muffled valve sounds or a new murmur suggests possible valve thrombosis.

Crs: In a study of pts > 75 yr old, reported 30-d hospital mortality was 7.5% (11/147); survival at 55 mon was 71%, and 81% of pts were assessed as functional class I/II (Chest 1997;112:885).

Cmplc: Thrombosis; dehiscence. Minor paravalvular leaks are not rare and require no rx if small and if infective endocarditis is not suspected.

Pts with left-sided prosthetic valve thrombosis have a 12% risk of cerebral embolus.

Lab: EKG, chemistries, CBC recommended 3-4 wk post-op; consider echocardiogram q yr

Marked increase in valve gradient by Doppler exam suggests possible valve thrombosis; TEE may demonstrate abnormal leaflet motion and/or thrombus size, shape, mobility

X-ray: CXR recommended 3-4 wk post-op

Rx: *Antithrombotic rx*

Warfarin for 3 mon after all valve replacement surgery	INR 2.0-3.0
Subsequent rx	
Warfarin for St. Jude valve in aortic position	INR 2.0-3.0
Warfarin for St. Jude or tilting disk valve in mitral position	INR 2.5-3.5
Warfarin for all caged ball/disk valves	INR 2.5-3.5 plus ASA 75-100 mg po qd
Warfarin for all bioprosthetic valves	ASA 75-100 mg

For pts who have an embolic event during adequate antithrombotic rx

If INR 2-3	Increase warfarin for INR of 2.5-3.5
If INR 2.5-3.5	Increase warfarin for INR of 3.5-4.5
Not on ASA	Add ASA 80-100 mg qd
Aspirin only	ASA 325 mg qd and/or warfarin for INR of 2-3
Warfarin + ASA 80-100 qd	INR 3.5-4.5 and/or ASA 325 mg qd

Antithrombotic rx in pts requiring noncardiac surgery/dental procedures: If procedure has a *low risk* of bleeding, continue rx. If pt has a *high risk* of thrombosis (especially with mechanical mitral valve), stop warfarin 72 hr before procedure, start heparin when INR < 2.0, start heparin 6 hr before procedure, resume after procedure, and continue until INR > 2.0. *Otherwise*, stop ASA 1 wk before procedure and warfarin 72 hr before procedure; resume after procedure.

Prosthetic valve thrombosis (PVT): Thrombolysis is acceptable for high-risk surgical candidates with left-sided PVT who are functional class III or IV. Absolute contraindications to thrombolysis include active internal bleeding, h/o hemorrhagic CVA, recent cranial trauma or neoplasm, BP > 200/120, and diabetic hemorrhagic retinopathy. Relative contraindications include gi bleeding or puncture of noncompressible vessel in past 10 d, major operation or trauma in past 2 wk, nonhemorrhagic CVA in past 2 mon, infectious endocarditis, uncontrolled HT, large thrombus on prosthesis or in LA, or known bleeding diathesis. Rx is streptokinase 250,000 U as iv bolus over 30 min, followed by 100,000 U/hr iv; assess with serial Doppler study (or TEE for nonobstructive thrombus); continue rx for 72 hr (24 hr if no improvement is seen), followed by heparin and then warfarin + ASA.

Surgery is recommended for pts who do not respond or who have mobile thrombus. For pts with nonobstructive PVT and class I or II sx, rx is heparin for 48 hr, followed by sc heparin **plus** warfarin (INR 2.5-3.5) for 1-3 mon (J Am Coll Cardiol 1997; 30:1521).

8.5 Infective Endocarditis

Circ 2005;111:3167; Lancet 2004;363:139

Cause: Infection of endothelial surface of heart valves, chordae tendinae, or mural surface. *S. aureus* is the most common agent in acute infective endocarditis (IE); streptococci, entercocci, coagulase-negative staphylococci, and the HACEK group are the major agents in subacute IE.

Epidem: Incidence 2-4 cases/100,000 population; more common in men; 55-75% of pts with native valve endocarditis have predisposing cardiac conditions (Jama 1985;254:1199); 65-75% of iv drug users who develop IE have right-sided valve involvement

Pathophys: Vegetation is composed of bacteria, platelets, and fibrin. Injury is caused by destruction of cardiac tissue and structures, pulmonary and systemic embolization of vegetation fragments, continuing bacteremia, and immune complex deposition. Large vegetations may also cause valvular obstruction.

Sx: Generally nonspecific—fever, chills, weight loss, anorexia, malaise, headache, arthralgia. Pts with acute IE generally appear toxic and acutely ill. Right-sided valve lesions can produce acute dyspnea and pleuritic chest pain.

Si: Duke criteria for d/o infective endocarditis

- Definite IE: 2 major criteria, or 1 major and 3 minor criteria, or 5 minor criteria (listed below)
- Not IE: Alternative dx found, resolution of illness with 4 d of antibiotic rx, or no evidence of IE found at surgery or autopsy
- Possible IE: Anything else
- Right-sided IE: Cough, hemoptysis of abrupt onset
- Major criteria: 2 separate blood cultures positive for *viridans* streptococci, *Streptococcus bovis*, HACEK group, community-acquired S. *aureus*, or enterococci (in the absence of primary focus); persistently positive blood cultures (2 positive cultures drawn > 12 hr apart or majority of 4 separate cultures); positive echocardiogram (vegetation, abscess, new partial dehiscence of prosthetic valve) or new valvular regurgitation
- Minor criteria: Predisposing heart condition or iv drug use; temperature ≥ 38°C; major arterial emboli, septic pulmonary infarcts, mycotic aneurysm, intracranial hemorrhage, conjunctival hemorrhages, or Janeway lesions; glomerulonephritis, Osler's nodes, Roth spots, or rheumatoid factor; positive blood cultures that do not meet major criteria or serological evidence of active infection with organism consistent with IE; echocardiographic findings consistent with IE but that do not meet major criteria

Crs: CHF may result from valvular destruction. 10-40% of pts with IE will have clinical evidence of embolization from vegetations.

Bacteremia may cause spread to CNS, spleen, kidneys, bone (especially vertebrae), or pericardium. 2-10% of pts will develop mycotic aneurysms, half of which will involve intracerebral arteries; 3-5% will develop splenic abscess; $< 15\%$ will develop immune complex glomerulonephritis.

Cmplc: Pts with prosthetic heart valves, *S. aureus* or fungal IE, prior h/o endocarditis, cyanotic congenital heart disease, prolonged symptoms, or poor response to rx are at high risk for complications of IE. The presence of abnormal mental status, moderate/severe CHF, etiology other than *S. viridans*, or medical rx without valve surgery is associated with increased 6-mon mortality (Jama 2003;289:1933). Conversely, surgery for pts with complicated left-sided native valve endocarditis and CHF show reduced 6-mon mortality (Jama 2003;290:3207).

Lab: *On admission:* CBC, urinalysis, protime, serum creatinine, liver panel, 3 blood cultures. If cultures are negative at 96 hr, ESR, repeat cultures (at least 2 for 2 d) and obtain circulating immune titer.

Echocardiogram: The sensitivity of TTE in detection of vegetations is only 45-75%; the sensitivity of TEE is 90-94%. Therefore, TTE is probably worth doing if blood cultures are positive at 24-48 hr; otherwise, TEE is the echo of choice and is also necessary if IE of prosthetic valve suspected. Echocardiogram and Doppler study can also assess the degree of valve dysfunction and extension of infection.

Surgery may be indicated if echocardiogram demonstrates persistence or progression of vegetation with rx; large vegetation of anterior mitral leaflet; acute AI or MR with CHF or CHF unresponsive to rx; perforation, rupture, or dehiscence; abscess; fistula; or extension of infection or new conduction disturbances.

Pathological criteria considered diagnostic of definite IE: Microorganisms demonstrated by culture or histology in a vegetation, in a vegetation that has embolized, or in an intracardiac abscess, or specimens of pathological lesions with vegetation or intracardiac abscess present, confirmed by histology showing active endocarditis

X-ray: Radiologic and other studies usually performed by radiology departments.

Right-sided vegetations may result in nodular infiltrates on CXR due to septic pulmonary infarcts

CT, MRI liver/spleen scan or ultrasound, or cerebral angiography may be required for assessment of extracardiac complications

Rx: *Prevention of bacterial endocarditis:* see Tables 8.1 and 8.2.

Table 8.1 Prophylactic Regimens for Dental, Oral, Respiratory Tract, or Esophageal Procedures

Situation	Agent	Regimen
Standard general prophylaxis	Amoxicillin	Adults: 2 gm; children: 50 mg/kg orally 1 hr before procedure
Unable to take oral medications	Ampicillin	Adults: 2 gm im or iv; children: 50 mg/kg im or iv within 30 min before procedure
Allergic to penicillin	Clindamycin or	Adults: 600 mg; children: 20 mg/kg orally 1 hr before procedure
	Cephalexin or cefadroxil or	Adults: 2 gm; children: 50 mg/kg orally 1 hr before procedure
	Azithromycin or clarithromycin	Adults: 500 mg; children: 15 mg/kg orally 1 hr before procedure
Allergic to penicillin and unable to take oral medications	Clindamycin or	Adults: 600 mg; children: 20 mg/kg iv within 30 min before procedure
	Cefazolin	Adults: 1 gm; children: 25 mg/kg im or iv within 30 min before procedure

Table 8.2 Prophylactic Regimens for Genitourinary/Gastrointestinal (Excluding Esophageal) Procedures

Situation	Agents	Regimen
High-risk patients	Ampicillin plus gentamicin	Adults: ampicillin 2 gm im or iv plus gentamicin 1.5 mg/kg (not to exceed 120 mg) within 30 min of starting procedure; 6 hr later, ampicillin 1 gm im/iv or amoxicillin 1 gm orally Children: ampicillin 50 mg/kg im or iv (not to exceed 2 gm) plus gentamicin 1.5 mg/kg within 30 min of starting the procedure; 6 hr later, ampicillin 25 mg/kg im/iv or amoxicillin 25 mg/kg orally
High-risk patients allergic to ampicillin/ amoxicillin	Vancomycin plus gentamicin	Adults: vancomycin 1 gm iv over 1–2 hr plus gentamicin 1.5 mg/kg iv/im (not to exceed 120 mg); complete injection/infusion within 30 min of starting procedure Children: vancomycin 20 mg/kg iv over 1–2 hr plus gentamicin 1.5 mg/kg iv/im; complete injection/infusion within 30 min of starting procedure
Moderate-risk patients	Amoxicillin or ampicillin	Adults: amoxicillin 2 gm orally 1 hr before procedure, or ampicillin 2 gm im/iv within 30 min of starting procedure Children: amoxicillin 50 mg/kg orally 1 hr before procedure, or ampicillin 50 mg/kg im/iv within 30 min of starting procedure
Moderate-risk patients allergic to ampicillin or amoxicillin	Vancomycin	Adults: vancomycin 1 gm iv over 1–2 hr; complete infusion within 30 min of starting procedure Children: vancomycin 20 mg/kg iv over 1–2 hr; complete infusion within 30 min of starting procedure

(Circ 1997;96:358)

Prophylaxis is recommended for pts with prosthetic valves, h/o endocarditis, congenital heart disease (*except* repaired or isolated secundum ASD, repaired VSD or PDA, or MVP without MR), acquired valve disease, MVP with MR, and hypertrophic cardiomyopathy. Prophylaxis is *not* needed for pts with prior CABG, RF without valve dysfunction, permanent pacemaker, AICD, or functional murmurs.

Procedures requiring endocarditis prophylaxis

- Dental: Extractions, periodontal procedures, dental implants, root canal, subgingival placement of antibiotic strips, initial placement of orthodontic bands, or cleaning (if bleeding is anticipated) but *not* restorative dentistry, local anesthetic injections, intracanal endodontic rx, placement of dams, suture removal, or placement of removable orthodontic appliances
- Respiratory tract: Tonsillectomy, adenoidectomy, surgery of respiratory mucosa, or rigid bronchoscopy but *not* endotracheal intubation, flexible bronchoscopy, or tympanostomy tube insertion
- Gi tract (recommended for high-risk pts, optional for medium-risk pts): Sclerosis of esophageal varices, esophageal dilation, endoscopic retrograde cholangiography with biliary obstruction, biliary tract surgery, or surgery involving intestinal mucosa but *not* endoscopy or TEE
- GU: Prostate surgery, cystoscopy, or urethral dilation but *not* vaginal hysterectomy or delivery, cesarean section, therapeutic abortion, sterilization procedures, insertion/removal of IUD, D & C, or urethral catheterization in the absence of infection

Prophylaxis is *not* required for cardiac catheterization, PTCA, or implantation of pacemaker, AICD, or coronary stent; incision/biopsy of surgically scrubbed skin; or circumcision.

Medical rx: See Table 8.3.

In pts with *S. aureus* IE involving aortic or mitral valves, anticoagulant rx is associated with death due to neurologic damage. Anticoagulation should be discontinued as soon as a

Table 8.3 Rx of Infective Endocarditis

Microorganism	Antibiotic	Dosage	Duration
Staphylococci	Nafcillin or oxacillin	2 gm iv q 4h	4–6 wk
Methcillin-susceptible	plus		
Native valve	Gentamicin (addition is optional)	1 mg/kg iv/im q 8h	3–5 d
Non-β-lactam–allergic pts	or		
	Vancomycin	15 mg/kg/24 hr iv bid; max 2 gm/24 hr	4–6 wk
Staphylococci	Cefazolin or other first-generation	2 gm iv q 8h or equivalent dosing	4–6 wk
Methcillin-susceptible	cephalosporin		
Native valve	plus		
β-lactam–allergic pts	Gentamicin (addition is optional)	1 mg/kg iv/im q 8h	3–5 days
	or		
	Vancomycin	15 mg/kg/24 hr iv bid; max 2 gm/24 hr	4–6 wk
Staphylococci	Vancomycin	15 mg/kg/24 hr iv bid; max 2 gm/24 hr	4–6 wk
Methcillin-resistant			
Native valve			
Staphylococci	Nafcillin or oxacillin	2 gm iv q 4h	≥ 6 wk
Methcillin-susceptible			
Prosthetic valve	May add rifampin	300 mg po q 8h	≥ 6 wk
Non-β-lactam–allergic pts	May add gentamicin	1 mg/kg iv/im q 8h	2 wk

Staphylococci Methcillin-susceptible Prosthetic valve	Cefazolin or other first-generation cephalosporin	2 gm iv q 8h or equivalent dosing	≥ 6 wk
β-Lactam allergic pts	May add rifampin	300 mg po q 8h	≥ 6 wk
	May add gentamicin	1 mg/kg iv/im q 8h	2 wk
Staphylococci Methcillin-resistant	Vancomycin	15 mg/kg/24 hr iv bid; max 2 gm/24 hr	≥ 6 wk
Prosthetic valve	May add rifampin	300 mg po q 8h	≥ 6 wk
	May add gentamicin	1 mg/kg iv/im q 8h	2 wk
HACEK group (*Hemophilis, Actinobacillis, Cardiobacterium, Eikenella, Kingella*)	Ceftriaxone or other third-generation cephalosporin	2 gm iv/im qd or equivalent dose	4 wk
	or		
	Ampicillin	12 gm/24 hr iv continuous infusion or in 6 divided doses	4 wk
	plus		
	Gentamicin (addition is optional)	1 mg/kg iv/im q 8h	4 wk
Fungal endocarditis	Amphotericin B	1 mg/kg/d iv; max dose 2-2.5 gm/d	6-8 wk
	May add flucytosine	150 mg/kg/d po in 4 divided doses	6-8 wk
Culture-negative endocarditis	Vancomycin	15 mg/kg/24 hr iv bid; max 2 gm/24 hr	6 wk
	plus		
	Gentamicin	1 mg/kg iv/im q 8h	6 wk

clinical dx is made until the septic phase of disease is over (Arch IM 1999;159:473).

Surgery for endocarditis

Native valve: Surgery required for acute AI with CHF or tachycardia and early mitral closure or MR with CHF, fungal endocarditis, abscess of mitral annulus or sinus of Valsalva, persistent infection or recurrent embolus after antibiotic rx, gram-negative endocarditis, and possibly for large mobile vegetations

Prosthetic valves: Surgery indicated for endocarditis within 2 mon of valve replacement, CHF with valve dysfunction, fungal endocarditis, staphylococcal endocarditis not responsive to rx, abscess, fistula, development of conduction disturbances, gram-negative endocarditis, persistent infection, recurrent embolus, and possibly for vegetation on prosthesis

Chapter 9

The Cardiomyopathies

9.1 Dilated Cardiomyopathy

Nejm 1994;331:1564

Cause: Dilated cardiomyopathy characterized by dilatation and impaired contraction of LV or both ventricles; may be idiopathic, familial/genetic, viral, immune, alcoholic, or toxic

A familial cause is identified in ~35% of cases; 16 chromosomal loci with altered cytoskeletal and nuclear transfer proteins have been implicated (J Am Coll Cardiol 2005;45:969; Lancet 2001;358:1627).

Ischemic cardiomyopathy: Dilated cardiomyopathy with impaired LV function not explained by extent of CAD or ischemic damage.

Valvular cardiomyopathy: LV dysfunction out of proportion to abnormal loading conditions.

Inflammatory cardiomyopathy: Myocarditis with cardiac dysfunction. Idiopathic, autoimmune, and infectious forms known include Chagas's disease and HIV, enterovirus, adenovirus, and cytomegalovirus infections.

Metabolic cardiomyopathy is associated with thyrotoxicosis, hypothyroidism, adrenal cortical insufficiency, pheochromocytoma, acromegaly, DM, hemochromatosis, glycogen storage disease, Hurler's syndrome, Refsum's syndrome, Niemann-Pick disease, Hand-Schüller-Christian disease, Fabry-Anderson disease, Morquio-Ullrich disease, disturbances of potassium metabolism, magnesium deficiency, kwashiorkor, anemia, beriberi, selenium deficiency, and familial Mediterranean fever.

Toxic cardiomyopathy may be produced by phenothiazines, reserpine, chloroquine, cobalt, lead, lithium, mercury, CO, EtOH, cocaine, snake venom, and cancer rx. Anthracyclines (doxorubicin, danorubicin) and imatinab are associated with the highest frequency of CHF, but CHF is also seen with mitoxantrone, cisplatin, cyclophosphamide, fosfamide, mitomycin, paclitaxel, bevacizumab, retinoic acid, and pentostatin (Circ 2001;109:3122).

Peripartum cardiomyopathy: Heterogeneous syndrome manifesting in last 6 wk of pregnancy or 5 mon thereafter. It is more common in women with multiple births or pre-eclampsia. Its incidence is 1 per 3000-4000 live births (Jama 2000;283:1183).

Epidem: Annual incidence: 5-8 cases/100,000 population. Blacks and males have a 2.5-fold increase in risk. Associated with HT, β-adrenergic agonist use, and alcohol consumption. Usually presents between ages 20 and 50. 75-85% of pts present with CHF, and 90% of these are already NYHA functional class III or IV.

20% of pts have a first-degree relative with decreased EF or cardiomegaly. Inheritance is usually autosomal dominant, although autosomal recessive, X-linked recessive, and mitochondrial inheritance have been reported (Nejm 1992;326:77).

Pathophys: 4-chamber cardiac enlargement with dilation frequently out of proportion to hypertrophy; histology in dilated cardiomyopathy is nonspecific and shows interstitial and perivascular fibrosis

Sx: Fatigue, diminished exercise capacity and exertional dyspnea (86% of pts), orthopnea, PND, palpitations (30%), peripheral edema (29%); asymptomatic cardiomegaly is detected in 4-13% of pts; abdominal distention, right-upper-quadrant pain, nausea, anorexia (with right-sided CHF). Exertional chest pain is the initial symptom in 8-20% and is present in ~35% of pts overall.

Si: JVD with prominent V wave, brisk Y descent; diffuse, laterally displaced apical impulse, S_4 (in pts in NSR); S_3; systolic murmur

(AV regurgitation). Syncope, S_3 gallop, and right-sided CHF indicate a poor prognosis.

Crs: Presentation is usually with CHF, often progressive. CHF is the cause of death in ~75% of pts. Arrhythmias, thromboembolism, and sudden death may occur at any stage. Reported mortality rates are 25-30% at 1 yr and 35-62% at 5 yr.

Predictors of poor outcome include male gender, age > 55 yr at diagnosis, class IV sx, syncope or h/o VT, cardiac arrest, EF < 20%, right-sided failure, and pulmonary HT. Pts with peripartum cardiomyopathy appear in general to have the best prognosis, while pts with HIV disease or h/o doxorubicin rx have a poor prognosis (Nejm 2000;342:1077).

Cmplc: Afib is seen in < 25% of cases.

Clinically apparent systemic and/or pulmonary emboli are the initial manifestations in 1.5-4% of cases; their overall incidence is 1-12%. Pts with severe LV ventricular dysfunction and pts with Afib, h/o thromboembolism, or echocardiographic evidence of thrombus or prothrombotic states of pregnancy are at greatest risk.

Lab: CBC, UA, glucose, creatinine, Ca^{++}, albumin, TSH level indicated

EKG: First-degree AV block, LBBB, left anterior fascicular block, and intraventricular conduction delays occur in > 80% of cases: first- or second-degree AV block RBBB is rare, but LBBB is a predictor of poor prognosis.

Echocardiogram: 4-chamber enlargement; global LV hypokinesis. Monitoring EF, fractional shortening, LV diastolic function, and abnormal response to iv dobutamine may be helpful in following pts receiving chemotherapy (Circ 2004;109:2122).

Stress test: For pts with chest pain, prior MI, or high probability of occult CAD

X-ray: CXR: Cardiomegaly; pulmonary venous redistribution; pulmonary edema

Rx: Treatment is that for CHF (see Chapter 6). Vasodilator rx is the standard initial rx (or hydralazine/isosorbide dinitrate) plus diuretics.

Digitalis is effective in controlling sx in pts in NSR. Its long-term benefits include improved EF and exercise capacity.

β-blockers (carvedilol or metoprolol) may also be of benefit.

Anticoagulation with warfarin is appropriate for pts with mural thrombi or h/o embolic phenomena; it is also frequently recommended for pts with EF < 0.30, even though evidence of efficacy from controlled clinical trials is lacking.

Antiarrhythmic drugs have not been shown to decrease mortality. AICD may be of benefit in pts with symptomatic VT or cardiac syncope (Jama 2004;292:2879).

Cardiac transplantation survival rates: 79% at 1 yr, 74% at 5 yr, 72% at 10 yr. Maximal O_2 uptake > 12 mL/kg/min characterizes those pts most likely to have improved survival after transplantation.

Doxorubicin-induced cardiomyopathy: Cardiotoxicity can be reduced by limiting the peak plasma concentration and overall cumulative dose. Echocardiography is recommended before every additional course up to a total dose of 300 mg/m^2. Radionuclide angiocardiography should also be performed if the pt is receiving > 400 mg/m^2 in one course. Echo should be repeated 3, 6, and 12 mon after completion of rx and q 2 yr thereafter, and radionuclide angiocardiography should be done after 12 mon and then q 5 yr (Nejm 1998;339:900).

In peripartum cardiomyopathy, persistence of LV dysfunction beyond 6-12 mon post-dx is a contraindication to subsequent pregnancy (Nejm 2001;344:1629).

9.2 Hypertrophic Cardiomyopathy

Lancet 2004;363:1881; J Am Coll Cardiol 2003;42:1687; Jama 2002;287:1308

Cause: Hypertrophic cardiomyopathy (HCM) characterized by LV and/or RV hypertrophy, usually asymmetric and involving intraventricular septum, with normal/decreased LV volume with or without systolic outflow gradient. Mutations in sarcomeric contractile protein genes cause disease; modifier genes and environmental factors influence phenotypic expression.

Epidem: HCM was identified in 0.29% of echocardiograms in a community study (J Am Coll Cardiol 1999;33:1590).

Familial disease with autosomal dominant inheritance predominates. Chromosome 14 is a common site of abnormality (Jama 1999;281:1746), but 10 genes and > 130 mutations have been identified as causing disease (Circ 2003;107:2227). Myosin-binding protein C, cardiac troponin T, and β-myosin heavy-chain genes account for the greatest number of identified mutations. A hereditary pattern is identifiable in ~50% of pts on family hx.

Pathophys: Morphological changes include myocyte hypertrophy and disarray surrounding areas of increased loose connective tissue. The pattern and extent of LVH vary widely among pts. 25% of Japanese pts have apical hypertrophy.

Septal hypertrophy and motion of the anterior mitral leaflet produce dynamic outflow gradient obstruction. Both diastolic relaxation and distensibility are abnormal.

HCM is a separate entity in hypertensive pts with LV hypertrophy and features of dilated or restrictive cardiomyopathy with CHF. It is more prevalent in elderly pts.

Sx: Fatigue, dyspnea, palpitations, angina (25% of pts), and syncope—but the majority of pts may be asymptomatic. In asymptomatic pts, obstruction is an important predictor of cardiac death (J Am Coll Cardiol 2005;45:1076).

Si: Systolic heave; S_4 gallop; harsh crescendo-decrescendo systolic murmur at left sternal border that increases with Valsalva maneuver (strain), standing, exercise, TNG or amyl nitrite, and that decreases with squatting, passive leg elevation, isometric hand grip, β-blockers

Crs: HCM shows extreme clinical and genetic heterogenicity, and it may present clinically at any point in life. The reported annual mortality is 1-3%, but cardiac mortality and incidence of sudden death for asymptomatic adult pts with HCM are very low (J Am Coll Cardiol 1999;33:206). In regionally selected populations, HCM did not significantly increase the risk of premature death or adversely affect overall life expectancy (Jama 1999;281:650). Major identified risk factors for sudden death in HCM include Vfib or spontaneous sustained VT, family h/o premature sudden death, unexplained syncope, septal wall thickness > 30 mm, and abnormal exercise BP response. All have low positive predictive value, but the absence of these findings in an asymptomatic pt with gradient < 30 mm Hg probably indicates low risk. In one study, cumulative risk 20 yr after initial evaluation was nearly 0% for pts with wall thickness ≤ 19 mm, and 40% for wall thicknesses ≥ 30 mm (Nejm 2000;342:1778); not all centers have confirmed the latter finding (J Am Coll Cardiol 2003;41:315; Lancet 2001;357:420). The presence of any gradient at rest can be a predictor of progression of sx or CHF (Nejm 2003;348:295). In North America, apical HCM had 10% incidence of MI and 12% incidence of Afib at 14 yr but was not associated with sudden death (J Am Coll Cardiol 2002;39:638).

Cmplc: Arrhythmias and premature/sudden death are over-represented in study populations. High-risk pts are those with family h/o HCM and/or sudden death and age < 30 yr at time of initial dx (Lancet 1997;350:127; Brit Hrt J 1994;72:S13)

Lab: *EKG:* LVH, T-wave abnormalities, Q waves (20-50% of pts) not diagnostic of MI (J Am Coll Cardiol 1990;16:375). SV arrhythmias occur in 25-50% of pts. Afib in 10% of pts frequently produces clinical deterioration due to loss of atrial kick (J Am Coll

Cardiol 1990;15:1279). 25% of pts have nonsustained VT; 15% of pts have normal EKGs.

Holter monitoring: In a study of 178 pts, 88% had PVC, 42% had ventricular couplets, 37% had SVT, and 31% had nonsustained VT. The presence of ventricular arrhythmias had low positive predictive value for sudden cardiac death (J Am Coll Cardiol 2005;45:697).

Stress test: Hypotensive BP response during exercise is seen in ~20% of pts with HCM and is associated with adverse long-term prognosis in patients < 50 yr old; normal BP response identifies a low-risk subset of pts (J Am Coll Cardiol 1999;33:2044). Exercise-induced abnormal BP response is related to subendocardial ischemia during exercise (J Am Coll Cardiol 1998;32:938). Metabolic exercise testing facilitates differentiation between physiologic LVH and HCM (J Am Coll Cardiol 2000;36:864).

Echocardiogram: Normal/small LV with asymmetric septal hypertrophy; narrowed outflow tract with gradient, systolic anterior motion (SAM) of mitral valve; diastolic dysfunction

Invasive electrophysiologic studies are not generally necessary or useful in identification of high-risk HCM pts (Jama 2002; 287:1308).

X-ray: CXR: Mild cardiomegaly, LA enlargement

Rx: Many patients achieve normal life expectancy without important symptoms even in the presence of substantial subaortic obstruction at rest with medication and do not require aggressive intervention.

Strenuous exercise and competitive sports should be avoided and are prohibited in pts with marked hypertrophy, resting gradient, or family h/o sudden death.

β-blockers improve angina, dyspnea, pre-syncope, and blunt exercise-related increase in LV outflow gradient. Verapamil up to 480 mg qd may also be used; adverse hemodynamic effects are a rare complication.

Digoxin should be avoided because of its positive inotropic effect; diuretics may be used cautiously (Am J Cardiol 1994; 73:312).

Disopyramide 300-600 mg qd improves sx in ~66% of pts (J Am Coll Cardiol 2005;45:1251). Negative inotropes eliminate obstruction by decreasing LV ejection acceleration, reducing hydrodynamic force on mitral leaflet, delaying mitral-septal contact, and lowering the pressure gradient (Circ 1998;97:41).

5% of HCM pts without obstruction develop LV dilation and systolic dysfunction. Their rx is similar to that for dilated cardiomyopathy.

Endocarditis prophylaxis is recommended for pts with evidence of LVOT obstruction. The usual site of vegetations is the anterior mitral leaflet.

Ventricular septal myotomy-myectomy is reserved for the management of pts with marked outflow gradient (> 50 mm Hg) and NYHA functional class III or IV sx of CHF refractory to medical rx (typically < 10% of pts). In a Mayo Clinic series, 89% of survivors were class I/II; 47% believed that they had 100% improvement at 1 yr; 67% of pts with dyspnea, 90% with angina, 86% with near-syncope, and 100% with syncope reported improvement; and 5-yr survival was 92%.

Overall, 70% of pts report symptomatic improvement for ≥ 5 yr after surgery. Basal outflow gradient is abolished or greatly reduced in > 90% of pts. Whether surgery prolongs survival or reduces risk of sudden cardiac death is unknown. LBBB is common after surgery but incidence of complete heart block requiring pacing is < 1-2%.

Dual-chamber pacing was originally reported to improve sx in pts with obstruction (Circ 1999;99:2927). Subsequent randomized studies have shown modest to no long-term decrease in gradient.

Infusion of ethanol into a major septal perforator branch of the LAD coronary artery has a mortality rate equal to that of myectomy (1-2%) and a 5-10% incidence of complete heart block. It usually reduces the resting gradient to < 25 mm Hg with an improvement in sx. Myocardial contrast echo is important for branch artery selection. The effect of alcohol ablation rx on sudden cardiac death is uncertain (Circ 2004;109:452; Thorac Cardiovasc Surg 1999;47:94; J Am Coll Cardiol 2000;36:852).

VT/Vfib appears to be the principal mechanism of sudden death in pts with HCM. AICD placement may be indicated in high-risk pts (Nejm 2000;342:365).

9.3 Restrictive Cardiomyopathy

Circ 2000;101:2490; Nejm 1997;336:267

Cause: Characterized by restrictive filling and reduced diastolic volume of LV and/or RV; systolic function and wall thickness usually normal. May be idiopathic, associated with familial cardiomyopathy, scleroderma, pseudoxanthoma elasticum, diabetic cardiomyopathy, infiltrative amyloidosis, sarcoidosis, Gaucher's disease, Hurler's disease, hemochromatosis, Fabry's disease, glycogen storage disease, endomyocardial fibrosis, hypereosinophilic syndrome, carcinoid heart disease, metastatic cancers, radiation, serotonin, methysergide, ergotamine, or busulfan.

Epidem: In U.S., ~85% of pts have primary systemic amyloidosis (monoclonal light chains). The heart is rarely involved in secondary amyloidosis, which is seen in rheumatoid arthritis, chronic inflammatory bowel disease (mainly Crohn's disease), tuberculosis, and leprosy. Idiopathic restrictive cardiomyopathy affects predominantly elderly pts.

Pathophys: Characteristic hemodynamic feature is deep, rapid early decline in ventricular pressure at onset of diastole with rapid rise and plateau ("square root sign"). LV pressure exceeds RV pressure by > 5 mm Hg. PA systolic pressure > 50 mm Hg.

Sx: Amyloidosis: Weakness, fatigue, light-headedness, change in voice

Si: Weight loss, edema and other signs of right-sided heart failure, paresthesias, syncope, dyspnea, purpura, bleeding, hepatomegaly without splenomegaly (25% of pts), macroglossia (10% of pts), orthostatic hypotension

Crs: Prognosis is variable, but the usual course is one of symptomatic progression. With amyloidosis, 25% of pts develop CHF. 50% of deaths are due to CHF or arrhythmias. Less than 10% of pts are alive 10 yr after the onset of sx.

Pts presenting with systemic and pulmonary venous congestion and Afib have a poor prognosis, particularly men > 70 yr old with LA diameter > 60 mm (Circ 2000;101:2490).

In sarcoidosis, autopsy data indicate cardiac involvement in 20-30% of cases, but only 5% of pts have sx ante-mortem.

Cmplc: Amyloid deposition leads to conduction disturbances (sinus arrest, SA exit block, AV block, ventricular conduction delays) and PVC. SV tachycardia can cause CHF, hypotension due to diastolic dysfunction, and restrictive cardiomyopathy.

Orthostatic symptoms and angina may occur (Nejm 1997;336). Nephrotic syndrome, renal failure, carpal tunnel syndrome, and sensorimotor peripheral neuropathy are also observed.

Lab: 90% of pts with immunoglobulin amyloidosis have monoclonal immunoglobulin protein in serum or urine. Serum protein electrophoretic pattern is abnormal in 50% of pts. Hypogammaglobulinemia is present in 20% of pts. Plasmacytosis is present in bone marrow > 50% of pts. M protein in serum or urine or monoclonal plasma cells in bone marrow are found in 98% of pts. Biopsy of abdominal fat or bone marrow is positive in 90% of pts. Anemia is an infrequent finding unless multiple myeloma, renal insufficiency, or gi bleeding is present. Thrombocytosis is observed in 10% of pts and reduced renal function in 50% of pts.

Hemochromatosis: elevated serum Fe level, normal/low Fe-binding capacity, elevated serum ferritin and transferrin saturation level

EKG: Cardiac amyloidosis may demonstrate a "pseudo-infarction" pattern (left-axis deviation; poor R-wave progression; Q waves in V_1, V_2); low voltages; Afib, complex ventricular arrhythmias; AV conduction disturbances; and sick sinus syndrome.

Echocardiogram: Increased thickness of the left and right ventricular walls, abnormal myocardial texture (granular sparkling), valvular thickening and regurgitation, atrial enlargement, and pericardial effusion; abnormal relaxation and restrictive hemodynamics in advanced disease; mural thrombi and AV valve regurgitation in hypereosinophilic syndrome

Biopsy: In suspected amyloidosis, abdominal fat pad aspirate is probably the most useful procedure to establish the dx.

Table 9.1 summarizes lab findings in restrictive cardiomyopathy and constrictive pericarditis.

X-ray: CXR may show hilar adenopathy in sarcoidosis. CT and MRI help distinguish constrictive pericarditis from restrictive cardiomyopathy.

Rx: In general, no specific rx is available for restrictive cardiomyopathy; therefore, primary rx is use of diuretics for relief of sx of congestion.

Hypereosinophilic syndrome (Loeffler's endocarditis) may respond well to steroids and hydroxyurea (Blood 1994;83:2759).

In pts with hemochromatosis, phlebotomy or chelation therapy with desferrioxamine is most helpful if begun before end-organ damage occurs.

Table 9.1 Restrictive Cardiomyopathy and Constrictive Pericarditis

Type of Evaluation	Restrictive Cardiomyopathy	Constrictive Pericarditis
Physical examination	Kussmaul's sign may be present Apical impulse may be prominent S3 may be present, rarely S4 Regurgitant murmurs common	Kussmaul's sign usually present Apical impulse usually not palpable Pericardial knock may be present Regurgitant murmurs uncommon
Electrocardiography	Low voltage (especially in amyloidosis), pseudo-infarction, left-axis deviation, Afib, conduction disturbances common	Low voltage ($< 50\%$)
Echocardiography	Increased wall thickness (especially thickened interatrial septum in amyloidosis) Thickened cardiac valves (amyloidosis) Granular sparkling texture (amyloid)	Normal wall thickness Pericardial thickening may be seen Prominent early diastolic filling with abrupt displacement of interventricular septum
Doppler studies	Decreased RV and LV velocities with inspiration Inspiratory augmentation of hepatic-vein diastolic flow reversal Mitral and tricuspid regurgitation common	Increased RV systolic velocity and decreased LV systolic velocity with inspiration Expiratory augmentation of hepatic-vein diastolic flow reversal
Cardiac catheterization	LVEDP often $>$ 5 mm Hg greater than RVEDP, but may be identical	RVEDP and LVEDP usually equal RV systolic pressure < 50 mm Hg RVEDP $> 1/3$ of RV systolic pressure
Endomyocardial biopsy	May reveal specific cause of restrictive cardiomyopathy	May be normal or show nonspecific myocyte hypertrophy or myocardial fibrosis
CT/MRI	Pericardium usually normal	Pericardium may be thickened

LVEDP = left ventricular end-diastolic pressure; RVEDP = right ventricular end-diastolic pressure.
Source: Reprinted with permission, Kusumoto, Fallon, Fuster, Medical Progress: Restrictive Cardiomyopathy, 1997;336:267–276, *New England Journal of Medicine.*

Arrhythmias and syncope are common in pts with cardiac involvement in sarcoidosis. Arrhythmias are frequently not controlled with drugs but pacing may provide symptomatic relief; the benefit from steroids is less certain (Chest 1994;106:988).

Liver transplantation can be beneficial in familial amyloidosis; it should be performed before symptomatic cardiac amyloidosis occurs. If CHF is present, cardiac transplant must be done before the liver transplant (Circ 1995;91:1269).

Chapter 10

Myocarditis, Pericardial Disease, and Cardiac Tumors

10.1 Acute Pericarditis

Nejm 2004;351;2195; Lancet 2004;363:717; Jama 2003;289:1150

Cause: Multiple; idiopathic most common in young adults, but causes include

Infections: Coxsackie A or B virus, echovirus, adenovirus, mumps virus, infectious mononucleosis, varicella, hepatitis B, HIV, tuberculosis, pneumococcus, staphylococcus, streptococcus, gram-negative septicemia, *Neisseria meningitidis*, *Neisseria gonorrhoea;* histoplasmosis, coccidioidomycosis, candida, blastomycosis, toxoplasmosis, amebiasis, mycoplasma, nocardia, actinomycosis, echinococcosis, Lyme disease

Acute MI

Uremia

Radiation injury

Autoimmune disorders: SLE, rheumatoid arthritis, seleroderma, mixed connective tissue disease, Wegener's granulomatosis, polyarteritis nodosa, acute rheumatic fever

Inflammatory disorders: sarcoidosis, amyloidosis, inflammatory bowel disease, Whipple's disease, temporal arteritis, Behcet's syndrome

Drugs: hydralazine, procainamide, phenytoin, isoniazid, phenylbutazone, dantrolene, doxorubicin, methysergide, penicillin
Neoplasm
Trauma
Dressler's syndrome; postpericardiotomy syndrome
Dissecting aortic aneurysm
Hypothyroidism
The cause in 9 out of 10 cases is either viral or unknown (Am J Cardiol 1995;75:378).

Epidem: Purulent pericarditis is most often seen as a complication of lung infection with staphylococcus, pneumococcus, or streptococcus. It may also be a life-threatening complication of infective endocarditis.

Histoplasmosis is the most common cause of fungal pericarditis. Coccidioidomycosis pericarditis is seen in the U.S. Southwest and San Joaquin Valley.

Although 60% of dialysis pts will develop pericardial effusion, clinical pericarditis is seen in < 20% of dialysis pts.

Breast and lung cancer, leukemia, Hodgkin's disease, and non-Hodgkin's lymphoma account for 80% of malignant pericarditis. Ovarian and gi malignancy, multiple myeloma, and melanoma are also associated with pericarditis.

12-48% of pts with SLE develop pericarditis (Mayo Clin Proc 1999;74:275), but it is frequently not clinically apparent and tamponade occurs in < 10% of pts. Approximately 25% of pts with RA develop pericarditis.

2-25% of pts with lupus-like syndrome from hydralzine or procainamide are reported to develop pericarditis.

10-40% of cardiac surgery pts develop postpericardiotomy syndrome 1-8 wk after the procedure.

Up to ⅓ of pts with myxedema develop pericardial effusion.

Pathophys: Inflammation can involve a superficial layer of myocardium. Fibrin deposits are particularly dense in tuberculous pericarditis, and virtually all untreated pts subsequently develop constrictive pericarditis.

Very large pericardial effusions can develop rapidly in histoplasmosis pericarditis.

Primary pericardial tumors are rare and are most frequently mesotheliomas.

Sx: Chest pain may be pleuritic, and may improve with sitting up and worsen when lying supine. Dyspnea is possible.

Bacterial pericarditis presents as acute illness with fever, chills, night sweats, and dyspnea.

Si: Pericardial friction rub may be evanescent. It is best heard at LLSB with the pt leaning forward. 85% of pts will have rub in course of the disease.

Crs: Idiopathic pericarditis is usually self-limited. Pain improves with rx in 1 wk and EKG findings resolve in 2-4 wk; < 20% of pts will have a recurrence within 6 mon.

Cmplc: Large pericardial effusion; constrictive pericarditis; up to 15% of pts with acute pericarditis will develop cardiac tamponade (Am J Cardiol 1985;56:623)

Lab: *EKG:* Sinus tachycardia; ST elevation (concave upward) in multiple leads, followed in hr/d by resolution of ST elevation; T-wave flattening followed by T-wave inversion. If the ratio of ST elevation (in mm)/T-wave inversion amplitude (in mm) in lead V6 > 0.24, acute pericarditis is likely (Circ 1982;65:1004).

Echocardiogram can demonstrate pericardial effusion but many pts with acute pericarditis will not have significant effusion.

Elevated ESR, leukocytosis, and mild elevation of CK-MB are observed. Plasma troponin I level is elevated in 35-50% of pts (J Am Coll Cardiol 2003;42:2144).

Tbc skin test, BUN, and creatinine tests are appropriate for all pts. Depending on the differential dx, ANA, rheumatoid factor, TSH, HIV test, blood cultures, and heterophile antibody may also be indicated.

Pericardial fluid analysis: Cell count, glucose, protein, LDH, bacterial culture, and cytology. Exudates are characterized by specific gravity > 1.015, fluid total protein > 3.0 g/dL, fluid/serum protein ratio > 0.5, fluid LDH ratio > 0.6, fluid/serum glucose ratio < 1.0. Cytologic study had a sensitivity of 92% and a specificity of 100% for malignant effusion (Chest 1997;111:1213). Cell cytology is diagnostic in 85% of pts with malignant pericarditis.

X-ray: CXR may be normal or show globular heart. 25% of pts will have pleural effusion.

Rx: ASA 2-4 gm po qd, ibuprofen 1600-3200 mg po qd, indomethacin 75-225 mg po qd for control of pain. If no response, give steroids (eg, prednisone 60-80 mg/d). Steroids may increase the risk of later recurrence.

Close observation for signs of developing tamponade and restriction of activity are required.

Warfarin should be avoided. If anticoagulation is mandatory, switch to iv heparin.

Diagnostic pericardiocentesis is reserved for pts with suspected purulent pericarditis or malignancy.

Colchicine 0.6 mg po bid may be a useful adjunct in prevention of recurrent idiopathic pericarditis (Circ 1998;97:2183).

Large idiopathic chronic pericardial effusion is usually well tolerated for long periods but tamponade can develop unexpectedly. Pericardiectomy should be considered whenever a large effusion recurs after pericardiocentesis (Nejm 1999;341:2054).

10.2 Constrictive Pericarditis

Cause: Fibrin deposition during acute pericarditis leads to fusion and thickening of visceral and parietal pericardium, resulting in chronic restriction of diastolic filling of heart

Epidem: TB was formerly the most common cause, but it now accounts for < 15% of cases in industrialized countries. Most cases are of unknown cause. Mediastinal radiation, post-surgical pericarditis, chronic renal failure, collagen vascular disease, and metastatic malignancy also are possible causes (Am Hrt J 1987;113:354).

Pathophys: Heavily fibrosed and calcified pericardium produces elevation and equilibration of diastolic pressures in all 4 cardiac chambers. Early diastolic filling of ventricles is relatively unimpaired, but filling comes to an abrupt halt for the remainder of diastole due to restriction by the pericardium.

Sx: Dyspepsia, anorexia; dyspnea, orthopnea; fatigue, weight loss, muscle wasting; chest pain

Si: Elevated jugular pulse with Kussmaul's sign (inspiratory increase in systolic jugular venous pressure—can be difficult to assess at bedside); diastolic pericardial knock (usually earlier and higher pitched than S_3 gallop); normal/diminished arterial pulses; pulsus paradoxicus is uncommon; pleural effusion; hepatomegaly, edema, ascites

Crs: Untreated, the course is one of progressive worsening of pericardial thickening and diastolic dysfunction with worsening of edema, ascites, weakness, and cardiac cachexia.

Lab: *EKG:* Low QRS voltages, nonspecific T-wave abnormalities, LA abnormality; Afib occurs in < 50% of pts

Echocardiogram: Dense immobile pericardium, early diastolic septal bounce in pt without LBBB, pacemaker, dilated hepatic veins, dilated IVC with loss of respiratory variation in diameter.

Doppler shows an abnormal tricuspid and hepatic-vein flow pattern variation with respiratory cycle (J Am Soc Echocardiogr 1997;10:246).

Cardiac catheterization: Shows ventricular early diastolic dip and plateau and helps differentiate constrictive pericarditis from constrictive cardiomyopathy

Liver enzymes, serum bilirubin, and serum albumen may be abnormal due to chronic passive engorgement of liver, kidneys, and gi tract.

X-ray: CXR: Cardiac silhouette may be normal or enlarged. Calcified pericardium is present in 50% of cases and pleural effusion in 60%.

CT and MRI can detect pericardial thickening.

Rx: Complete surgical resection of pericardium. Operative mortality is 6-25%; 90% of survivors of surgery report improvement in sx and 50% have complete relief; 5-yr survival is 74-87% (Eur J Cardiothorac Surg 1994;8:487). Pts with severe debility, renal insufficiency, extensive calcification of pericardium, or prior radiation have a poorer prognosis.

Pts with tuberculous pericarditis require drug rx.

Pts with mild disease benefit from diuretic administration and avoidance of β-blockers and slowing Ca^{++}-channel blockers (Am J Cardiol 1993;72:615).

10.3 Cardiac Tamponade

Nejm 2005;349:684

Cause: Any form of pericarditis that can cause rapid accumulation of pericardial fluid

Epidem: In 2 hospital series, 32-58% of cases of tamponade were seen in pts with malignancy, 14% in pts with idiopathic pericarditis, 9-14% in pts with uremia, 9% in pts with acute MI and anticoagulation, 7.5% in pts with cardiac perforation, 5-7.5% in pts with purulent pericarditis, 1-5% in pts with tbc, 4% in pts with radiation rx, 4% in pts with myxedema, and 4% in pts with dissection aortic aneurysm (J Am Coll Cardiol 1991;17:59; Circ 1981; 64:633).

Pathophys: The pericardial space normally contains 15-50 cc fluid; it can accommodate > 1 L if fluid accumulates slowly. Rapid accumulation of 200 cc can increase intrapericardial pressure, causing equalization of intracardiac filling pressures. When pressure ≥ atrial pressure, diastolic filling falls and stroke volume and CO decline; atrial naturetic peptide release is reflexly inhibited, decreasing urinary Na^{++} excretion

Sx: Dyspnea and/or "air hunger"; pts may also report chest pain, weakness, fatigue, anorexia

Si: JVD (100% of pts), tachypnea (80%), tachycardia (77%), hypotension (64%), diminished heart sounds (34%), pericardial rub (29%), rapid decline in BP (25%) (Circ 1981;64:633)

Pulsus paradoxicus should be suspected if systolic BP decreases by 15 mm Hg during inspiration. It can be difficult to detect in the presence of Afib, hypotension, or pericardial adhesions. It is absent in pts with ASD, severe aortic regurgitation, or pulmonary HT.

Crs: Fatal if not treated

Cmplc: Risk of life-threatening complications from pericardiocentesis < 5%

Lab: *EKG:* May show ST elevations of pericarditis, decreased QRS voltages, nonspecific T-wave flattening, electrical alternans (regular variation in R-wave amplitude) due to swinging of heart

Echocardiogram: Shows pericardial effusion, thrombus, fibrin strands or tumor in pericardial space; localization of fluid distribution; and loculation. RA or RV collapse in diastole is a marker for elevated intrapericardial pressures and tamponade physiology. In 25% of pts, LA may also collapse.

X-ray: CXR: Normal or enlarged cardiac silhouette

Rx: Pts with echocardiographic findings and no JVD, tachycardia, or pulsus paradoxicus require careful monitoring and observation. Those with hypotension and/or suspected cardiac perforation/rupture require immediate pericardiocentesis or surgery.

β-blockers and slowing Ca^{++}-channel blockers are contraindicated in suspected tamponade because reflex tachycardia is an important compensatory mechanism in the face of falling CO.

Pericardiocentesis provides a dx in 29% of cases, pericardial biopsy in 54% (Am J Cardiol 1985;56:623).

Pericardiocentesis with catheter drainage should be guided by echocardiogram (Mayo Clin Proc 1998;73:647). Right heart catheterization should document elevation of right-sided pressures and their improvement with drainage. Pericardiocentesis with extended catheter drainage is safe and effective for pts with malignant pericardial effusion (Mayo Clin Proc 2000;75:248).

Pericardiocentesis is often complicated or ineffective in pts with effusion < 200 mL, traumatic hemopericardium, or purely posterior or loculated effusion, or in pts with fibrin/clot in the pericardial space.

Pericardiectomy or balloon pericardiotomy may be needed for recurrent pericardial effusion and tamponade or for pts with suspected purulent or tuberculous pericarditis.

Mechanical ventilation with positive airway pressure should be avoided in tamponade because of the potential for reduction in cardiac output.

10.4 Myocarditis

Nejm 2000;343:1388; Nejm 1994;330:1129

Cause: Inflammation produced by infectious agent (see Table 10.1), either through direct infection, effect of myocardial toxin, or

Table 10.1 Infectious Agents Associated with Myocarditis

Type	Example
Bacterial	Streptococcus
	Staphylococcus
	Pneumococcus
	Meningococcus
	Hemophylis
	Gonococcus
	Brucellosis
	Diphtheria
	Salmonella
	Tuberculosis
	Tularemia
Spirochetal	Syphilis
	Leptospirosis (Weil disease)
	Lyme disease
Fungal	Aspergillosis
	Actinomycosis
	Blastomycosis
	Candidiasis
	Coccidiodomycosis
	Cryptococcus
	Histoplasmosis
Parasitic	Schistosomiasis
	Toxoplasmosis
	Trichiosis
	Trypanosomiasis (Chagas's disease)
Rickettsial	Rocky Mountain spotted fever
	Q fever
	Typhus
Viral	Coxsackie virus
	Cytomegalovirus
	Encephalomyocarditis virus
	Hepatitis
	HIV
	Infectious mononucleosis
	Influenza
	Mumps
	Mycoplasma pneumonia

continues

Table 10.1 continued

Type	Example
Viral	Poliomyelitis Psittacosis Respiratory syncytial virus Rabies Rubella Rubeola Varicella Yellow fever

immunologically mediated injury of myocardium. Idiopathic, familial, and postpartum forms have also been identified. Myocarditis accompanies cardiac allograft rejection. Collagen vascular disease, sarcoidosis, and drug allergy may be associated with giant cell myocarditis.

Epidem: In North America, viruses are the most likely causative agent. In South America, Chagas's disease is a common cause.

In a study of 952 asymptomatic HIV-positive pts followed 60 mon, the mean annual incidence rate of dilated cardiomyopathy (diagnosed by echocardiogram) was 15.9 cases/1000 pts; 83% of these pts had a histologic dx of myocarditis (Nejm 1998;339: 1093).

Pathophys: Myocardial contractility is impaired by cell-mediated injury or local release of cytokines. Myocardial involvement is typically patchy with random distribution of lesions.

Giant cell myocarditis is a rare, rapidly fatal disease of unknown cause affecting young or middle-aged adults.

Sx: Many pts may be asymptomatic. Symptomatic pts may note fatigue, dyspnea, palpitations, chest discomfort, or sx of overt CHF.

Si: Tachycardia, S_3 gallop, apical systolic murmur

Crs: The survival rate in a group of pts with a histopathological dx of myocarditis and LVEF < 0.45 was 20% at 1 yr and 56% at 4.3 yr (Nejm 1995;333:269).

Fulminant vs nonfulminant myocarditis: 93% of pts with fulminant myocarditis were alive without having received a heart transplant 11 yr after biopsy as compared with 45% of pts with acute myocarditis (Nejm 2000;342:690). Pts with fulminant myocarditis are sicker but have a better long-term prognosis if they survive the acute episode.

Cmplc: Pts with either symptomatic or asymptomatic myocarditis may develop dilated cardiomyopathy after a long latency period.

Lab: *EKG:* ST-T abnormalities, ventricular arrhythmias, AV and IV conduction abnormalities

Echocardiogram: Regional or global LV dysfunction, LV thrombi, impaired LV diastolic function. Pts with fulminant myocarditis have near-normal LV diastolic dimensions but increased septal thickness on echocardiogram, while pts with acute myocarditis have increased diastolic dimensions and normal septal thickness. At 6 mon, only pts with fulminant myocarditis had improvement in fractional shortening (J Am Coll Cardiol 2000;36:227).

X-ray: CXR may show normal or enlarged heart. Frank pulmonary edema is seen in fulminant cases.

Rx: Limitation of physical activity is recommended.

CHF is treated with routine management. Pts with myocarditis may have increased sensitivity to digitalis.

Heart block and arrhythmias may be transient but can be the cause of sudden death.

Rx of myocarditis with cyclosporine or azathioprine did not improve LV function or survival; ventricular function improved regardless of whether pts received immunosuppressive rx (Nejm 1995;333:269).

In a group of pts with giant cell myocarditis, median survival was 5.5 mon from the onset of sx. Pts treated with corticosteroids and cyclosporine, azathioprine, or both survived for an average of 12.3 mon. When 34 pts underwent heart transplantation, 9 (26%) had giant cell infiltrate in the transplanted heart (Nejm 1997;336:1860).

10.5 Cardiac Tumors

Nejm 1995;333:1610

Cause: Myxomas originate in primitive subendocardial mesenchymal cells through benign neoplasia. Fibroelastomas may develop secondary to endocardial trauma (Am Hrt J 1975;89:4). 25% of cardiac tumors are malignant.

Epidem: The incidence of cardiac tumors found at autopsy is 0.017-0.28% (Am J Cardiol 1996;77:107). Myxomas are particularly frequent between 3rd and 6th decades of life. They account for 30-50% of benign tumors in adults, lipomas 20%, and papillary fibroelastoma 15%. Angiosarcomas account for 33% of malignant tumors in adults, rhabdomyosarcomas 21%, mesotheliomas 16%, and fibrosarcomas 11%.

Approximately 10% of pts with myxomas have an autosomal dominant pattern of familial myxomas.

Angiosarcomas are twice as common in men as in women.

Pathophys: 6-8% of myxomas in ventricles, 75% in LA, 15-20% in RA. Most arise from the intra-atrial septum at the border of the fossa ovalis.

Constitutional sx are likely due to tumor production of interleukin-6 (J Thorac Cardiovasc Surg 1992;103:599).

Sx: DOE (> 75% of pts), fever (50%), PND (25%), weight loss (25%), dizziness/syncope (20%), hemoptysis (15%), sudden death (15%); cachexia, malaise. Sx may occur with a change in body position.

Si: Mitral murmur (75% of pts), pulmonary HT (70%), right-sided CHF (70%), tumor plop (early diastolic sound that may be mistaken for S_3 gallop; 33%), Afib (15%), Raynaud's phenomenon (< 5%) (Cardiovasc Rev Rep 1983;9:1195); widely split S_1 due to late closure of mitral valve, S_4 gallop

A left atrial myxoma may mimic rheumatic valvular disease, pulmonary HT, COPD, endocarditis, myocarditis, vasculitis, or CVA. A right atrial myxoma can be confused with findings of Epstein's anomaly, ASD, pulmonary embolus, pericarditis, carcinoid heart disease, or cardiomyopathy.

Crs: Myxomas recur in 1-5% of pts (Thorac Cardiovasc Surg 1989;37:226). Life expectancy after discovery of a malignant cardiac tumor is typically 1-24 mon. 75% of pts with malignant cardiac sarcomas have metastatic disease at time of death.

Cmplc: Embolism occurs in 30-40% of pts with myxomas. Involvement of cerebral and retinal arteries occurs in a majority of cases.

Lab: 33% of pts with myxomas will have anemia or elevated ESR; 10% will have hypergammaglobulinemia.

Arrhythmias on EKG are common. Angiomas and mesotheliomas are associated with development of heart block.

Echocardiography and TEE are the primary means for dx of cardiac tumors.

X-ray: MRI gives the best images of cardiac tumor anatomy. Coronary arteriography is recommended in pts > 40 yr to rule out concomitant CAD.

Rx: Operative excision is the rx of choice for benign tumors. The major operative risk is embolization.

Surgery is generally not effective for malignant tumors. Partial resection, chemotherapy, and radiation may provide palliation.

Chapter 11

Hypertension

11.1 Systemic Hypertension in Adults

Circ 2004;109:2953,3081; HT 2003;42:1206; Lancet 2003;362:1527; NIH Publications 03-5233, 98-4080

Cause: 15-18% of adults in the U.S. are hypertensive. Essential HT represents 90-94% of all cases seen. Other causes include chronic renal disease (chronic nephritis, polycystic kidney disease, diabetic nephropathy, hydronephrosis), renovascular disease, coarctation of aorta, Cushing's syndrome, primary aldosteronism, pheochromocytoma, acromegaly, hyperthyroidism, hyperparathyroidism, cardinoid syndrome, increased intracranial pressure of any cause, acute porphyria, lead poisoning, Guillain-Barré syndrome, use of oral contraceptives, NSAIDs, ETOH, cocaine, PCP, steroids, cyclosporine, tacrolimus, erythropoietin, and licorice (also found in some chewing tobacco and ephedra; Lancet 2003;361:1629).

A study of 297 hypertensive pts undergoing angiography found 19.2% incidence of renal artery stenosis > 50%; 7% had stenosis > 70%, and 3.7% had bilateral renal artery stenosis (Mayo Clin Proc 2002;77:309).

Epidem: HT is reported to be 2-3 times more common in women taking oral contraceptives, especially in obese and older women, than in those not taking oral contraceptives. Postmenopausal estrogen replacement is not associated with a significant increase in BP.

Among Americans ≥ age 60, elevated BP is found in 60% of non-Hispanic whites, 71% of non-Hispanic African Americans, and 61% of Mexican Americans.

HT is associated with obesity, sleep apnea, physical inactivity, cigarette smoking, ETOH (> 3 oz spirits/d), polycythemia, and hyperuricemia.

Sleep-disordered breathing may be a risk factor for HT in the general population (Nejm 2000;342:1378).

Pathophys: The mechanisms of essential HT are unknown.

Sx: Uncomplicated HT is usually asymptomatic. Sx frequently attributed to HT (headache, facial flushing, tinnitus, lightheadedness) are equally prevalent in the normotensive population.

Si: Possible physical exam findings: hypertensive retinopathy (arteriolar narrowing, focal arteriolar constrictions, arteriovenous crossing changes, hemorrhages and exudates, disc edema); carotid bruits, distended veins, irregular or rapid heartbeat, cardiomegaly, precordial heave, clicks, murmurs, S_3, S_4; rales; abdominal bruits, abnormal aortic pulsation; diminished/absent peripheral arterial pulsations, bruits, edema. Headache, palpitations, pallor, and perspiration suggest pheochromocytoma. Delayed/absent femoral arterial pulses and decreased BP in lower extremities suggest aortic coarctation. Truncal obesity with purple striae is seen in Cushing's syndrome.

Crs: Individuals normotensive at age 55 have a 90% lifetime risk for development of HT. BP of 130-139/85-89 is associated with increased risk of CVD (Nejm 2001;345:1291) and may progress to stage 1 HT over the next 4 yr (Lancet 2001;358:1682). In the Framingham Heart Study, all-cause mortality was lower among men with long-term rx of HT (31% vs 43%), and CVD mortality was less than half (13% vs 28%). Among treated women, all-cause mortality was 21% vs 34%, and CVD mortality was 9% vs 19% (Circ 1996;93:697). Rx of HT is associated with reduction in stroke incidence of 35-40%, MI 20-25%, and CHF > 50%.

Pts with adequate BP control on captopril, HCTZ, and atenolol showed reduction of LV mass after 1 yr; pts on diltiazem, clonidine, or prazosin did not (Circ 1997;95:2007). In a meta-analysis, ACEIs were more potent than β-blockers and diuretics in the reduction of LV mass index (Jama 1996;275:1507).

Cmplc: The risk of CVD doubles with each increment of 20/10 mm Hg beginning with a BP of 115/75. 50% of pts with untreated HT die of ASHD/CHF, 33% die of CVA, and 10-15% die of renal failure. HT is the major cause of LV failure in the U.S. (Framingham Heart Study).

Lab: For all pts: EKG, serum glucose, electrolytes, Ca^{++}, creatinine, CBC, UA; consider thyroid function studies, especially in elderly; lipid profile for risk stratification

If pt age, hx, severity of HT, or initial labs suggest secondary HT, or if BP is unresponsive to rx or begins to increase, or if the onset of HT is sudden, test for pheochromocytoma (24-hr urine for total catecholamines or metanephrine/vanillylmandelic acid) or mineralocorticoid abnormalities (plasma renin activity, plasma aldosterone, urine aldosterone and Na^{+}); for latter, pt must be on a high-salt diet in the absence of β- and Ca^{++}-channel blockers, ACEIs, or thiazide diuretics; control BP with clonidine or α-blockers

The metanephrine/creatinine ratio is a sensitive and specific test for pheochromocytoma, but acute events may increase urinary metanephrine excretion (Ann IM 1996;125:300).

X-ray: CXR if cardiac disease suspected; captropril renal scan, renal duplex US if likelihood of renovascular HT is moderate (abdominal bruit, age < 20 yr, HT refractory to standard rx, pt with occlusive vascular disease); renal arteriography for pts with high likelihood (malignant HT, Grade 4 HT with progressive renal insufficiency)

Rx: JNC-7 classifies BP as normal or ideal, prehypertensive or non-ideal, stage 1, stage 2 (Table 11.1)

Table 11.1 Classification and Management of Blood Pressure for Adults[1]

				Initial Drug Therapy	
BP Classification	**SBP[1] (mm Hg)**	**DBP[1] (mm Hg)**	**Lifestyle Modification**	**Without Compelling Indication**	**With Compelling Indications**
Normal	< 120	and < 80	Encourage		
Prehypertension	120-139	or 80-89	Yes	No antihypertensive drug indicated.	Drug(s) for compelling indications.[3]
Stage 1 hypertension	140-159	or 90-99	Yes	Thiazide-type diuretics for most. May consider ACEI, ARB, β-blocker, Ca^{++}-channel blocker, or combination.	Drug(s) for compelling indications.[3] Other antihypertensive drugs (diuretics, ACEI, ARB, β-blocker, Ca^{++}-channel blocker) as needed.
Stage 2 hypertension	≥ 160	or ≥ 100	Yes	Two-drug combination for most[2] (usually thiazide-type diuretic and ACEI or ARB or β-blocker, or Ca^{++}-channel blocker).	

1. Treatment determined by highest BP category.
2. Initial combined therapy should be used cautiously in those at risk for orthostatic hypotension.
3. Treat patients with chronic kidney disease or diabetes to BP goal of < 130/80 mm Hg.
(JNC-7)

Initial BP follow-up recommendations (JNC-6): < 130 mm Hg systolic or < 85 mm Hg diastolic, recheck in 2 yr; if 130-139 or 85-89, recheck 1 yr; 140-159 or 90-99, confirm within 2 mon; 160-179 or 100-109, evaluate or refer to source of care within 1 mon; > 180 or > 110, evaluate or refer to source of care immediately or within 1 wk, depending on clinical situation

Diet: Avoid high intake of NaCl; increase intake of fruits, vegetables, and fat-free and low-fat dairy products (Nejm 1997;336:1117; 2001;344:3). For the general population, AHA recommends average daily consumption of NaCl by adults < 6 gm (Circ 1998;98:613). However, in 58 trials of hypertensive persons, the effect of reduced Na^+ intake on SBP was 3.9 mm Hg and on DBP was 1.9 mm Hg (Jama 1998;279:1383). In prevention trials, change in BP was more convincingly related to change in weight than to change in dietary salt.

Other lifestyle measures: Lose weight if overweight; limit alcohol intake to 1 oz qd, 0.5 oz ETOH qd for women and lighter-weight people; increase aerobic physical activity; reduce Na^+ intake to 2.4 g Na^+/6 gm NaCl qd; maintain adequate intake K^+, Ca^{++}, Mg^+; stop smoking.

Table 11.2 Lifestyle Modifications to Manage Hypertension

Modification	Recommendation	Approximate SBP Reduction (Range)
Weight reduction	Maintain normal body weight (body mass index 18.5-24.9 kg/m^2).	5-20 mm Hg/10 kg weight loss
Adopt DASH eating plan	Consume a diet rich in fruits, vegetables, and low-fat dairy products with a reduced content of saturated and total fat.	8-14 mm Hg
Dietary sodium reduction	Reduce dietary sodium intake to no more than 100 mmol per day (2.4 gm sodium or 6 gm sodium chloride).	2-8 mm Hg
Physical activity	Engage in regular aerobic physical activity such as brisk walking (at least 30 min per day, most days of the week).	4-9 mm Hg
Moderation of alcohol consumption	Limit consumption to no more than 2 drinks (1 oz or 30 mL ethanol; eg, 24 oz beer, 10 oz wine, or 3 oz 80-proof whiskey) per day in most men and to no more than 1 drink per day in women and lighter-weight persons.	2-4 mm Hg

DASH, Dietary Approaches to Stop Hypertension.
For overall cardiovascular risk reduction, stop smoking.
The effects of implementing these modifications are dose and time dependent, and could be greater for some individuals.
(JNC-7)

Review of trials (16,164 pts ≥ 60 yr): Diuretic rx is effective in preventing CVA/TIA, CAD, cardiovascular, and all-cause mortality. β-blockers in these studies reduced the odds for CVA/TIA but did not prevent CAD or reduce cardiovascular and all-cause mortality (Jama 1998;279:1903).

Thiazide diuretics are effective initial rx in most pts. The primary focus is attaining the systolic BP goal. The diastolic BP goal is usually reached once systolic BP is controlled. In older pts with systolic HT, chlorthalidone is protective against CHF; in pts with prior MI, the risk is reduced 80% (Jama 1997;278:212). Rx of systolic HT in pts > age 60 is most effective in those at high risk for CAD (Circ 2001;104:1923).

ARBs are recommended for pts with type II diabetes. ACEIs are preferred as initial rx in hypertensive pts with type I diabetes; they are more effective than other antihypertensive agents in reducing the development of end-stage nondiabetic renal disease (Arch IM 2004;164:1850).

Use of nondihydropyridine Ca^{++}-channel blockers may reduce reinfarction in pts with ASHD but mortality is not reduced. Long-acting formulas may decrease strokes and arrhythmias in hypertensive pts and decrease CHF in pts with dilated, but not ischemic, cardiomyopathy. Short-acting agents (primarily those that increase HR) may increase CAD events in hypertensive pts (J Am Coll Cardiol 1997;29:1414). In a study of 3539 pts with HT, no differences in mortality were found among subjects using a Ca^{++}-channel antagonist compared with those who were not (Arch IM 1998;158:1882).

There is no increase in risk of serious hypoglycemia with any class of antihypertensive agents in elderly pts who require insulin or sulfonylureas (Jama 1997;278:40).

The BP goal for pts with renal insufficiency and > 1 gm per day is 125/75 mm Hg. For those with less proteinuria, the goal is 130/80 mm Hg.

In acute CVA, BP of 106/100 is appropriate. BP rx with ACEIs plus thiazide diuretics reduces the recurrent CVA rate (Lancet 2001;358:1033).

Orthostatic hypotension occurs in > 50% of elderly nursing home residents; it has a relationship with elevated BP, but not antihypertensive medication (Jama 1997;277:1299). Midodrine 10 mg po tid improved standing systolic BP and reported sx in pts with neurogenic orthostatic hypotension; the main adverse effects were urinary retention and supine HT (Jama 1997;277:1046).

In pts with HT and renal artery stenosis, angioplasty was reported to offer little advantage over antihypertensive drug rx (Nejm 2000;342:1007).

Medical management of aldosterone-producing adenomas is a viable option for controlling BP and serum K^+ concentration (Ann IM 1999;131:105).

Sublingual absorption of nifedipine is poor, and most of the drug is absorbed by the intestinal mucosa. Because of the serious adverse effects (cerebrovascular ischemia, CVA, severe hypotension, acute MI, conduction disturbances, fetal distress, death) reported, use of nifedipine capsules for hypertensive emergencies should be abandoned (Jama 1996;276:1328).

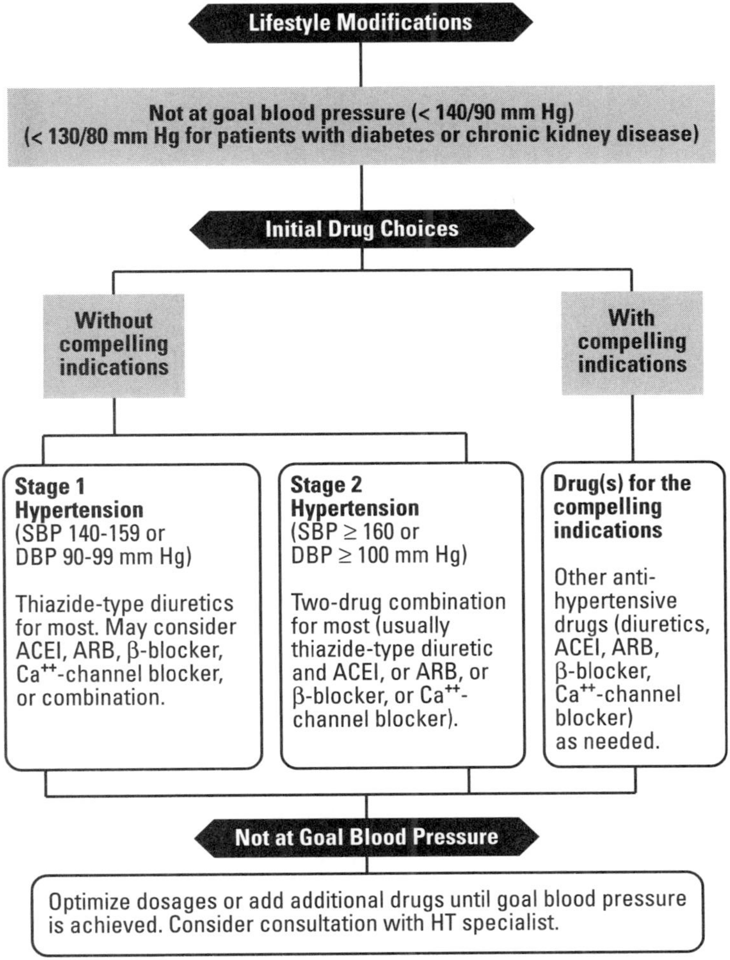

Figure 11.1 Algorithm for rx of hypertension. (JNC-7)

Table 11.3 Compelling Indications for Individual Drug Classes

	Recommended Drugs						
Compelling Indication[1]	**Diuretic**	**β-Blocker**	**ACEI**	**ARB**	**Ca^{++}-Channel Blocker**	**Aldo ANT[2]**	**Clinical Trial Basis[3]**
Heart failure	•	•	•	•		•	ACC/AHA Heart Failure Guideline, MERIT-HF, COPERNICUS, CIBIS, SOLVD, AIRE, TRACE, ValHEFT, RALES
Postmyocardial infarction		•	•			•	ACC/AHA Post-MI Guideline, BHAT, SAVE, Capricorn, EPHESUS
High coronary disease risk	•	•	•		•		ALLHAT, HOPE, $ANBP_2$, LIFE, CONVINCE
Diabetes	•	•	•	•	•		NKF-ADA Guideline, UKPDS, ALLHAT
Chronic kidney disease			•	•			NKF Guideline, Captopril Trial, RENAAL, IDNT, REIN, AASK
Recurrent stroke prevention	•		•				PROGRESS

1. Compelling indications for antihypertensive drugs are based on benefits from outcome studies or existing clinical guidelines; the compelling indication is managed in parallel with the BP.
2. Aldo ANT = aldosterone antagonist.
3. Conditions for which clinical trials demonstrate benefit of specific classes of antihypertensive drugs.
(JNC-7)

Table 11.4 Oral Antihypertensive Drugs[1]

Class	Drug (Trade Name)	Usual Dose Range, mg/day (Daily Frequency)
Thiazide diuretics	Chlorothiazide (Diuril)	125-500 (1)
	Chlorthalidone (generic)	12.5-25 (1)
	Hydrochlorothiazide (Microzide, HydroDIURIL[2])	12.5-50 (1)
	Polythiazide (Renese)	2-4 (1)
	Indapamide (Lozol[2])	1.25-2.5 (1)
	Metolazone (Mykrox)	0.5-1.0 (1)
	Metolazone (Zaroxolyn)	2.5-5 (1)
Loop diuretics	Bumetanide (Bumex[2])	0.5-2 (2)
	Furosemide (Lasix[2])	20-80 (2)
	Torsemide (Demadex[2])	2.5-10 (1)
Potassium-sparing diuretics	Amiloride (Midamor[2])	5-10 (1-2)
	Triamterene (Dyrenium)	50-100 (1-2)
Aldosterone receptor blockers	Eplerenone (Inspra)	50-100 (1-2)
	Spironolactone (Aldactone[2])	25-50 (1-2)
β-Blockers	Atenolol (Tenormin[2])	25-100 (1)
	Betaxolol (Kerlone[2])	5-20 (1)
	Bisoprolol (Zebeta[2])	2.5-10 (1)
	Metoprolol (Lopressor[2])	50-100 (1-2)
	Metoprolol extended release (Toprol XL)	50-100 (1)
	Nadolol (Corgard[2])	40-120 (1)
	Propranolol (Inderal[2])	40-160 (2)
	Propranolol long-acting (Inderal LA[2])	60-180 (1)
	Timolol (Blocadren[2])	20-40 (2)
β-Blockers with intrinsic sympathomimetic activity	Acebutolol (Sectral[2])	200-800 (2)
	Penbutolol (Levatol)	10-40 (1)
	Pindolol (generic)	10-40 (2)
Combined α- and β-blockers	Carvedilol (Coreg)	12.5-50 (2)
	Labetalol (Normodyne, Trandate[2])	200-800 (2)
ACE inhibitors	Benazepril (Lotensin[2])	10-40 (1-2)
	Captopril (Capoten[2])	25-100 (2)
	Enalapril (Vasotec[2])	2.5-40 (1-2)
	Fosinopril (Monopril)	10-40 (1)

continues

HYPERTENSION

Table 11.4 continued

Class	Drug (Trade Name)	Usual Dose Range, mg/day (Daily Frequency)
	Lisinopril (Prinivil, Zestril[2])	10-40 (1)
	Moexipril (Univasc)	7.5-30 (1)
	Perindopril (Aceon)	4-8 (1-2)
	Quinapril (Accupril)	10-40 (1)
	Ramipril (Altace)	2.5-20 (1)
	Trandolapril (Mavik)	1-4 (1)
Angiotensin II antagonists	Candesartan (Atacand)	8-32 (1)
	Eprosartan (Tevetan)	400-800 (1-2)
	Irbesartan (Avapro)	150-300 (1)
	losartan (Cozaar)	25-100 (1-2)
	Olmesartan (Benicar)	20-40 (1)
	Telmisartan (Micardis)	20-80 (1)
	Valsartan (Diovan)	80-320 (1)
Ca^{++}-channel blockers: nondihydropyridines	Diltiazem extended release (Cardizem CD, Dilacor XR, Tiazac[2])	180-420 (1)
	Diltiazem extended release (Cardizem LA)	120-540 (1)
	Verapamil immediate release (Calan, Isoptin[2])	80-320 (2)
	Verapamil long acting (Calan SR, Isoptin SR[2])	120-360 (1-2)
	Verapamil—Coer (Covera HS, Verelan PM)	120-360 (1)
Ca^{++}-channel blockers: dihydropyridines	Amlodipine (Norvasc)	2.5-10 (1)
	Felodipine (Plendil)	2.5-20 (1)
	Isradipine (Dynacirc CR)	2.5-10 (2)
	Nicardipine sustained release (Cardene SR)	60-120 (2)
	Nifedipine long-acting (Adalat CC, Procardia XL)	30-60 (1)
	Nisoldipine (Sular)	10-40 (1)
α_1-Blockers	Doxazosin (Cardura)	1-16 (1)
	Prazosin (Minipress[2])	2-20 (2-3)
	Terazosin (Hytrin)	1-20 (1-2)

Table 11.4 continued

Class	Drug (Trade Name)	Usual Dose Range, mg/day (Daily Frequency)
Central α_2-agonists and other centrally acting drugs	Clonidine (Catapres[2])	0.1-0.8 (2)
	Clonidine patch (Catapres-TTS)	0.1-0.3 (1 wkly)
	Methyldopa (Aldomet[2])	250-1000 (2)
	Reserpine (Generic)	0.05[3]-0.25 (1)
	Guanfacine (generic)	0.5-2 (1)
Direct vasodilators	Hydralazine (Apresoline[2])	25-100 (2)
	Minoxidil (Loniten[2])	2.5-80 (1-2)

1. These dosages may vary from those listed in the *Physicians' Desk Reference.*
2. Are now or will soon become available in generic preparations.
3. A 0.1 mg dose may be given every other day to achieve this dosage.
(JNC-7)

Table 11.5 Antihypertensive Combination Medications

Combination Type	Fixed-Dose Combination (mg)[1]	Trade Name
ACEI and Ca^{++}-channel blocker	Amlodipine/benazepril hydrochloride (2.5/10, 5/10, 5/20, 10/20)	Lotrel
	Enalapril maleate/felodipine (5/5)	Lexxel
	Trandolapril/verapamil (2/180, 1/240, 2/240, 4/240)	Tarka
ACEI and diuretic	Benazepril/hydrochlorothiazide (5/6.25, 10/12.5, 20/12.5, 20/25)	Lotensin HCT
	Captopril/hydrochlorothiazide (25/15, 25/25, 50/15, 50/25)	Capozide
	Enalapril maleate/hydrochlorothiazide (5/12.5, 10/25)	Vaseretic
	Lisinopril/hydrochlorothiazide (10/12.5, 20/12.5, 20/25)	Prinzide
	Moexipril HCl/hydrochlorothiazide (7.5/12.5, 15/25)	Uniretic
	Quinapril HCl/hydrochlorothiazide (10/12.5, 20/12.5, 20/25)	Accuretic

continues

Table 11.5 continued

Combination Type	Fixed-Dose Combination (mg)[1]	Trade Name
ARB and diuretic	Candesartan cilexetil/hydrochlorothiazide (16/12.5, 32/12.5)	Atacand HCT
	Eprosartan mesylate/hydrochlorothiazide (600/12.5, 600/25)	Teveten/HCT
	Irbesartan/hydrochlorothiazide (150/12.5, 300/12.5)	Avalide
	Losartan potassium/hydrochlorothiazide (50/12.5, 100/25)	Hyzaar
	Telmisartan/hydrochlorothiazide (40/12.5, 80/12.5)	Micardis/HCT
	Valsartan/hydrochlorothiazide (80/12.5, 160/12.5)	Diovan/HCT
β-Blocker and diuretic	Atenolol/chlorthalidone (50/25, 100/25)	Tenoretic
	Bisoprolol fumarate/hydrochlorothiazide (2.5/6.25, 5/6.25, 10/6.25)	Ziac
	Propranolol LA/hydrochlorothiazide (40/25, 80/25)	Inderide
	Metoprolol tartrate/hydrochlorothiazide (50/25, 100/25)	Lopressor HCT
	Nadolol/bendrofluthiazide (40/5, 80/5)	Corzide
	Timolol maleate/hydrochlorothiazide (10/25)	Timolide
Centrally acting drug and diuretic	Methyldopa/hydrochlorothiazide (250/15, 250/25, 500/30, 500/50)	Aldoril
	Reserpine /chlorothiazide (0.125/250, 0.25/500)	Diupres
	Reserpine/hydrochlorothiazide (0.125/25, 0.125/50)	Hydropres
Diuretic and diuretic	Amiloride HCl/hydrochlorothiazide (5/50)	Moduretic
	Spironolactone/hydrochlorothiazide (25/25, 50/50)	Aldactone
	Triamterene/hydrochlorothiazide (37.5/25, 50/25, 75/50)	Dyazide, Maxzide

1. Some drug combinations are available in multiple fixed doses.
(JNC-7)

Table 11.6 Individualizing Antihypertensive Rx

Indication	Drug Rx
Compelling Indications Unless Contraindicated	
Diabetes mellitus (type I) with proteinuria	ACEI
Heart failure	ACEI, diuretics
Isolated systolic HT (older patients)	Diuretics (preferred), calcium antagonist (long-acting dihydropyridine)
Myocardial infarction	β-Blockers (non-intrinsic sympathomimetic activity), ACEI (with systolic dysfunction)
May Have Favorable Effects on Comorbid Conditions	
Angina	β-Blockers, calcium antagonist
Atrial tachycardia and fibrillation	β-Blockers, calcium antagonist, (nondihydropyridine)
Cyclosporine-induced HT (caution with the dose of cyclosporine)	Calcium antagonist
Diabetes mellitus (types I and II) with proteinuria	ACEI (preferred), calcium antagonist
Diabetes mellitus (type II)	Low-dose diuretics
Dyslipidemia	α-Blockers
Essential tremor	β-blockers noncardioselective
Heart failure	Carvedilol, losartan potassium
Hyperthyroidism	β-Blockers
Migraine	β-Blockers (noncardioselective), calcium antagonist (nondihydropyridine)
Myocardial infarction	Diltiazem hydrochloride, verapamil hydrochloride
Osteoporosis	Thiazides
Preoperative HT	β-Blockers
Prostatism (BPH)	α-Blockers
Renal insufficiency (caution in renovascular HT and creatinine ≥ 265.2 μmol/L [3 mg/dL])	ACEI

continues

HYPERTENSION

Table 11.6 continued

Indication	Drug Rx
May Have Unfavorable Effects on Comorbid Conditions[1]	
Bronchospastic disease	β-Blockers[2]
Depression	β-Blockers, central alpha-agonists, reserpine[2]
Diabetes mellitus (types I and II)	β-Blockers, high-dose diuretics
Dyslipidemia	β-Blockers (non-intrinsic sympathomimetic activity), diuretics (high-dose)
Gout	Diuretics
2° or 3° heart block	β-Blockers[2], calcium antagonist (nondihydropyridine)[2]
Heart failure	β-Blockers (except carvedilol), calcium antagonist (except amlodipine besylate, felodipine)
Liver disease	Labetalol hydrochloride, methyldopa[2]
Peripheral vascular disease	β-blockers
Pregnancy	ACEI,[2] angiotensin II receptor blockers[2]
Renal insufficiency	Potassium-sparing agents
Renovascular disease	ACEI, angiotensin II receptor blockers

1. These drugs may be used with special monitoring unless contraindicated.
2. Contraindicated.
(JNC-6)

Table 11.7 Emergency Iv Rx of Hypertensive Crisis[1]

Drug	Dose	Onset of Action	Duration of Action	Adverse Effects[2]	Special Indications
Vasodilators					
Sodium nitroprusside	0.25-10 μgm/kg per min as iv infusion[3] (maximal dose for 10 min only)	Immediate	1-2 min	Nausea, vomiting, muscle twitching, sweating, thiocyanate and cyanide intoxication	Most hypertensive emergencies; caution with high intracranial pressure or azotemia
Nicardipine hydrochloride	5-15 mg/hr iv	5-10 min	1-4 hr	Tachycardia, headache, flushing, local phlebitis	Most hypertensive emergencies except acute heart failure; caution with coronary ischemia
Fenoldopam mesylate	0.1-0.3 μgm/kg per min iv infusion	< 5 min	30 min	Tachycardia, headache, nausea, flushing	Most hypertensive emergencies; caution with glaucoma
Nitroglycerin	5-100 μgm/min as iv infusion[3]	2-5 min	3-5 min	Headache, vomiting, methemoglobinemia, tolerance with prolonged use	Coronary ischemia
Enalaprilat	1.25-5 mg every 6 hr iv	15-30 min	6 hr	Precipitous fall in pressure in high-renin states; response variable	Acute left ventricular failure; avoid in acute myocardial infarction

continues

Table 11.7 continued

Drug	Dose	Onset of Action	Duration of Action	Adverse Effects[2]	Special Indications
Hydralazine hydrochloride	10-20 mg iv 10-50 mg im	10-20 min 20-30 min	3-8 hr	Tachycardia, flushing, headache, vomiting, aggravation of angina	Eclampsia
Diazoxide	50-100 mg iv bolus repeated, or 15-30 mg/min infusion	2-4 min	6-12 hr	Nausea, flushing, tachycardia, chest pain	Now obsolete; when no intensive monitoring available
Adrenergic Inhibitors					
Labetalol hydrochloride	20-80 mg iv bolus every 10 min 0.5/2.0 mg/min iv infusion	5-10 min	3-6 hr	Vomiting, scalp tingling, burning in throat, dizziness, nausea, heart block, orthostatic hypotension	Most hypertensive emergencies except acute heart failure
Esmolol hydrochloride	250-500 μgm/kg/min for 1 min, then 50-100 μgm/kg/min for 4 min; may repeat sequence	1-2 min	10-20 min	Hypotension, nausea	Aortic dissection, perioperative
Phentolamine	5-15 mg iv	1-2 min	3-10 min	Tachycardia, flushing, headache	Catecholamine excess

1. These doses may vary from those in the *Physicians' Desk Reference* (51st edition).
2. Hypotension may occur with all agents.
3. Require special delivery system.

Table 11.8 Antihypertensive Drug Interactions

Class of Agent	Increase Efficacy	Decrease Efficacy	Effect on Other Drugs
Diuretics	• Diuretics that act at different sites in the nephron (eg, furosemide + thiazides)	• Resin-binding agents • NSAIDs • Steroids	• Diuretics raise serum lithium levels • Potassium-sparing agents may exacerbate hyperkalemia due to ACEIs
β-Blockers	• Cimetidine (hepatically metabolized β-blockers) • Quinidine (hepatically metabolized β-blockers) • Food (hepatically metabolized β-blockers)	• NSAIDs • Withdrawal of clonidine • Agents that induce hepatic enzymes, including rifampin and phenobarbital	• Propranolol hydrochloride induces hepatic enzymes to increase clearance of drugs with similar metabolic pathways • β-blockers may mask and prolong insulin-induced hypoglycemia • Heart block may occur with nondihydropyridine calcium antagonists • Sympathomimetics cause unopposed α-adrenoceptor-mediated vasoconstriction • β-blockers increase angina-inducing potential of cocaine
ACE inhibitors	• Chlorpromazine or clozapine	• NSAIDs • Antacids • Food decreases absorption (moexipril)	• ACEIs may raise serum lithium levels • ACEIs may exacerbate hyperkalemic effect of potassium-sparing diuretics

continues

HYPERTENSION

Table 11.8 continued

Class of Agent	Increase Efficacy	Decrease Efficacy	Effect on Other Drugs
Calcium antagonists	• Grapefruit juice (some dihydropyridines) • Cimetidine or ranitidine (hepatically metabolized calcium antagonists)	• Agents that induce hepatic enzymes, including rifampin and phenobarbital	• Cyclosporine levels increase[1] with diltiazem hydrochloride, verapamil hydrochloride, mibefradil dihydrochloride, or nicardipine hydrochloride (but not felodipine, isradipine, or nifedipine) • Nondihydropyridines increase levels of other drugs metabolized by the same hepatic enzyme system, including digoxin, quinidine, sulfonylureas, and theophylline • Verapamil hydrochloride may lower serium lithium levels
α-Blockers			• Prazosin may decrease clearance of verapamil hydrochloride

Central α_2-agonists and peripheral neuronal blockers		• TCAs (and probably phenothiazines) • MAO inhibitors • Sympathomimetics or phenothiazines antagonize guanethidine monosulfate or guanadrel sulfate • Iron salts may reduce methyldopa absorption	• Methyldopa may increase serum lithium levels • Severity of clonidine hydrochloride withdrawal may be increased by β-blockers • Many agents used in anesthesia are potentiated by clonidine hydrochloride

1. This is a clinically and economically beneficial drug–drug interaction because it both retards progression of accelerated atherosclerosis in heart transplant recipients and reduces the required daily dose of cyclosporine.
(JNC-6)

Table 11.9 Antihypertensive Drugs Used in Pregnancy[1]

The report of the NHBPEP Working Group on High Blood Pressure in Pregnancy permits continuation of drug therapy in women with chronic HT (except for ACEIs). In addition, angiotensin II receptor blockers should not be used during pregnancy. In women with chronic HT with diastolic levels of 100 mm Hg or greater (lower when end-organ damage or underlying renal disease is present) and in women with acute HT when levels are 105 mm Hg or greater, the following agents are suggested.

Suggested Drug	Comments
Central α-agonists	Methyldopa (C) is the drug of choice recommended by the NHBPEP Working Group.
β-Blockers	Atenolol (C) and metoprolol (C) appear to be safe and effective in late pregnancy. Labetalol (C) also appears to be effective (α- and β-blockers).
Calcium antagonists	Potential synergism with magnesium sulfate may lead to precipitous hypotension. (C)
ACE inhibitors, angiotensin II receptor blockers	Fetal abnormalities, including death, can be caused, and these drugs should not be used in pregnancy. (D)
Diuretics	Diuretics (C) are recommended for chronic HT if prescribed before gestation or if patients appear to be salt sensitive. They are not recommended in preeclampsia.
Direct vasodilators	Hydralazine (C) is the parenteral drug of choice based on its long history of safety and efficacy. (C)

1. There are several other antihypertensive drugs for which there are very limited data. The U.S. FDA classifies pregnancy risk as follows: C, adverse effects in animals; no controlled trials in humans; use if risk appears justified; D, positive evidence of fetal risk.
(JNC-6)

11.2 Hypertension in Children

Nejm 1996;335:1968

Cause:

In neonates and young infants: Renal artery thrombosis after umbilical artery catheterization, coarctation of aorta, congenital renal disease, renal artery stenosis; less commonly, bronchopulmonary dysplasia, patent ductus arteriosus, intraventricular hemorrhage

Age 1-10: Renal disease, coarctation of the aorta; less commonly, renal artery stenosis, hypercalcemia, neurofibromatosis, neurogenic tumors, pheochromocytoma, mineralocorticoid excess, primary hyperaldosteronism, 11β-hydroxylase deficiency, 17α-hydroxylase deficiency, Liddle's syndrome, glucocorticoid-remediable aldosteronism, hyperthyroidism, transient HT after urologic surgery, HT induced by immobilization (traction), sleep apnea-associated HT

Adolescence: All of the above plus essential HT

Epidem: BP is slightly higher in boys than in girls during the first decade; the difference widens around puberty. A direct relation between weight and BP is present from age 5; it becomes more prominent in the second decade. Height is also independently related to BP at all ages. No significant differences in BP are observed among whites, blacks, Hispanics, and Southeast Asians until adolescence.

There is a significant correlation in BP and cardiovascular risk factors between parents and their children. A greater correlation in BP exists between mothers and their children than between fathers and their children.

Pathophys: HT in infants is usually related to renal or vascular disease. An underlying cause can be found in most children 1-10 yr old with HT (most common cause is renal disease).

Sx: In neonates and young infants: Failure to thrive, irritability, feeding problems, cyanosis, respiratory distress, cardiac failure, seizures; HT is frequently "silent" after infancy

Si: Blood pressures outside of established normal range (see Figures 11.2 and 11.3)

Crs: Limited data relating BP in childhood or adolescence to cardiovascular risk in adulthood

Cmplc: A significant correlation exits between BP and fasting insulin levels in grade-school children and adolescents. Higher insulin levels can be associated with Na^+ sensitivity and increased vascular reactivity.

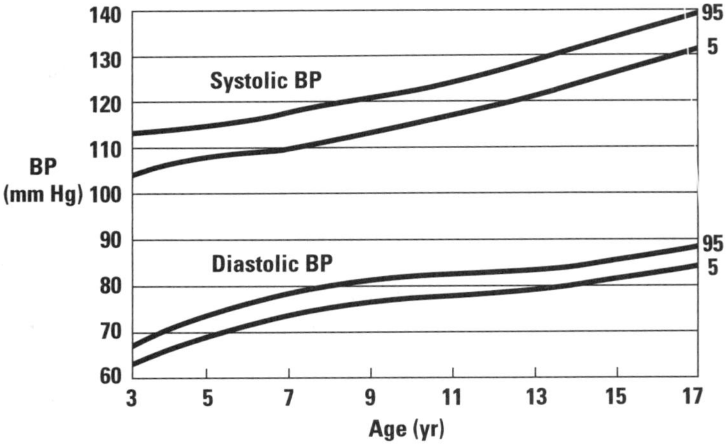

Figure 11.2 Normal blood pressure in boys. 95th percentile blood pressure standards for age, gender, and 5th and 95th percentiles for height. Data derived from CDC growth charts and NHANES 1999-2000.

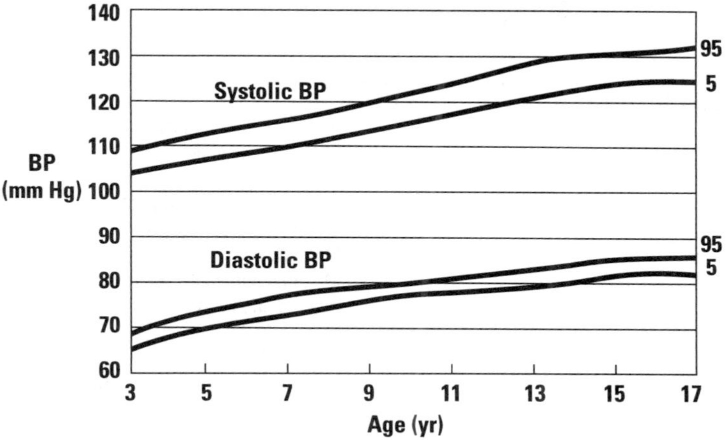

Figure 11.3 Normal blood pressure in girls. 95th percentile blood pressure standards for age, gender, and 5th and 95th percentiles for height. Data derived from CDC growth charts and NHANES 1999-2000.

HYPERTENSION

Lab: Initial evaluation: CBC, serum electrolytes, creatinine, BUN, nitrogen, calcium, uric acid, cholesterol, plasma renin activity, UA and culture; may also require echocardiography, urine collection for catecholamines, measurement of plasma and urinary steroids

X-ray: Renal ultrasonography; may also require isotopic renography with administration of captopril or renal arteriography

Rx: Conservative management recommended as initial rx for essential HT: diet, wt reduction, exercise. Sodium restriction is usually not feasible.

Table 11.10 Drug Rx for Hypertension in Children

Drug	Dosage
Long-Term RX	
Captopril	Initial dose: 1.5 mg/kg/day Maximum dose: 6 mg/kg/day
Enalapril	Initial dose: 0.15 mg/kg/day
Nifedipine (extended release)	Initial dose: 0.25 mg/kg/day Maximum dose: 3 mg/kg/day
Propranolol	Initial dose: 1 mg/kg/day Maximum dose: 8 mg/kg/day
Atenolol	Initial dose: 1 mg/kg/day Maximum dose: 8 mg/kg/day
Prazosin	Initial dose: 0.05-0.1 mg/kg/day Maximum dose: 0.5 mg/kg/day
Minoxidil	Initial dose: 0.1-0.2 mg/kg/day Maximum dose: 1 mg/kg/day
HCTZ	Initial dose: 1 mg/kg/day Maximum dose: 2-3 mg/kg/day
Furosemide	Initial dose: 1 mg/kg/day Maximum dose: 12 mg/kg/day
Bumetanide	Initial dose: 0.02-0.05 mg/kg/day Maximum dose: 0.3 mg/kg/day
Hypertensive emergencies	
Nitroprusside	Initial dose: 0.5 μgm/kg/min iv Maximum dose: 8 μgm/kg/min iv
Labetolol	Initial dose: 1 mg/kg/hr iv Maximum dose: 3 mg/kg/hr iv

(Nejm 1996;336:1968)

Chapter 12
Syncope

12.1 Syncope

Nejm 2005;352:1004; 2000;343:1856; Lancet 2001;357:348; Ann IM 1997;126:989; 1997;127:76

Cause: Neurocardiogenic syncope; orthostatic hypotension; decreased CO; neurologic disorders (uncommon)

Epidem: Framingham: The incidence of syncope is 6.2/1000 person-yr (Nejm 2002;347:878). 30% of pts with obstructive hypertrophic cardiomyopathy, 30% of pts with pulmonary HT, 10-15% of pts with acute pulmonary embolus, and 25-70% of pts with sick sinus syndrome have syncope. The overall prevalence of causes of syncope reported in different series is vasovagal, 8-37%; cough/micturation, 1-8%; orthostatic hypotension, 4-10%; medication side effect, 1-7%; neurologic causes, 3-32%; organic heart disease, 1-8%; arrhythmia, 4-38%; and unknown, 13-41%.

Pathophys: Neurocardiogenic syncope: Compensatory response to upright posture is replaced by a paradoxical decrease of sympathetic activity and an increase in parasympathetic (vagal) activity, producing vasodilatation and bradycardia. The hypothesized mechanism is excessive activation and/or hypersensitivity of cardiac mechanoreceptors.

Decreased cardiac output: Aortic, pulmonary, or mitral stenosis; obstructive hypertrophic cardiomyopathy; pulmonary embolus; atrial myxoma; arrhythmias; and tamponade can all produce impairment of cardiac flow and syncope.

Orthostatic hypotension may occur in Shy-Drager syndrome (primary autonomic failure), diabetes, amyloid, SLE, Guillain-Barré syndrome, porphyria, Fabry's disease, vitamin B_{12} deficiency, multiple sclerosis, and drugs (phenothizines, MAO inhibitors, TCAs, clonidine, hydralazine, prazosin, guanethidine, α-methyldopa, ACEIs).

Sx: Hx and physical exam identify possible cause of syncope in ~45% of pts (Ann IM 1997;126:989).

Si: Syncope occurring with use of an upper extremity raises the possibility of subclavian steal syndrome, as does a pulse pressure difference of > 20 mm Hg between arms. The occurrence of diplopia, dysarthria, or signs of brain stem ischemia suggest possible TIA or basilar artery migraine. Syncope with exertion is seen in AS, MS, pulmonary HT, HCM, and CAD.

Crs: Up to 45% of pts with severe aortic stenosis will develop syncope. Life expectancy after onset of syncope is 2-3 yr without valve replacement. The overall 1-yr mortality for pts with syncope of cardiac origin is 18-33%.

Framingham: Pts with syncope of unknown cause had increased rate of death from all causes.

Overall recurrence rate is 34% at 3 yr (Am J Med 1987;83:700).

Lab: See Figure 12.1.

EKG is rarely diagnostic by itself (< 5% of pts); it may document arrhythmias.

Holter monitoring: In one study, 4% of pts with syncope had arrhythmias and sx, 17% had sx but no arrhythmias, and the remaining 79% were asymptomatic but 13% had arrhythmias (Ann IM 1990;113:53). 48-hr monitoring does not increase the yield of symptomatic arrhythmias (Arch IM 1990;150:1073).

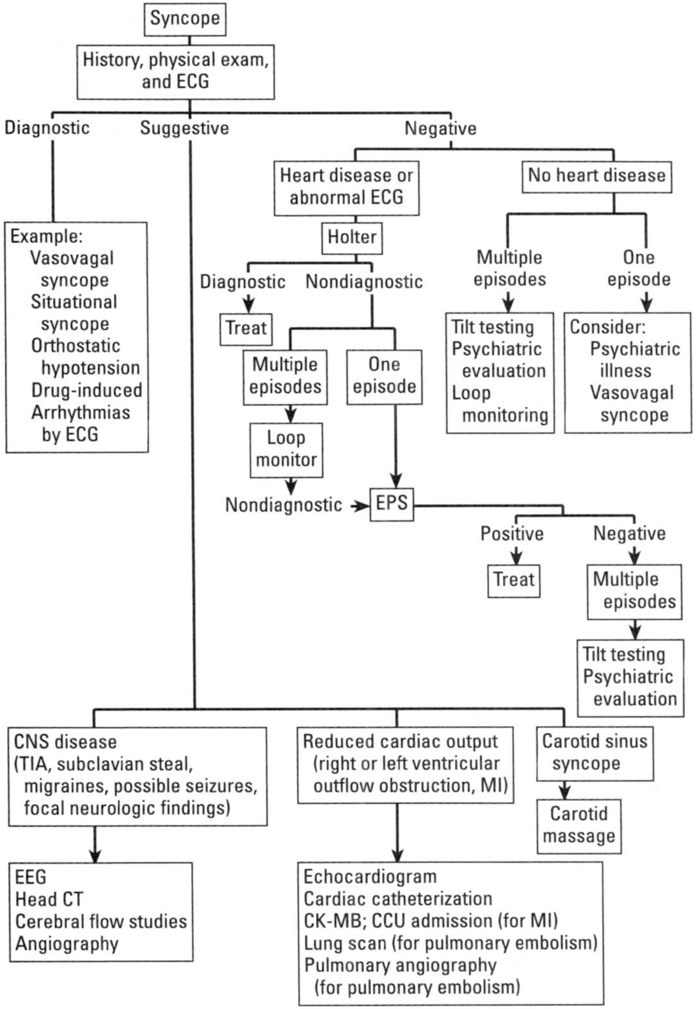

Figure 12.1 Evaluation of syncope. *Source:* Reprinted with permission, Syncope: diagnostic algorithm for, Goldman et al: Primary Cardiology, © 1998 Elsevier, Inc., p. 149.

Event (loop) monitoring: Symptomatic arrhythmias are found in 8-20% of pts; 12-27% have sx without associated arrhythmia (Am J Cardiol 1990;66:214).

EEG: ~1% of pts with syncope have EEG abnormalities of seizure disorder (Arch IM 1990;50:2027). EEG is not recommended for routine screening.

Echocardiogram: Useful if organic heart disease with obstruction to flow suspected

Exercise stress testing: Very low yield (< 1%) in identifying cause of syncope; primary value is identification of possible ischemia heart disease in pts with documented arrhythmias

Tilt-table test: For dx of vasovagal syncope. Fasting but nondehydrated pt is given a 20-45 min supine equilibration period, then tilted upright at 60-80° for 30-45 min with EKG and BP monitoring. The endpoint is hypotension or bradycardia with reproduction of sx. If negative, may place pt prone and infuse iv isoproterenol at 1-3 μgm/min until HR increases by 20% and repeat upright tilt (Nejm 2005;352:1004). The test is positive in 39-87% of pts and has a reported sensitivity of 67-83% and specificity of ~90% but with a range of 0-100% (Am J Med 1994;97:78).

Invasive electrophysiologic testing: Yield is ~50% in pts with structural heart disease or EKG abnormalities (prior MI, BBB, pre-excitation), 10% in those without (J Am Coll Cardiol 1999;34:1082).

X-ray: Head CT scan, angiography may be indicated in pts with suspected neurologic disease

Rx: Drug rx is reserved for pts with recurrent episodes of idiopathic vasovagal syncope. Reports of efficacy are mostly case series reports. Drugs used include β-blockers (metoprolol 50 mg po qd or bid), fludrocortisone (0.1-1 mg qd), fluoxetine (20-40 mg qd), scopolamine patch, theophylline (6-12 mg/kg/day), and midodrine 2.5-10 mg po tid (Circ 1999;100:1242).

Chapter 13

Pulmonary Vascular Disease

13.1 Pulmonary Embolus

Lancet 2004;363:1295; Circ 2003;108:2726,2834

Cause: Thrombi from deep veins of the legs, pelvis, or arms embolize to the pulmonary arteries, producing pulmonary arterial obstruction

Nurses' Health Study: Highest rates of PE seen in nurses > 60 yr old who were in highest quintile of body mass index; cigarette smoking, high BP also risk factors; hormone replacement rx doubles risk of venous thromboembolism and hence of PE; surgery increases risk of PE

Epidem: Up to 40% of pts with DVT will have evidence of PE on lung scan; 29% of pts with PE have abnormal scans of leg veins (Jama 1994;271:223; Ann IM 1997;12:775).

Among patients ≥ 50 yr old, incidence of PE was higher among women. Only a trivial difference in incidence was observed among African Americans compared to whites (Chest 1999;116:909).

Pathophys: Thrombi produce pulmonary arterial obstruction and hypoxic vasoconstriction. Release of vasoactive agents also increases pulmonary vascular resistance. An increase in alveolar dead space and redistribution of blood flow impair gas exchange. Reflex bronchoconstriction augments airway resistance. Edema decreases pulmonary compliance, and RV afterload increases. RV enlargement shifts intraventricular septum, impairing LV diastolic function.

If patent foramen ovale or ASD is present, paradoxical embolism and/or right to left shunting and further hypoxemia can occur.

Sx: Dyspnea is the most frequent sx. Pleuritic chest pain, cough, hemoptysis, syncope, and cyanosis may also occur. In data from a multicenter registry, sx were acute in 63% of pts.

The differential dx includes acute MI, CHF, dilated cardiomyopathy, pericarditis, pneumonia, asthma, primary pulmonary HT, pneumothorax, malignancy, rib fx, and costochondritis.

Si: JVD, parasternal lift, increased P_2, systolic murmur of TR at LLSB that increases in intensity during inspiration

Crs: The reported 3-mon mortality rate after PE is 13-17.5%. 30-day case fatality rates in Medicare pts with PE were 13.7% for men and 12.8% for women, 16.1% for blacks and 12.9% for whites (Nejm 1998;33:93).

Lab:

ABGs: Hypoxemia raises suspicion for PE, but ABGs alone are neither sensitive nor specific enough to confirm or disprove the dx by themselves.

EKG: Anterior T-wave inversion is most frequent abnormality. Occasionally new RBBB, $S_1Q_3T_3$ pattern, T-wave inversion in leads V1-V4, or Afib is observed.

Echocardiogram: RV hypokinesis is seen in ~ 40% of pts and is associated with a twofold increase in the 14-d mortality rate and a 1.5-fold increase at 3 mon (Circ 1997;96:I-159). Normotensive pts with acute PE who present with RV dysfunction have a 10% rate of PE-related shock and 5% in-hospital mortality, while normotensive pts without echocardiographic RV dysfunction have a benign short-term prognosis (Circ 2000;101:2817). Other nonspecific echo signs include RV dilation, abnormal septal motion, dilated PA, tricuspid regurgitation, and decreased/absent collapse of IVC during inspiration. Echo may be useful in excluding other conditions, such as acute MI or pericardial tamponade.

In a study of 1177 pts with suspected PE, a D-dimer assay had a sensitivity of 85%, but a specificity of 69%; this suggests that a negative test is useful in excluding PE in pts with a low pretest probability of this condition (Mayo Clin Proc 2004;79:164; J Am Coll Cardiol 2002;40:1475; Ann EM 2002;39:144). Levels of D-dimer are elevated in acute MI, pneumonia, CHF, malignancy, and after surgery. The latex agglutination test is less sensitive than immunosorbent assay.

X-ray: CXR may show enlarged pulmonary arteries with pulmonary HT. Lung scan: In the PIOPED study, 933 pts were studied prospectively. Few had negative lung scans; 88% of pts with high-probability scans, 33% of pts with intermediate-probability scans, and 12% of pts with low-probability scans had PE by angiogram, but a minority of the pts with PE by angiogram had high-probability scans (sensitivity, 41%; specificity, 97%). Hence, a high-probability scan makes PE likely, but the absence of a high-probability scan does not exclude PE (Jama 1990;263:2753).

The frequency of silent PE is 40-50% in pts with DVT. A baseline lung scan may detect PE in these pts but is not useful for predicting early thromboembolic recurrences (Arch IM 2000; 160:159).

Recommendations are based on these data: Consider VQ scan confirmatory if either normal or high probability; otherwise, treat as PE if lower-extremity venous US is positive for thrombus; consider serial venous studies or pulmonary angiogram if leg scan is negative (Nejm 1998;33:93; Arch IM 1995;155: 2101).

Spiral CT is best suited for identifying PE in proximal pulmonary vascular tree; third-generation scanners have 1 mm resolution and are replacing VQ scan as the diagnostic test of first choice (Circ 2004;109:2160; Lancet 2002;360:1914). Withholding anticoagulants in pts with low/intermediate clinical probability of PE and negative spiral CT and leg vein ultrasonography is safe (Lancet 2002;360:1914). The incidence of fatal PE with negative CT scan was 0.3% at 3 mon (Mayo Clin Proc 2002;77:130).

The sensitivity and specificity of MRI pulmonary angiography are under investigation (Circ 2004;109:Suppl 1,I-15).

Pulmonary angiogram remains the gold standard.

Rx: Pts with a moderate/high clinical likelihood of PE: Heparin 5000 U bolus followed by a continuous infusion of 18 U/kg/hr (100 U/hr max), adjusted for a target PTT of 60-80 sec. Heparin without oral anticoagulation may be used in pregnancy or with metastatic cancer (oral anticoagulation usually fails to prevent recurrent thrombosis).

LMW heparin was no less effective and probably more effective than dose-adjusted iv unfractionated heparin in reduction of mortality and prevention of recurrent venous thromboembolism in pts with PE and associated proximal DVT (Nejm 2001;344:626; Arch IM 2000;160:229).

Fondaparinux, a synthetic Factor Xa inhibitor, is as effective and safe as IV unfractionated heparin in the initial Rx of hemodynamically stable pts with PE (NEJM 2003;349:1695)

Warfarin is started once PTT is in the therapeutic range. At least 5 days of continuous iv heparin is recommended because true anticoagulation requires depletion of factor II (thrombin). The initial target is INR = 3 because administration of unfractionated heparin usually prolongs INR by 0.5.

The duration of anticoagulation after PE remains uncertain; 6 mon has been standard rx. An indefinite period of anticoagulation may be necessary for pts with recurrent PE, but even pts with low risk of bleeding major hemorrhages are at risk (Nejm 1997; 336:393). Lower-limb venography demonstrates 82% prevalence of residual DVT in patients with angiography-proven PE (Chest 1999;116:903).

Thrombolysis provides no additional benefit in unselected pts with PE (J Am Coll Cardiol 2002;40:1660). It typically has been reserved for pts with massive PE, cardiogenic shock, or hemodynamic instability. Current indications may also include normotensive pts with RV hypokinesis. Rx may be efficacious for 14 d after presentation (Am J Cardiol 1997;80:184).

In pts receiving primary thrombolytic rx within 24 hr of dx, 30-d mortality is lower (4.7% vs 11.1%), the rate of recurrent PE is lower (7.7% vs 18.7%), and frequency of major bleeding is higher (21.9% vs 7.8%). Factors associated with a higher death rate were syncope, hypotension, h/o CHF, and COPD (Circ 1997;96:882; Chest 1999;115:1695), but disparities have been noted between results in clinical trials and those in "real-life" practice.

In a trial of 400 pts with DVT, IVC filters plus anticoagulation did not reduce the 2-yr mortality rate compared with anticoagulation alone (Nejm 1998;338:409), and filter placement has been associated with a 2.6-fold increase in the likelihood of rehospitalization for venous thrombosis within 1 yr (Arch IM 2000;160:2033). Filters may be indicated in pts with PE and active hemorrhage, absolute contraindication to anticoagulation, or recurrent embolism despite intensive anticoagulation.

13.2 Pulmonary Hypertension

Nejm 2004;351:1425,1655; Lancet 2003;361:1533

Cause: WHO classification of pulmonary arterial HT:

Group 1: Idiopathic; familial; collagen vascular disease, congenital L-to-R shunt, portal HT, HIV disease, anorexigens, rapeseed oil, tryptophan, methamphetamine, and cocaine; thyroid disorders, glycogen storage disease, Gaucher's disease, hereditary hemorrhagic telangiectasia, hemoglobinopathies, myeloproliferative disorders, splenectomy; pulmonary veno-occlusive disease, pulmonary capillary hemangiomatosis; persistent pulmonary HT of the newborn

Group 2: Left-sided atrial/ventricular cardiac and valvular heart disease

Group 3: COPD, interstitial lung disease, sleep apnea, alveolar hypoventilation disorders, chronic exposure to altitude

Group 4: Thromboembolic obstruction of proximal or distal pulmonary arteries; nonthrombotic pulmonary embolism (tumor, parasites, foreign material)

Group 5 (miscellaneous): Sarcoidosis, pulmonary Langerhans cell histiocytosis, lymphangiomatosis, compression of pulmonary vessels

Epidem: The most common cause of chronic cor pulmonale in North America is COPD.

Use of derivatives of fenfluramine was associated with increased risk of primary pulmonary HT in a case-control study (Nejm 1996;335:609).

Pathophys: Pulmonary heart disease can result from disease affecting the walls of pulmonary resistance vessels (interstitial fibrosis, granulomatous disease), thromboembolic disease, diseases of the chest wall (kyphoscoliosis), neuromuscular apparatus, or alveoli. Major mechanisms are alveolar hypoxemia leading to pulmonary vasoconstriction and subsequent structural change in vessels and/or actual destruction of vessels.

Sx: Dyspnea on exertion; syncope

Si: Weight gain secondary to fluid retention, distended neck veins, peripheral cyanosis, clubbing of digits, ascites, peripheral edema, RUQ tenderness, hepatojugular reflux, RV lift, widely split S_2

with increased P_2, S_3 gallop, murmur of tricuspid and/or pulmonary regurgitation

Crs: Median survival in 1980s reported to be 2.8 yr; prospective studies showed 68-77% survival at 1 yr, 40-56% survival at 3 yr; 22-38% survival at 5 yr

Lab: EKG is specific but insensitive; findings include P pulmonale, right axis deviation, R/S > 1 in lead V1, S_1Q_3 or $S_1S_2S_3$ pattern.

Echo may demonstrate RA, RV enlargement, or abnormal septal motion resulting from RV pressure overload. Doppler assessment of tricuspid regurgitation permits calculation of RV and PA systolic pressures.

X-ray: Heart size normal or RV enlargement; dilated main PA with underperfusion of peripheral PA branches

Rx: O_2 rx improves survival in pts with cor pulmonale and COPD (Ann IM 1980;93:931).

Digoxin is controversial; it is reserved for pts with concomitant LV failure.

Low-salt diet, diuretics, and phlebotomy may be needed to correct fluid retention and increased blood viscosity secondary to chronic hypoxemia.

Nitrates, hydralazine, nifedipine and felodipine, prazosin, captopril, and prostaglandins have all been used as vasodilator rx with mixed results. In pts who reseponded to short-term testing with epoprostenol, survival was prolonged by use of Ca^{++}-channel blockers plus warfarin. Retrospective studies report that < 7% of pts had a sustained benefit.

Continuous infusion of epoprostenol (prostacyclin) is reported to have decreased PA pressures and improved survival compared to historical controls (J Am Coll Cardiol 1997;30:343) as well as in a 12-wk prospective, randomized trial (Nejm 1998; 338:273; 1996;334:296). It requires continuous iv infusion with periodic increases in dose to circumvent tachyphylaxis. Side effects include nausea and gi upset, jaw pain, rash, headache, local infections, sepsis, and depression. Epoprostenol rx improved exercise capacity, cardiopulmonary hemodynamics, and survival in pts with pulmonary HT due to the scleroderma spectrum of disease (Circ 2002;106:1477; J Am Coll Cardiol 2002;40:780; Ann IM 2000;132:425).

Aerosolized iloprost, a prostacyclin analog, is reported to have sustained effects on exercise capacity and pulmonary hemodynamics in pts with primary pulmonary HT. It is not yet approved in the U.S. (Nejm 2002;347:322; 2000;342:1866). Trepostinil is a prostacycline analog that can be administered sc (Chest 2002;121:1561).

Bosentan is an approved endothelin receptor antagonist that has shown encouraging 1-yr results. It requires monthly liver function testing (Nejm 2002;346:896; Lancet 2001;358:1119).

Lung transplantation may be necessary and is associated with high surgical mortality rates. Epoprostenol may obviate the need for transplantation in some pts (Chest 1998;114:1269).

Chapter 14

Aortic and Peripheral Vascular Disease

14.1 Thoracic and Abdominal Aortic Aneurysm

Circ 2005;111:816; Nejm 2003;348:1895; 1993;328:1167

Cause: Thoracic aortic aneurysms result from cystic medial degeneration and are seen in Marfan syndrome (fibrillin-1 gene mutations), familial TAA syndrome, bicuspid aortic valve, syphilis, Turner syndrome, Takayasu's arteritis (15% of pts), and giant cell arteritis (18% of pts). Factors in development of AAA include familial clustering, genetically predisposed and acquired biochemical alterations in the structural matrix of the aortic wall, and hemodynamic mechanical factors. Atherosclerosis may be secondary response to wall injury. Smoking is the strongest independent risk factor for AAA (Lancet 1998;352:1649).

Epidem: Prevalence of AAA is ~5% in men > 55 yr old, and is 18% in male siblings (age > 60 yr) of pts with AAA (Ann IM 1999;130:637). Men are 10 times more likely than women to have AAA > 4 cm (J Vasc Surg 1996;23:724). The Mayo Clinic reported an increase in the incidence of detected AAA from 12.2/100,000 to 36.2/100,000 between 1951 and 1980.

Pathophys: Annual expansion rates are 0.2- 0.4 cm/yr. Aneurysms > 5-6 cm in diameter expand more rapidly, but the expansion rate is unpredictable in a given pt.

Sx: Usually asymptomatic. Aneurysms of ascending aorta may produce AI with murmur. Large thoracic aneurysms may produce cough, wheezing, and dyspnea. Rupture of AAA may be associated with abdominal pain radiating to back and hypotension (may be seen in only 50% of pts); the sx of rupture are frequently mistaken for renal colic, diverticulitis, or gi hemorrhage.

Si: Pulsatile abdominal mass; abdominal bruit

Crs: The natural h/o of TAA is not well defined. The growth rate is greatest for descending TAA and pts with Marfan syndrome; the annual growth rate is 2% for TAA < 5 cm, 3% for 5-5.9 cm, 7% for TAA > 6 cm diameter (Ann Thorac Surg 2002;73:17). AAAs with diameter < 4 cm have a 0.3% risk of rupture, while 4-4.9 cm AAAs have a 1.5% risk, and 5-5.9 cm AAAs have a 6.5% risk (J Vasc Surg 1996;23:724); 25-41% of aneurysms > 5 cm rupture within 5 yr. Up to 62% of pts with ruptured aneurysms die before reaching the hospital. Annual rates of rupture for TAA and AA are 3/1000 and 9/1000 pts, respectively (Mayo Clin Proc 2004;79:176).

The aneurysm growth rate is not predicted by either size or initial growth rate (Arch IM 1997;157:2064).

Most aneurysms rupture into the retroperitoneum, producing hypovolemic shock but not exsanguination, due to the tamponade effect of the retroperitoneum.

Cmplc: Dissection with TAA; ASHD common in pts with AAA: severe CAD identified in 31%; CAD accounted for 39% of deaths within 5 yr of operation in 1 study, and 37% of early post-op deaths were due to MI.

Lab: Exercise stress testing in pts with AAA seems to be safe and is associated with a low incidence of acute adverse events (Ann IM 1998;129:628).

X-ray: US, contrast CT, and MRI angiography have 100% sensitivity in dx. Ultrasonography is used for aneurysm detection and sequential follow-up. CT is used when ultrasonography is not possible or precise sizing is required.

Aortography can provide anatomical information useful for aortic reconstruction; it is necessary for suspected suprarenal/juxtarenal aneurysms, renovascular HT, ischemic nephropathy, mesenteric artery stenosis, and iliofemoral arterial occlusive disease. MRI can also provide detailed anatomical data.

Rx: Consider screening pts at high risk for AAA: age 60-80 with CAD risk factors, HT, pts > 50 yr old with family h/o of AAA (J Vasc Surg 2004;39:267).

β-Blockade and rx to lower systolic BP to 105-120 mm Hg

Aerobic exercise is safe if BP is controlled.

Surveillance: Image aneurysms 3-3.4 cm q 3 yr; 3.5-3.9 cm q 2 yr; 4-4.4 cm q 1 yr; 4.5-4.9 cm q 6 mon

Repair symptomatic aneurysms and asymptomatic TAA > 5.5-6 cm and AAA > 5-5.5 cm diameter in men and 4-4.5 cm in women. Contraindications to elective surgical repair include recent MI, intractable CHF or angina, severe COPD with dyspnea at rest, severe chronic renal insufficiency, incapacitating residual effects from stroke, and life expectancy < 2 yr.

In an unstable pt with suspected ruptured AAA, immediate operation without confirmatory testing or full resuscitation is mandatory.

The reported operative mortality rate for nonruptured ascending TAA is 3-5%; AAA repair, 1.4-6.5%; ruptured aneurysm, 23-69%. Survival after repair is 92% at 1 yr, 67% at 5 yr. Descending TAA has a 5-6% incidence of post-op paraplegia and surgical mortality of 5-14%.

Early complications of AAA after elective surgery include cardiac ischemia, arrhythmia, CHF (15%), pulmonary insufficiency (8%), renal injury (6%), bleeding (4%), distal thromboembolism (3%), and infection (2%). Rare complications include ischemic colitis and stroke/paraplegia. Late (3-5 yr post-op) complications include graft infection, graft occlusion, anastomotic aneurysms, and aortoenteric fistula.

Endovascular stent grafts are an alternative approach to exclude and stabilize both TAA and AAA (Nejm 2004;351:1607); they may have lower short-term mortality than open repair (Lancet 2004;364:843).

14.2 Aortic Dissection

Circ 2003;108:628,772; 1995;92:113

Cause: Atherosclerotic plaque with ulceration (moderate atherosclerosis of aorta present in 15-20% of pts > 50 yr old); blunt/penetrating trauma; HT; bicuspid aortic valve; coarctation; thoracic aortic aneurysm due to Marfan, Ehler-Danlos syndromes; cystic medial necrosis; infection; inflammation (Takayasu's arteritis, Behcet's syndrome); familial aortic dissection

Epidem: 10-20 cases/1 million population/yr; 36-72% of untreated pts die within 48 hr of dx, 62-91% die within 7 d

Pathophys: Tear in intima produces dissection of layers of aortic media; resulting column of blood may rupture back into lumen of aorta

Stanford classification: Type A dissection involves ascending aorta with or without involvement of arch, descending aorta; type B dissection involves descending aorta with or without involvement of arch, ascending aorta

Sx: Chest pain radiating into back, neck, jaw, abdomen; hoarseness, stridor, dysphagia, dyspnea can be caused by impingement on mediastinal structures

In a retrospective study of 464 pts, murmur of AI and pulse deficit were noted in only 31.6% and 15.1% of pts, respectively; no abnormalities were noted in initial CXR and EKG in 12.4% and 31.3% of pts, respectively (Jama 2000;283:897).

Si: Compression of coronary arteries and branches of aorta can produce acute MI, neurological deficits, renal failure, and ischemia of limbs or intestine.

Crs: Type A dissection has 1-2%/hr early mortality rate after onset (Jama 2000;283:897), 20% mortality at 24 hr, and 40% mortality by d 7. More than 90% of pts with untreated type A dissection die within 3 mon. Mortality is more variable in type B dissection. Death is due to aortic rupture obstruction of coronary, brachiocephalic, or visceral arteries.

X-ray: Mediastinal widening on CXR (but 17% of pts have normal CXR)

CT scan requires contrast, will image all of aorta, may be limited in identifying entry/exit tear; has overall sensitivity of 94%, specificity of 87%

TEE does not require contrast, can visualize entry site, provides information about heart and valves, can be performed in OR, has "blind spots"; has overall sensitivity of 98%, specificity of 77%

MRI does not require contrast, can visualize entire aorta and identify entry site; cannot be used with pts on ventilators or who have pacemakers; has overall sensitivity of 98%, specificity of 98%

Aortography requires contrast; has sensitivity of 88%, specificity of 94%; usually required for elective surgery

Rx: Type A acute dissections: Immediate surgical intervention to avert death due to cardiac tamponade, aortic regurgitation, MI. Type B dissections: Antihypertensive drugs and β-blockers; surgery is reserved for pts with progression of dissection retrograde extension into ascending aorta, impending rupture, refractory HT, localized false aneurysm, continued pain, or end-organ ischemia. Mortality rates for surgical repair of acute type A and B dissections are 29% and 35%, respectively. The surgical mortality rate > 50% for acute dissection complicated by end-organ ischemia. The mortality rate with medical rx is 20%.

Operative mortality rates for pts with chronic aortic dissection = 27%. Earlier operative year, HT, cardiac tamponade, renal dysfunction, and older age are determinants of operative death. In 1 series, freedom from reoperation was 84%, 67%, and 57% at 5, 10, and 15 yr, respectively (Circ 1995;92:113).

Overall 30-d mortality after repair of aortic valve and root in patients with Marfan syndrome is ~2% but is ~12% among pts who required emergency surgery. Survival rates are 84% at 5 yr, 75% at 10 yr, and 59% at 20 yr. More than 10 of pts in 1 study required additional surgery on the distal aorta or died of dissection or rupture of the residual aorta (Nejm 1999;340:1307).

Endovascular stent-grafts placed across the primary entry tear for management of acute dissections originating in descending thoracic aorta are currently evolving (Nejm 1999; 340:1546).

14.3 Arterial Insufficiency of Lower Extremities

Nejm 2001;344:1608; Lancet 2001;358:1257

Cause: Atherosclerosis is the most common cause of chronic arterial occlusive disease of the lower extremities. 50% of pts with lower extremity arterial disease have hyperlipidemia.

Cigarette smoking is the most significant independent risk factor for development of chronic peripheral arterial occlusive disease and is associated with progression of established disease and higher likelihood of disabling claudication, limb-threatening ischemia, amputation, and/or need for intervention.

Epidem: Adult prevalence in U.S. adults > 40 yr old is 4.3% (Circ 2004;110:758). Age, sex, serum cholesterol, HT, cigarette smoking, diabetes, and CAD are associated with an increased risk for claudication (Framingham) (Circ 1997;96:44).

Up to 5% of men and 2.5% of women ≥ 60 yr old have sx of intermittent claudication. Prevalence is at least threefold higher when sensitive noninvasive tests are used to make a dx in asymptomatic and symptomatic individuals.

Pts with diabetes have a different distribution of arterial disease with greater involvement of the more distal (ie, tibial) arteries.

Pathophys: Superficial femoral and popliteal arteries are the vessels most commonly affected. The distal aorta and its bifurcation are the next most frequent sites.

Sx: Pain in calf, thigh, buttocks with exertion, progressing to rest pain

Si: Abnormal pedal pulses, unilaterally cool extremity, femoral bruit, abnormal femoral pulse, lower-extremity bruits, foot discoloration, atrophic skin (Arch IM 1998;158:1357). Pts who are older, male, or diabetic are more likely to have asymptomatic peripheral arterial disease (Arch IM 1999;159:387).

Crs: Slow progression: After 5-10 yr, > 70% of pts report no change/improvement in sx, 20-30% progress and require intervention, < 10% need amputation

Cmplc: Compared with age-matched controls, pts with intermittent claudication have a threefold increase in cardiovascular mortality

Lab: Total cholesterol/HDL-C ratio and hs CRP are the biomarkers with the greatest predictive value for development of PAD (Jama 2001;285;2481).

Ankle-brachial index (ABI): Systolic BP measured at ankle divided by systolic BP at brachial artery. Normal values 0.95-10. Lower-extremity arterial disease is present when ABI ≤ 0.9 (incidence in pts age 55-74 ≈10%).

ABI may be of less value in pts with diabetes, who have higher incidence of calcification of the tibial and peroneal arteries, because there is no relation between calcification and extent of ASPVD in these vessels.

Abnormal ABI is also an independent predictor of all-cause and cardiovascular mortality.

Exercise testing (2 mi/hr with 12° grade for 5 min) in pts with claudication: Ankle systolic pressure usually falls precipi-

AORTIC AND PERIPHERAL VASCULAR DISEASE

tously, will not return to baseline for several min.

Level of arterial disease can be estimated by measuring pressures at multiple levels (ankle, calf, above knee, upper thigh).

X-ray: Duplex US scanning can identify stenotic segments. It is used when the pt is scheduled for balloon angioplasty or direct arterial surgery and in follow-up studies after femoropopliteal or distal saphenous vein grafting; 20-30% of such pts may develop myointimal hyperplastic lesions that can be detected by duplex scanning before graft failure occurs.

Rx: Exercise and risk factor modification (especially smoking cessation) are the initial management of all pts with nondisabling intermittent claudication.

ASA 75-325 mg qd may improve a natural h/o claudication. The benefit is likely due to prevention/retardation of platelet thrombogenesis on the surface of atherosclerotic plaque. ASA may also reduce the associated risk of MI and CVA.

Lipid-lowering therapy (HMG-COA reductase inhibitors) are recommended for pts with intermittent claudication and elevated serum cholesterol to reduce the risk associated with generalized atherosclerosis. Their impact on symptoms of peripheral arterial insufficiency is not established.

Controlled trials have documented that vasodilators failed to increase blood flow or relieve sx.

Pentoxifylline is reported to improve abnormal erythrocyte deformability, reduce blood viscosity, and decrease platelet reactivity and plasma hypercoagulability. Several studies demonstrated that pentoxifylline is more effective than placebo in improving treadmill walking distances, but no consistent benefit was found in 6 trials. Pts treated with placebo also had significant improvement; actual improvement was often unpredictable. This drug may permit some pts to undertake a walking program.

Selective/intra-arterial thrombolytic rx may be used for acute thrombotic/embolic occlusion of the native artery or a prosthetic graft, provided that there is a low risk of myonecrosis developing during the time needed to achieve revascularization. The usual contraindications to use of thrombolytic agents apply.

PTA, stenting, and surgery are indicated for incapacitating claudication, limb salvage in pts with limb-threatening ischemia (pain at rest, nonhealing ulcers/infection/gangrene), or vasculogenic impotence.

Revascularization surgery is indicated to relieve symptoms of limb-threatening ischemia (ischemic pain at rest, ischemic ulcers, gangrene) and to remove or bypass and exclude sources of atheroemboli. The choice of surgical procedure depends on the level of arterial disease. Surgical revascularization may provide salvage of unselected limbs threatened by ischemia in 85-90% of cases.

Coronary revascularization before elective vascular surgery in pts with both CAD and PVD does not affect long-term outcomes (Nejm 2004;351:2795).

Mortality and morbidity results of nonrandomized but concurrently performed amputation and revascularization procedures: Operative mortality, hospital stay, and long-term survival superior in the revascularization group; advantage over the amputation group greatest in pt subgroups with the highest predicted operative risk

Review of controlled studies: Chelation therapy not superior to placebo (Circ 1997;96:1031)

14.4 Deep Venous Thrombosis

Circ 1996;93:2212; Nejm 1996;335:1815

Cause: Risk factors include age > 60 yr; previous venous thromboembolism; fx of pelvis, femur, or tibia; hip, knee, or major orthopedic surgery; immobility; surgery for malignant disease; post-op sepsis; major medical illness; CHF; IBD; sepsis; MI

Symptomatic upper-extremity deep venous thrombophlebitis is associated with central venous catheters, thrombophilic states, or previous leg vein thrombosis. Pulmonary embolism is a common complication (Arch IM 1997;157:57).

Epidem: Conditions associated with increased risk of thrombosis: Activated protein C resistance, factor V Leiden mutation, antithrombin III deficiency, protein C deficiency, protein S deficiency (Ann IM 1998;128:8), malignancy, antiphospholipid antibody, paroxysmal nocturnal hemoglobinuria, myeloproliferative syndrome, nephrotic syndrome, estrogen rx for infertility, chemotherapy for cancer, reduction in post-op fibrinolytic activity

High levels of factor XI are a risk factor for DVT, with a doubling of the risk at levels that are present in 10% of the population (Nejm 2000;342:696). Pts with a high plasma level of factor VIII have an increased risk of recurrent VTE (Nejm 2000;343:457). Use of estrogen plus progestin in postmenopausal women doubles the risk of DVT (Jama 2004;292:1573).

Pathophys: Post-thrombotic syndrome caused by venous HT resulting from recanalization of venous thrombi valves (patent but incompetent) or persistent outflow obstruction; increased venous pressure produces progressive incompetence of valves, edema, and ulceration

41-43% of pts have unilateral proximal DVT, 10% have bilateral proximal DVT, 25-27% have DVT isolated to calf, 10% have proximal and calf involvement (Am Hrt J 1996;132:1010)

Sx: Sensation of tightness, tenderness in lower calf

Si: Swelling of thigh and calf, especially swelling of calf to 3 cm greater than on symptomless side (measured 10 cm below tibial tuberosity); pitting edema; dilated superficial veins (nonvaricose) in symptomatic leg; erythema; palpable cord

Differential dx includes acute/chronic venous insufficiency, cellulitis, hematoma, ruptured Baker's cyst

Crs: Pulmonary emboli detected (perfusion lung scan) in ~50% of pts with documented DVT; asymptomatic venous thrombosis is found in ~70% of pts with confirmed symptomatic PE

Pts with symptomatic DVT have a high risk for recurrent venous thromboembolism that persists for many years; post-thrombotic syndrome occurs in ~1/3 of pts and is strongly related to ipsilateral recurrent DVT (Ann IM 1996;125:1)

Lab: Screening for hereditary disorders and conditions listed above

X-ray: Venous ultrasonography is the diagnostic method of choice in most patients with clinically suspected venous thrombosis. IPG and venography also have good accuracy.

Rx: Prophylaxis: Low-dose subcutaneous heparin (NEJM 2003;348: 1425); intermittent pneumatic compression of the legs, oral anti-coagulants, adjusted doses of subcutaneous heparin, graduated compression stockings, LMW heparin, and fondaparinux for pts undergoing general surgery, hip or knee replacement, prolonged bed rest; antiplatelet agents less effective for preventing VTE; low-dose heparin (5000 U bid) or intermittent pneumatic compression is the rx of choice for neurosurgery, urogenital surgery, pts with high risk of hemorrhage; LMW heparin for pregnant women with h/o pulmonary embolism or DVT

In pts with acute VTE who receive an iv bolus of 5000 U, followed by a starting dose of at least 1250 U/hr of heparin, a subtherapeutic PTT response during the first 48 hr of rx is not associated with a large increase in risk of recurrent VTE (Arch IM 1999;159:2029).

LMW heparin is at least as effective and safe as standard heparin, has a lower incidence of heparin-induced thrombocytopenia, and may be safe in pregnancy (it does not cross the placenta) (Ann IM 1999;130:800).

Fondaparinux, a synthetic Factor Xa inhibitor, is effective in the prevention of asymptomatic and symptomatic venous thromboembolism in older acute medical pts (BMJ 2006;332:325). In addition fondaparinux has not been reported to be associated with heparin-induced thrombocytopenia (NEJM 2006;355:809)

For confirmed DVT, IV heparin for a 4-5 d course (7-10 d for pts with large iliofemoral vein thrombi or major PE); fondaparinux 5.0 mg (<50 kg), 7.5 mg (50 kg-100 kg), 7.5 mg (>100 kg) for 5-9 d; give warfarin for 6 wk-3 mon if pt has reversible risk factors, 3-6 mon for idiopathic venous thrombosis, longer (? for life) in pts with inherited molecular abnormalities, lupus anticoagulant, anticardiolipin antibody.

In pts in whom heparin-induced thrombocytopenia (HIT/HITT) is diagnosed, immediate discontinuation of heparin infusions and elimination of heparin from all flushes and ports are mandatory. Direct thrombin inhibitors constitute the current standard for patients with HIT (Chest 2004:126(3);311S).

Indication for vena caval filter: Anticoagulant-induced bleed-ing or anticipation of hemorrhagic complications in pts with predisposing lesions (bleeding peptic ulcer, gi malignancy, recent in-tracranial operation) or failure of anticoagulation rx. After the cessation of anticoagulation, filters do not seem to prevent PE and may actually predispose pts to symptomatic DVT (Nejm 1998;338:409).

Heparin is the anticoagulant of choice for rx of VTE during pregnancy. If warfarin is used, it should be restricted to the 2nd and early 3rd trimesters and avoided between 6 and 12 wk of gestation and near term. Pts receiving long-term warfarin before pregnancy should be treated with sc heparin q 12 hr throughout pregnancy in doses to prolong the 6-hr post-injection PTT to 1.5-2.5 times control.

Elective surgery should be avoided in the 1st mon after an acute episode of venous thromboembolism. If this is not possible, iv heparin should be given before and after procedure while the INR < 2 and stopped 6 hr prior to surgery. Heparin should not be restarted until 12 hr after major surgery and restarted without bolus. If the risk of bleeding during iv heparin rx is unacceptable, a vena caval filter should be inserted (NEJM 1997;336:1506).

Dental extractions can be performed with minimal risk in pts who are at or above therapeutic levels of anticoagulation (Arch IM 1998;158:1610).

Chapter 15

Congenital Heart Disease in Adults

15.1 Atrial Septal Defect

Nejm 2000;342:256

Cause:

ASD: 75% ostium secundum defects (fossa ovalis); 15% ostium primum defects (lower intra-atrial septum); 10% sinus venosus defects (upper intra-atrial septum); most often due to spontaneous mutations

10-20% of pts with secundum ASD are reported to have mitral valve prolapse (Am J Cardiol 1976;38:167).

Lutembacher's syndrome: ASD plus (rheumatic) mitral stenosis

Epidem: The population of U.S. adults with surgically corrected or uncorrected congenital heart disease is increasing 5%/yr. ASD represents 1/3 of all cases of congenital heart disease detected in adults; it is 2-3 times more common in women.

AV canal defects (endocardial cushion defects) are seen with trisomy 21 (Down's syndrome).

Pathophys: A shunt from the LA to RA produces increased pulmonary blood flow and dilatation of the RA, RV, pulmonary arteries, and LA; defects < 0.5 cm in diameter are usually not hemodynamically significant. Mitral valve prolapse is associated with ostium secundum defects; cleft anterior mitral leaflet is seen with ostium primum defects. Partial anomalous drainage of pulmonary veins can accompany sinus venosus defects.

Sx: Most pts asymptomatic for years; exertional dyspnea; fatigue; palpitations, paradoxical emboli likely after age 60

Si: S_1 normal; fixed splitting of S_2 (phasic changes in venous return to RA with respiration matched by changes in volume of LA to RA shunt), soft mid-systolic ejection murmur (pulmonary valve) or diastolic flow murmur across tricuspid valve may also be present

Pansystolic murmur of mitral regurgitation present with cleft mitral valve accompanying ostium primum defect

Crs: Pts with secundum ASD survive into adulthood but have shortened life expectancy (50% survival past age 40). Those with large shunts die of RV failure or arrhythmia in the 4th-5th decades.

Pts with secundum or sinus venosus ASD who are minimally symptomatic in the 3rd decade do not develop severe pulmonary HT and do well with medical management (Brit Hrt J 1994; 71:224).

Symptomatic pts have near-normal life expectancy and morbidity when surgery is performed before age 25 (Nejm 1990;323: 1645). Surgery in older pts improves survival but not the incidence of atrial arrhythmias (which are related to atrial dilation) and thromboembolic events compared with medical rx (Nejm 1995;333:469).

Cmplc: Pts develop at least mild/moderate pulmonary HT after age 40; 10-15% develop severe pulmonary HT with shunt reversal and resultant cyanosis. 15% of pts develop mitral fibrosis and mitral regurgitation.

Lab:

EKG: IRBBB; left axis deviation with ostium primum defect; Afib, SVT are common after age 30

Echocardiogram: Dilated atria and RV; ostium primum/secundum defects may be visible directly or detected via contrast study;

TEE superior for detection of ASD and anomalous pulmonary venous drainage

Cardiac catheterization: To measure magnitude of shunt and presence of pulmonary HT and for detection of CAD in older pts

X-ray: *CXR:* Prominent pulmonary arteries with peripheral pulmonary vascular pattern well defined ("shunt vasculature" pattern); anomalous pulmonary veins may be visible

Rx: Surgical closure for pulmonary/systemic flow ≥ 1.8; surgery not recommended for pts with irreversible pulmonary vascular disease and pulmonary HT; endocarditis prophylaxis not recommended unless valve disease also present

Pts with ostium primum ASD and cleft mitral valve may require valve repair/replacement

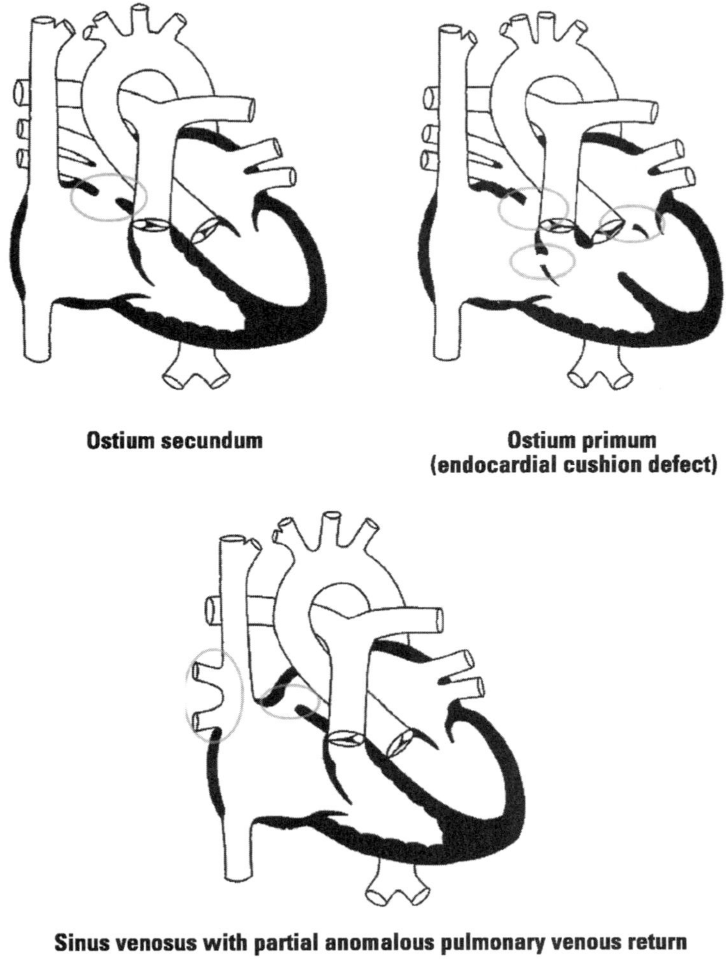

Figure 15.1 ASD

15.2 Ventricular Septal Defect

Nejm 2000;342:256

Cause: 70% of VSDs are located in membranous septum; 20% in the muscular septum; 5% below aortic valve and cause AI; 5% near mitral/tricuspid valves (AV canal defects)

Epidem: Adult survivors either have had spontaneous closure/near closure or develop increased pulmonary vascular resistance with systemic right-sided pressures and relief of persistent LV volume overload (Eisenmenger's syndrome)

Pathophys: VSD initially produces shunt from LV to RV. With large defects, pressures eventually equalize or reverse as pulmonary HT worsens.

Sx: Cyanosis with R-to-L shunting; decreased exercise tolerance and DOE; palpitations (due to Aflut or Afib); visual disturbances, fatigue, headache, dizziness, paresthesias if hyperviscosity syndrome develops with Eisenmenger's syndrome. Adults with a shunt ratio $< 2:1$ are usually asymptomatic; with a ratio of 3:1, exertional dyspnea is likely after age 30.

Si: Cyanosis; clubbing; normal/split S_2; S_3; holosystolic murmur loudest at lower LSB ± palpable thrill with restrictive defect; mid-diastolic rumble; murmur of AI if VSD near aortic annulus; with muscular VSD, murmur may end in mid/late systole as muscle contracts; murmur diminishes/disappears as flow decreases; murmur of pulmonary regurgitation (Graham Steell murmur) may appear

Crs: 25-40% close spontaneously by age 2; 90% of defects that close do so by age 10. Adults with small defects are usually asymptomatic and unlikely to develop pulmonary HT. In adults diagnosed with VSD, 10-yr survival ≈75%. Those presenting with cardiomegaly, pulmonary HT, or impaired exercise capacity have poorer prognosis.

Cmplc: Even a small VSD still carries an increased risk for infective endocarditis. With a large shunt, development of Eisenmenger's syndrome is associated with risk of hemoptysis due to pulmonary infarction or rupture of dilated pulmonary arteries/arterioles. CVA may result from paradoxical embolization, venous thrombosis of cerebral vessels, or intracranial hemorrhage. Brain abscess, syncope, and sudden death have also been reported.

Lab:

EKG: LAE and LVH with large defect; right axis shift and RAE with pulmonary HT

Echocardiogram: VSD may be visible directly or detected via contrast study or TEE; Doppler study can usually provide an estimate of PA systolic pressure

Cardiac catheterization: To measure magnitude of shunt and presence of pulmonary HT

X-ray: *CXR:* Normal with small VSD; LV enlargement and "shunt vascularity" with large defect; enlargement of proximal pulmonary arteries, rapid tapering of peripheral pulmonary arteries, and oligemic lung fields with pulmonary HT

Rx: Small VSD requires antibiotic prophylaxis for infective endocarditis; adults with large defects will have CHF and pulmonary HT, and should have surgical closure if pulmonary/systemic vascular resistance < 0.7, QP:QS $> 1.5:1$

At 25 yr after surgery, the cumulative incidence of infective endocarditis is 2.7% in pts with isolated VSD.

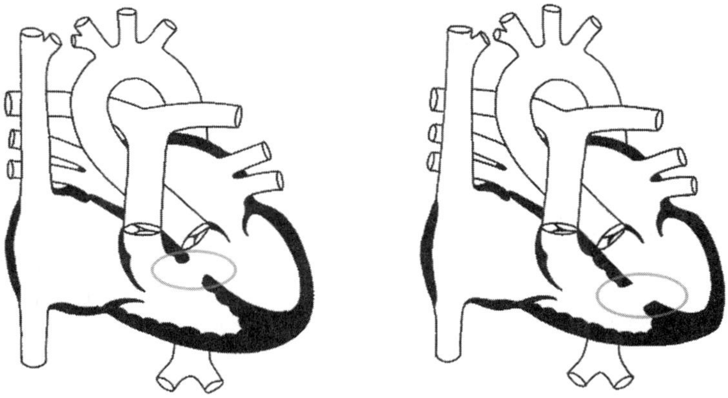

Membranous septum **Muscular septum**

Figure 15.2 VSD

15.3 Patent Ductus Arteriosus

Cause: Failure of closure of ductus arteriosus (connects proximal descending aorta to main PA bifurcation or left pulmonary artery distal to the left subclavian artery). In a fetus, pulmonary arterial blood flows into the descending aorta for oxygenation in the placenta; failure to close produces a L-to-R shunt from the aorta to the pulmonary artery.

Epidem: PDA accounts for ~10% cases of congenital heart disease. Increased incidence is noted in premature infants or in pregnancies complicated by persistent perinatal hypoxemia or maternal rubella infection.

Pathophys: In the absence of increased pulmonary vascular resistance, blood is shunted from the aorta to the pulmonary artery throughout the cardiac cycle, producing left-sided volume overload.

Sx: Small PDA causes no sx. If sx develop, they usually do so in the 1st year of life. Fatigue, dyspnea, or palpitations are the most common sx reported.

Si: With moderate/large shunt: Bounding peripheral pulses and widened pulse pressure; hyperdynamic LV impulse; "machinery" murmur in 2nd LICS may obscure S_2 and continues into diastole but shortens/disappears as pulmonary HT develops; flow murmurs across mitral and aortic valves; pulmonary ejection click and diastolic murmur of pulmonary regurgitation with pulmonary HT

Development of Eisenmenger's physiology can produce "differential cyanosis" and clubbing of toes but not of fingers.

Crs: Spontaneous closure of PDA after infancy is rare; normal life expectancy with small defect, but increased risk of infective endocarditis (pulmonary side) and/or septic pulmonary emboli; LV failure, pulmonary vascular obstruction, and severe pulmonary HT; aneurysmal dilation, calcification, rupture of PDA may also occur

Cmplc: Risk of infective endocarditis exceeds that of CHF by 2nd decade; risk of endarteritis ≈ 0.45% annually after age 20

~1/3 of pts with unrepaired PDA die from CHF, pulmonary HT, or endarteritis by age 40; 2/3 by age 60

Lab:

EKG: Normal, or LAE and LVH with large shunt; RVH if pulmonary HT develops

Echocardiogram: Ductus arteriosus occasionally visualized; continuous and increased flow in the pulmonary trunk seen on Doppler

Cardiac catheterization: To demonstrate ductus, quantify shunt, and allow calculation of pulmonary vascular resistance

X-ray: *CXR:* Normal with small PDA; large shunt produces dilated LA and LV, pulmonary vascular engorgement, dilation of proximal PA; prominent ascending aorta; ductus may be seen as an opacity at junction of aortic knob and descending aorta

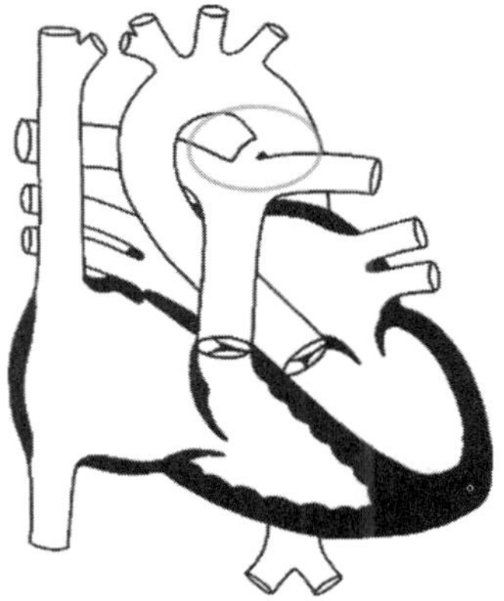

Figure 15.3 PDA

Rx: Perioperative mortality for ligation of PDA < 0.5% without cardiopulmonary bypass. Surgical ligation or percutaneous closure is contraindicated if severe pulmonary vascular obstructive disease has developed.

Small PDA may be able to be closed with an intravascular device, but data on long-term follow-up are still pending.

Closure of a PDA eliminates the risk of infective endocarditis.

15.4 Congenital Aortic Stenosis

Cause: Bicuspid aortic valve is the most common pathological finding in pts with symptomatic AS < age 65. The valve has a single fused commissure and an eccentrically oriented orifice (Circ 2002;106:900).

Supravalvular stenosis and discrete subvalular aortic stenosis are also seen in childhood.

Epidem: Congenital bicuspid valve is found in 2-3% of the population. It is four times more common in males than in females.

20% of pts with a bicuspid aortic valve have an associated cardiovascular abnormality (PDA, coarctation of aorta).

Pathophys: Bicuspid valve is subject to abnormal hemodynamic stress, which leads to thickening and calcification of leaflets. Coexisting conditions (fibrillin-1 and endothelial NOS gene abnormalities) predispose to dilatation of aortic root.

Sx: See **aortic stenosis:** Angina, syncope/near-syncope; CHF

Si: See **aortic stenosis:** With severe AS, delayed carotid; decreased S_2; S_4 gallop; aortic ejection click disappears as valve becomes calcified; harsh late systolic murmur; aortic regurgitation common with subaortic stenosis

Crs: Asymptomatic adults have normal life expectancy. AS becomes hemodynamically significant when the valve area is reduced to ~1 sq cm. Median survival is 5 yr after angina develops, 3 yr after syncope occurs, 2 yr after CHF develops.

Cmplc: Pts with bicuspid aortic valve have an increased incidence of cystic medial necrosis of the aortic root with aneurysm formation and aortic regurgitation or aortic dissection (J Am Coll Cardiol 1992;19:283).

Lab:

EKG: LVH

Echocardiogram: Will show aortic stenosis; Doppler allows assessment of valve area; TEE is superior in dx of subaortic and supravalvular stenosis

Cardiac catheterization: To determine the severity of AS in cases where echo is unsatisfactory and to determine whether CAD is also present

X-ray: CXR is usually normal

Rx: Management and valve replacement criteria in adults are the same as for AS of other causes.

Pts with bicuspid aortic valve should have close monitoring for dilation of the ascending aorta (Clin Cardiol 1998;21:439). Pts with 4-5 cm aorta should have surgical replacement of the valve and aortic root (Ann Thorac Surg 1999;67:1834).

25% of pts treated in childhood with valvotomy will require repeat surgery over the next 25 yr (Circ 1993;87:I-16).

At 25 yr after surgery, the cumulative incidence of infective endocarditis is 13.3% for valvular aortic stenosis. Pts should receive antibiotic prophylaxis against infective endocarditis.

15.5 Pulmonary Stenosis

Cause: Obstruction of RV outflow is valvular in 90% of pts, supravalvular (narrowed pulmonary trunk or peripheral branches) or subvalvular (narrowed right ventricular infundibulum/subinfundibulum, usually in association with VSD) in the remainder

Supravalvular PS can coexist with valvular pulmonary stenosis, ASD, VSD, PDA, tetralogy of Fallot, Williams syndrome (infantile hypercalcemia, elfin facies, mental retardation)

Valvular pulmonary stenosis usually an isolated abnormality, but can be associated with VSD; valve leaflets usually normal with fused commissures, but 10-15% of pts have dysplastic leaflets

~⅔ of pts with Noonan's syndrome have PS due to valve dysplasia

Epidem: PS accounts for 10-12% of cases of congenital heart disease in adults.

Pathophys:

Mild PS: Valve area > 1 cm^2/m^2 (normal is 2 cm^2/m^2), transvalvular gradient < 50 mm Hg, or peak RV pressure < 75 mm Hg systolic

CONGENITAL HEART DISEASE IN ADULTS

Moderate PS: Valve area 0.5-1 cm^2/m^2, gradient 50-80 mm Hg, or RV pressure 75-100 mm Hg systolic

Severe PS: Valve area < 0.5 cm^2/m^2, gradient > 80 mm Hg, or RV pressure > 100 mm Hg systolic

Sx: Adults are often asymptomatic. Sx are determined by the severity of stenosis, RV systolic function, and tricuspid valve competence. With severe PS, pts develop fatigue, DOE, peripheral edema, and ascites with RV failure; cyanosis and clubbing occur when right to left shunt develops with severe pulmonary HT.

Si: Moderate/severe PS: RV heave at the LSB; thrill 2nd LICS; widely split S_2 with normal respiratory variation and decreased P_2; ejection click (softens or disappears with inspiration); crescendo-decrescendo systolic murmur along LSB (increases with inspiration). Murmur peaks occur later in systole and the ejection click moves closer to S_1 as stenosis worsens.

Crs: Only 5% of pts with gradient < 25 mm Hg develop sx vs 20% of pts with gradient 25-49 mm Hg and 76% of pts with gradient 50-79 mm Hg.

94% of adults with mild valvular disease are alive 20 yr after the initial dx, but 60% of pts with severe PS require intervention by 10 yr after dx.

If stenosis is relieved in childhood, long-term survival is similar to that of controls (Circ 1994;89:243); ~50% of pts develop mild/moderate pulmonary regurgitation.

Cmplc: RV failure is the most common cause of death from PS. Infective endocarditis is a risk for pts with moderate/severe PS.

Lab:

EKG: Right axis deviation; RVH; RAE

Echocardiogram: RVE; RVH; paradoxical septal motion; site of obstruction frequently visualized; increased flow velocities in PA on Doppler study

X-ray: *CXR:* Normal cardiac silhouette with post-stenotic dilatation of main PA and decreased pulmonary vascular markings; right-sided CHF produces an enlarged cardiac silhouette

Rx: Pts with valvular PS require antibiotic prophylaxis against infective endocarditis

Patients with moderate PS (gradient 40-60 mm Hg) have an excellent prognosis with either medical or interventional rx. Balloon valvuloplasty is the procedure of choice if gradient > 60 mm Hg and the valve is mobile and pliant. Long-term results are good, and secondary hypertrophic subpulmonary stenosis usually regresses after successful valvuloplasty.

Valve replacement is required if the leaflets are dysplastic or calcified or if marked pulmonary regurgitation is present.

No children with PS had infective endocarditis after surgery in 20-yr follow-up. Endocarditis prophylaxis is recommended only for those with murmur and residual stenosis or insufficiency (Jama 1998;279:599).

15.6 Aortic Coarctation

Cause: Discrete ridge extending distal to the left subclavian artery at the site of the aortic ductal attachment (ligamentum arteriosum) or proximal to the left subclavian artery

Epidem: Coarctation is 2-5 times more common in males than in females. It occurs in conjunction with Turner's syndrome (gonadal dysgenesis), bicuspid aortic valve (up to 80% of pts), VSD, PDA, congenital MS/MR, aneurysms of circle of Willis, and mitral valve abnormalities. The frequency of intracranial aneurysms in pts with coarctation is increased fivefold compared with the general population (Mayo Clin Proc 2003;78:1491).

Pathophys: Extensive collateral arterial circulation develops through internal thoracic, intercostal, subclavian, and scapular arteries

Sx: Sx usually present in infancy or after age 30; many adults asymptomatic; reported sx include headache, epistaxis, dizziness, palpitations, leg fatigue, or claudication

Si: Widened pulse pressure with systolic BP in arms > legs (coarctation distal to left subclavian); BP in right arm > left arm (coarctation proximal to left subclavian); diastolic pressures similar in all limbs; weak femoral pulses; systolic thrill in suprasternal notch; systolic ejection click and murmur if bicuspid aortic valve also present (30% of pts); harsh late systolic ejection murmur along LSB radiating to back secondary to increased collateral flow; bicuspid aortic valve, if present, may produce systolic murmur

Crs: If coarctation is not corrected surgically, the mortality rate is 50% by age 30, 75% by age 50, and 90% by age 60; ⅔ of pts over age 40 develop CHF.

Cmplc: HT; CHF; aortic dissection (peak incidence in 3rd-4th decades; pregnant pts and women with Turner's [XO] syndrome are at higher risk); ASHD; infective endocarditis (of bicuspid valve) or endarteritis (at site of coarctation); CVA if associated intracerebral aneurysm present

50% of pts who undergo surgery after age 40 have persistent HT. With repair in childhood, 90% of pts are normotensive 5 yr later, 50% are normotensive 20 yr later, and 25% are normotensive 25 yr later.

Lab:

EKG: LVH

Echocardiogram: Coarctation may occasionally be imaged from suprasternal notch; bicuspid aortic valve can be identified

X-ray:

CXR: Symmetric notching of posterior third of the 3rd-8th ribs, usually symmetric; indentation of aorta; pre- and/or post-stenotic dilatation of aorta produces "reversed-3" sign on barium swallow

CT, MRI, contrast aortography: To assess location and length of the coarctation, to assess collateral circulation or presence of aneurysm

Rx: Surgical repair recommended for pts with gradient > 30 mm Hg across coarctation

After surgical repair during childhood, 89% of pts are alive 15 yr later; 83% survive 25 yr. If repair is performed at age 20-40, 25-yr survival is 75%. When repair is performed after age 40, 15-yr survival is 50%.

Postoperatively, 3% of pts require repeat surgery for recurrent coarctation at 20-yr follow-up; saccular aneurysm may also develop (J Am Coll Cardiol 1995;26:266). Up to 10% of pts will require surgery for aortic valve disease.

Balloon dilatation is reported to have a higher incidence of aortic aneurysm and recurrent coarctation than surgery. In one series (74 pts), optimal results (post-procedure gradient < 20 mm Hg) were obtained acutely in 88% of pts; 72% of pts with early optimal results remained free from reintervention (J Am Coll Cardiol 1997;30:811).

Although experience is limited, stents may be useful adjuncts to balloon angioplasty in rx of isthmic hypoplasia and tortuous segments (J Am Coll Cardiol 1997;30:1853).

HT is likely to persist and to require rx in pts receiving surgical rx after age 10.

At 25 yr after surgery, the cumulative incidence of infective endocarditis was 3.5%; prophylaxis is indicated (Jama 1998; 279:599).

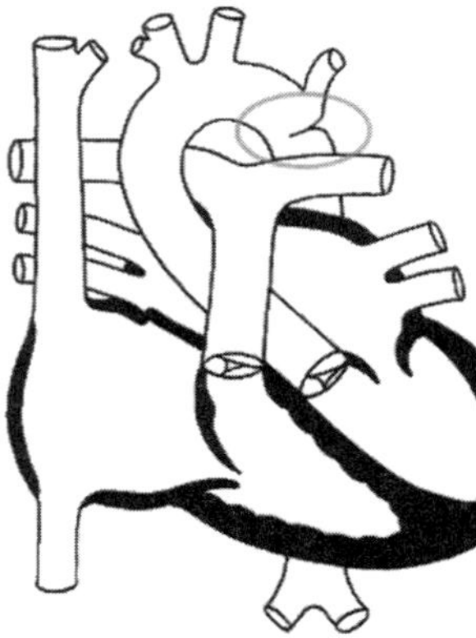

Aortic coarctation

Figure 15.4 Coarctation of aorta.

15.7 Tetralogy of Fallot

Cause: VSD plus overriding aorta plus RVOT obstruction (subvalvular, valvular, supravalvular, or in pulmonary arterial branches) plus RVH; right-sided aortic arch is present in 10% of cases

Epidem: Most common cyanotic congenital heart defect after infancy; 25% of pts also have right aortic arch, 10% also have ASD; 10% have anomalous coronary arteries

Pathophys: R-to-L shunt due to VSD and increased resistance at RV outflow produces cyanosis and equalization of pressures in RV and LV

Sx:

Adults: Dyspnea; decreased exercise tolerance
Childhood: Cyanosis, tachypnea, hyperpnea, seizures

Si: Cyanosis, clubbing; RV lift; systolic thrill (produced by RV outflow tract flow); normal S_1; single S_2; aortic ejection sound; systolic ejection murmur along LSB (due to PS) that shortens and diminishes as severity of RV outflow obstruction worsens

After total repair, murmurs of residual PS and of pulmonary regurgitation may be noted.

Crs: Without surgical intervention, the survival rate is 66% at age 1 yr, 40% at 3 yr, 11% at 20 yr, 6% at 30 yr, and 3% at 40 yr.

In one series, the rate of survival 32 yr after surgery was 86% among pts with repaired tetralogy, and 96% in an age-matched control population. Complications after repair include pulmonary regurgitation and RV dysfunction, RV outflow aneurysm or obstruction, residual VSD (10-20% of cases), RBBB, and aortic regurgitation.

Cmplc: Erythrocytosis, hyperviscosity, abnormalities of hemostasis, cerebral abscesses or stroke, endocarditis; Aflut, Afib, venticular arrhythmias (seen in 40-50% of pts s/p repair; more frequent in pts who are older at the time of surgical repair, moderate/severe pulmonary regurgitation, systolic and diastolic ventricular dysfunction, prolonged cardiopulmonary bypass, QRS > 180 ms)

The main sources of morbidity in adult pts after surgical correction are atrial arrhythmias, which can be present in 1/3 of pts (Circ 1995;91:2214).

Lab:

EKG: RVH, right axis deviation; after primary repair, RBBB and/or AV block may be present

CBC: Erythrocytosis

Echocardiogram: VSD, overriding aorta; RV outflow obstruction; RVH. Doppler study can assess the severity of RVOT obstruction and R-to-L shunting across VSD.

Cardiac catheterization: Determine location and magnitude of shunt and severity of LVOT obstruction and origin and course of the coronary arteries and pulmonary artery anatomy

X-ray: *CXR:* Heart size normal or small and "boot-shaped" (concave main PA segment); diminished lung markings; right-sided aortic arch may be present

Rx: Complete surgical correction (closure of VSD, relief of RVOT obstruction) has mortality < 3.0% in children, 2.5-8.5% in adults

Older surgical procedures included Waterston operation (side-to-side anastomosis of the ascending aorta and right PA), Potts operation (side-to-side anastomosis of the descending aorta to left PA), Blalock-Taussig operation (end-to-side anastomosis of the subclavian artery to PA); frequently resulted in pulmonary HT, LV volume overload

In a group of 115 pts undergoing repair at an average age of 4 yr, electrophysiologic studies 1 yr post-op induced ventricular arrhythmia in 4%. Phenytoin rx resulted in no sudden deaths in a 12-yr follow-up period (J Am Coll Cardiol 1997;30:1384).

Pts require infectious endocarditis prophylaxis before and after surgical correction. 25 yr after surgery, the cumulative incidence of infective endocarditis was 1.3% (Jama 1998;279:599).

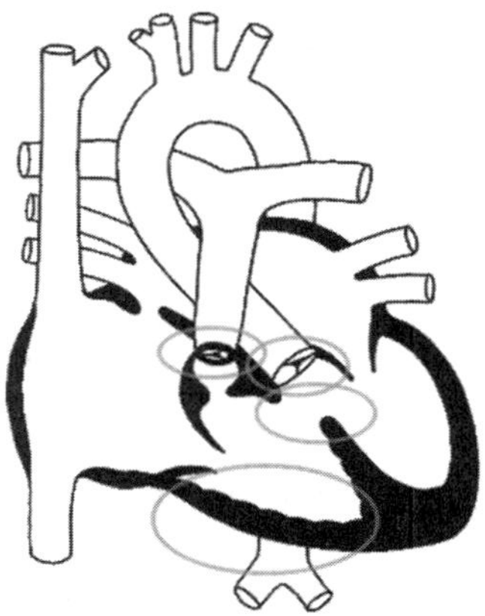

Tetralogy of Fallot

Figure 15.5 Tetralogy of Fallot.

15.8 Ebstein's Anomaly

Cause: Malformed anterior leaflet of tricuspid valve has abnormal attachment to RV wall. Septal leaflets (and sometimes posterior leaflets) are displaced a variable amount into the RV, so that a portion of the RV located on the atrial side of the tricuspid valve and functional RV is small. The tricuspid valve is regurgitant. 80% of pts have ASD/PDA.

Epidem: Most common congenital cause of significant tricuspid regurgitation

Pathophys: Pts with mild apical displacement of tricuspid leaflets have normal valve function. Severe displacement and valve dysfunction produce elevated RA pressures and R-to-L shunt across the septum.

Sx: Dyspnea; atypical chest pain; palpitations; syncope

Si: Cyanosis (depends on degree of R-to-L shunt); widely split S_1 and S_2; systolic click; S_3 or S_4 may be present; systolic murmur at lower LSB (due to TR); hepatomegaly

Children with Ebstein's anomaly frequently present as incidental murmur; adolescents/adults present with SV arrhythmia.

Crs: Most important predictors of outcome in adults: NYHA functional class, heart size, presence of cyanosis or SVT

Cmplc: Right-sided CHF; SVT; pts with interatrial communication are at risk for paradoxical embolization, brain abscess, sudden death

Lab:

EKG: Tall/broad P waves; first-degree AV block, RBBB; type B WPW pattern in 20% of pts

Echocardiogram: Confirms displacement of the tricuspid valve leaflets and can assess degree of RA enlargement, severity of tricuspid regurgitation/stenosis, presence and severity of interatrial shunting, and presence of associated cardiac abnormalities

Electrophysiologic evaluation: Indicated for atrial tachyarrhythmias

CONGENITAL HEART DISEASE IN ADULTS

X-ray: *CXR:* Heart and pulmonary vasculature normal in mild cases; RA enlargement, decreased pulmonary vascular markings in moderate/severe disease

Rx: CHF is treated with digoxin and diuretics.

Prophylaxis against infective endocarditis is recommended.

Atrial arrhythmias are treated pharmacologically. Catheter ablation can be undertaken if an accessory pathway is present, but the success rate is lower and the incidence of arrhythmia recurrence is higher than in pts with accessory pathways and normal tricuspid valves.

Repair/replacement of the tricuspid valve and closure of the interatrial communication are recommended for older pts with refractory sx or cardiac enlargement. This approach usually improves RV function and eliminates the risk of paradoxical emboli and reentrant arrhythmias.

Operative complications include complete heart block and persistence of SVT or tricuspid regurgitation.

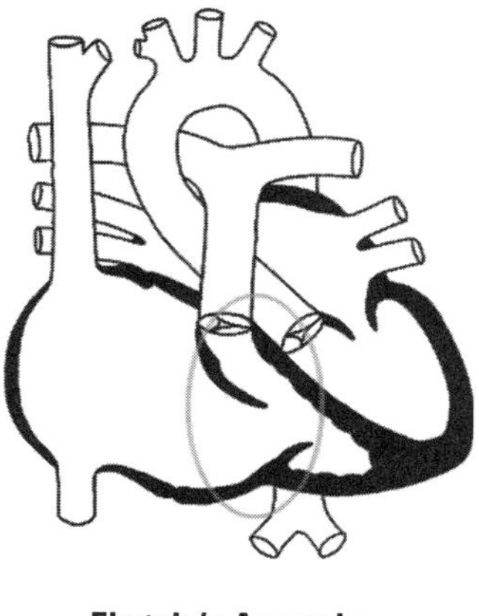

Ebstein's Anomaly

Figure 15.6 Ebstein's anomaly.

15.9 Eisenmenger's Syndrome

Cause: Most common cause of cyanosis in adults with congenital heart disease; seen in pts with ASD, VSD, PDA with large L-to-R shunt with the development of pulmonary vascular disease

Epidem: Matches that of predisposing congenital abnormalities

Pathophys: The pulmonary vasculature reponse to increased flow and pressure is medial hypertrophy of pulmonary arterioles, intimal proliferation and fibrosis, and occlusion of capillaries and small arterioles (potentially reversible), followed by irreversible necrotizing arteritis and obliteration of the pulmonary vascular bed. The process is irreversible once pulmonary vascular resistance reaches ~70% of systemic vascular resistance.

Sx: Dyspnea, fatigue, syncope, chest pain, palpitations, headache, hemoptysis

Si: Cyanosis; RV heave; pulmonary ejection sound or increased S_2; S_4; murmurs usually quiet/absent as L-to-R shunting diminishes

Crs: Survival after diagnosis 80% at 10 yr, 77% at 15 yr, 42% at 25 yr (Circ 1993;87:I-38); causes of death include arrhythmia, CHF, pulmonary infarction, brain abscess; sudden death common

Lab: Findings associated with underlying congenital lesion plus decreased O_2 saturation and polycythemia

X-ray: *CXR:* RV enlargement, prominent pulmonary arteries with peripheral oligemia

Rx: Avoidance of volume depletion, heavy exertion, high altitude, vasodilator use, pregnancy

Surgical closure of defects contraindicated when shunt reversal is present

No rx proven beneficial for pulmonary HT; use of iv epoprostenol under investigation

Phlebotomy indicated for severe sx of hyperviscosity

Heart-lung transplant or lung transplant with repair of cardiac defect for symptomatic pts with RV failure, syncope, ventricular arrhythmias has had limited success (Nejm 1999;340:1081)

Table 15.1 Exercise Guidelines for Pts with Congenital Heart Disease

No Restrictions
ASD, VSD, or PDA, small or operated on and without residual pulmonary HT
Pulmonary stenosis, gradient < 50 mm Hg
Aortic stenosis, peak gradient < 25 mm Hg
Aortic coarctation, treated and without gradient or significant HT
Tetralogy of Fallot, repaired without residue
Transposition of great vessels s/p arterial switch
Low-Intensity Sports
ASD, VSD, PDA, moderate
Pulmonary stenosis, gradient > 50 mm Hg
Aortic stenosis, peak gradient 25-49 mm Hg
Aortic coarctation, differential < 20 mm Hg
Unoperated/palliated cyanotic heart disease
Tetralogy of Fallot, repaired, with mild RV pressure/volume overload
Transposition of great vessels s/p atrial switch
Anomalous left coronary artery
Marfan's syndrome
No Competitive Sports
ASD, VSD, PDA with CHF or Eisenmenger's syndrome
Pulmonary stenosis, severe with symptoms
Aortic stenosis, peak gradient > 50 mm Hg
Aortic coarctation, differential > 20 mm Hg
Tetralogy of Fallot, repaired, with severe residua

Source: Adapted from the American College of Cardiology, J Am Coll Cardiol 1994;24:867.

Chapter 16

Heart Disease in Women

16.1 Coronary Artery Disease

Nejm 1996;334:1311

Despite its limited prognostic value, chest pain is the most common initial manifestation of ASHD in women. The risk of death due to ASHD in women is similar to that of men 10 yr younger. Death rates are 34% higher for black women than for white women. Smoking remains the leading preventable cause of ASHD in women; > 50% of MIs among middle-aged women are attributable to tobacco. Diabetes is associated with a 3- to 7-fold elevation in ASHD risk among women (Circ 1997;96:2468).

Elevated total cholesterol and LDL are only weakly associated with CAD in women (Nejm 1995;332:1758). HDL and triglycerides have greater predictive value (Atherosclerosis 1994;108:S73).

An increase in cholesterol precedes natural menopause by 3 yr and occurs at the time of surgical menopause (Circ 1996;94:61). During average follow-up of 4.1 yr, rx with oral conjugated estrogen plus medroxyprogesterone did not reduce the overall rate of coronary events in postmenopausal women with established CAD. Because more events occurred in the hormone group in yr 1 and fewer in yr 4 and 5, it could be appropriate for women already receiving this rx to continue it (HERS trial) (Jama 1998;280:605). A population-based case-control study concluded that low-dose oral contraceptives did not increase the risk of MI in women (Circ 1998;98:1058).

Estrogen and estrogen/medroxyprogesterone acetate produced reductions in LDL and increases in HDL cholesterol levels but did not alter the progression of coronary atherosclerosis in postmenopausal women with established disease (Nejm 2003;349:535; 2000;343:522). Estrogen plus progesterone did not protect against CAD in healthy postmenopausal women (Nejm 2003;349:523).

Among pts presenting to the ER with acute cardiac ischemia, gender is not an independent predictor of hospital mortality. Women tend to have higher mortality from AMI but are older and have greater frequency of diabetes and higher Killip class on presentation (J Am Coll Cardiol 1997;29:1490). Women with ACS are older than men and have more comorbidity. The outcome with unstable angina and non–Q-wave MI is related to severity of illness and not gender, and mortality associated with revascularization for unstable angina and non–Q-wave MI is similar for women and men (TIMI IIIb) (J Am Coll Cardiol 1997;30:141). After MI, younger women—but not older women—have higher rates of death during hospitalization than men of the same age; the younger the age of the pts, the higher the risk of death among women relative to men (NRMI 2 registry) (Nejm 1999;341:217).

Female survivors of cardiac arrest are less likely to have underlying CAD, but ASHD status is the most important predictor of survival in women, while impaired LV function is the most important predictor in men (Circ 1996;93:1170).

Although the unadjusted mortality rate suggests that women and men undergoing CABG and PTCA have a similar 5-yr mortality, women have higher risk profiles. Consequently, female sex is an independent predictor of improved 5-yr survival (Circ 1998;98:1279).

Treadmill testing without imaging is reported to have higher false-positive rates in women than in men (38-67% vs 7-44%); the false-negative rate in women is 12-22% (Am J Cardiol 1995;75:865). Radionuclide treadmill imaging has sensitivity of 71-93% and specificity of 85-91%. Dobutamine stress echocardiography reliably detects multivessel stenosis in women but is usually negative in single-vessel stenosis (WISE Study) (J Am Coll Cardiol 1999;33:1462).

ASA 100 mg po qd lowered the risk of CVA in women > 45 yr old but did not reduce the risk of MI or of death from CV causes (Nejm 2005;352:1293).

Cardiac Syndrome X: Chest pain with normal coronary angiograms; usually not associated with increased mortality or risk of CV events; may represent 20% of pts with chest pain and abnormal exercise EKGs; associated with reduced coronary microvascular dilatory response and increased coronary resistance along with subendocardial hypoperfusion on cardiac MRI in response to iv adenosine administration (Nejm 2002;346:1948; Am J Cardiol 1988;61:1338). Pts with microvascular angina secondary to systemic disease (DM, HT, amyloidosis, myeloma) and/or LBBB have a poor prognosis (Circ 2004;109:452). Rx includes imipramine for analgesia, aminophylline (adenosine receptor antagonist), TENS or spinal cord stimulation, and physical training.

16.2 Other Forms of Heart Disease

Aortic regurgitation: Indications for surgical correction of aortic regurgitation were established mostly in men. Unadjusted LV diameter surgical criteria result in criteria irrelevant to women, who often undergo surgery after developing severe sx and exhibit excess late mortality. Surgery should be performed even in asymptomatic pts if EF < 55% or if end-systolic dimension ≥ 55 mm. Whether smaller end-systolic dimension should be recommended in women is still in question (Circ 1996;94:2472).

Valvular disease in pregnancy: Mid-systolic murmurs develop in most women during pregnancy due to increased blood volume and CO. Lesions with low maternal and fetal risk include

- Asymptomatic AS with gradient < 50 mm Hg and normal LV function

- AI with NYHA class 1 or class II sx and normal LV function
- MR with NYHA class 1 or class II sx and normal LV function
- MVP with mild/moderate MR and normal LV function
- MS with valve area > 1.5 cm^2 and without severe pulmonary HT
- Mild/moderate PS

High-maternal-risk lesions include

- EF < 40%
- H/o CHF
- H/o TIA/CVA

High-maternal- and fetal-risk lesions include

- Severe AS
- AI with class III or class IV sx
- MS with class III or class IV sx
- MR with class III or class IV sx
- Any valvular disease with severe pulmonary HT
- Aortic or mitral valve disease with EF < 40% (Nejm 2003; 349:52)

Prosthetic heart valves and pregnancy: Pts with mechanical valves require close monitoring of warfarin rx. Pts with bioprosthetic valves do not require anticoagulation but have increased risk of structural valve deterioration during and after pregnancy. The reported risk of warfarin embryopathy is 0-7.6%; it is lowest in women who require ≤ 5 mg warfarin qd. Use of iv heparin for first 6-12 wk and last 2 wk of pregnancy may reduce the risk of warfarin embryopathy (Chest 2004;126:627S; Circ 2003;107:1240).

HCM: Increases maternal mortality in high-risk women during pregnancy, but development of sx, Afib, or syncope is uncommon (J Am Coll Cardiol 2002;40:1864)

Dilated cardiomyopathy: In pts with end-stage CHF, 60% NYHA class IV, LVEF 18 ± 4.9%, women appear to have better survival than men; finding is strongest among pts with a nonischemic etiology of CHF (FIRST study) (Circ 1999;99:1816)

Athletes: In highly trained women athletes, 8% had absolute LV cavity size exceeding normal limits. Absolute LV wall thickness was within normal limits for all women athletes. Clinical differentiation of athlete's heart and hypertrophic cardiomyopathy is a diagnostic dilemma limited to male athletes (Jama 1996; 276:211).

16.3 Stroke

The incidence of stroke is ~19% higher in men than in women. Among older adults, gender differences disappear after adjustment for age. The incidence of ischemic stroke for persons with h/o TIA is higher in women than in men. Risk factors uniquely associated with stroke in women include fibromuscular dysplasia, choriocarcinoma, mitral annular calcification, pregnancy, migraine, mitral valve prolapse, antiphospholipid syndrome, Takayasu's arteritis, retinocochleocerebral vasculopthathy, and SLE (Circ 1997;96:2468).

Estrogens: In a population-based case-control study, overall risk for stroke and for particular types of stroke was not increased among current users of low-dose oral contraceptives (Ann IM 1997;127:596).

Risks of cerebral infarction and intracerebral hemorrhage are increased in the 6 wk after delivery but not during pregnancy itself (Nejm 1996;335:768).

16.4 Hypertension and Vascular Disease

In the HERS trial, estrogen/progesterone rx did increase the rate of thromboembolic events.

In a retrospective cohort study, the risk for venous thromboembolism was increased eightfold in women with an inherited deficiency of antithrombin, protein C, or protein S (Ann IM 1996;125:955). Among users of low-dose oral contraceptives, disease occurred mainly in smokers and women with predisposing factors (Ann IM 1998; 128:467).

Unopposed estrogen rx is associated with the Raynaud phenomenon in postmenopausal women; this association was not found in women receiving combined hormone therapy (Ann IM 1998;129:208).

Pulmonary embolism: In a prospective study based on questionnaires with 16-yr follow-up, obesity, cigarette smoking, and HT were associated with increased risk of PE in women (Jama 1997; 277:642).

Excess weight and adult weight gain increased the risk for HT, and weight loss reduced the risk for HT in a cohort of 82,473 U.S. female nurses (Ann IM 1998;128:81).

Although use of oral contraceptives is associated with increased risk of HT, only 41.5 cases/10,000 person-years could be attributed to oral contraceptive use, and risk decreased quickly with cessation of oral contraceptives (Circ 1996;94:483).

16.5 Pregnancy

Normal pregnancy is associated with a reversible fall in contractility. Systolic function is preserved by a fall in afterload but decreases near term and early postpartum as a result of decreased contractility and diminished preload (Circ 1996;94:667).

Pts with h/o a single episode of DVT have low incidence of recurrence antepartum and may not require prophylactic heparin (Nejm 2000;343:1439). The safety of ASA during the 1st trimester is still a subject of debate. For other cardiac drugs, see Table 16.1.

Hypertension: Gestational HT usually appears in the 3rd trimester and is mild. Preeclampsia typically appears after 20 wk of gestation, can be mild or severe, and is characterized by proteinuria and (in severe cases) by hemoconcentration, thrombocytopenia, and hepatic dysfunction. Maternal and neonatal outcomes are usually good among pregnant women with mild chronic HT or gestational HT. Preeclampsia is potentially dangerous for both mother and fetus and does not respond well to conventional antihypertensive rx; med-

Table 16.1 Cardiovascular Drugs in Pregnancy

Drug	Potential Fetal Adverse Effects	Safety
Warfarin	Crosses placental barrier, fetal hemorrhage in utero, embryopathy, CNS abnormalities	Unsafe
Heparin	None reported	Probably safe
Digoxin	Low birth weight	Safe
Quinidine	Toxic dose may induce premature labor and cause damage to fetal 8th cranial nerve	Safe
Procainamide	None reported	Safe
Disopyramide	May initiate uterine contractions	*
Lidocaine	High blood levels and fetal acidosis may cause CNS depression	Safe
Mexiletine	Fetal bradycardia, IUGR, low Apgar score, neonatal hypoglycemia, neonatal bradycardia, and neonatal hyperthyroidism	*
Flecainide	1 reported fetal death	*
Propafenone	None reported	*
Adenosine	None reported; use during 1st trimester limited to a few pts	Safe
Amiodarone	IUGR, prematurity, hypothyroidism	Unsafe
Calcium-channel blocking agents	Fetal distress due to maternal hypotension	*
β-Adrenergic blocking agents	IUGR, apnea at birth, bradycardia, hypoglycemia, hyperbilirubinemia; β_2-blockade blocking agents may initiate uterine contractions	Safe
Hydralazine	None reported	Safe
Sodium nitroprusside	Potential thiocyanate toxicity with high dose, fetal mortality with nitroprusside in animal studies	Potentially unsafe

continues

Table 16.1 continued

Drug	Potential Fetal Adverse Effects	Safety
Organic nitrates	Fetal heart rate deceleration and bradycardia	*
ACE inhibitors	Skull ossification defect, IUGR, premature deliveries, low birth weight, oligohydramnios, neonatal renal failure, anemia and death, limb contractures, patent ductus arteriosus	Unsafe
Diuretic agents	Impairment of uterine blood flow and danger of placental hypoperfusion, thrombocytopenia, jaundice hyponatremia, bradycardia	Potentially unsafe

IUGR = intrauterine growth retardation.
*To date, only limited information is available, and safety during pregnancy cannot be established.
Source: Reprinted with permission, Braunwald: Heart Disease, 5/E, © 1997 Elsevier, Inc.

ical supervision and timely delivery are the keys to rx (Nejm 1996; 335:257). Use of β-blockers during pregnancy may lower infant birth weight. ACEIs are associated with urogenital defects, intrauterine gestational retardation, and fetal death and are contraindicated during pregnancy.

Calcium supplementation during pregnancy can reduce systolic and diastolic BP and preeclampsia. More data are needed to confirm calcium's impact on maternal and fetal morbidity (Jama 1996;275:1113).

In a retrospective study, postpartum interval was associated with an increase in risk for cardiac events among pts with long QT syndrome; prophylactic rx with β-blockers is recommended (Circ 1998;97:451).

In pts with known heart disease, poor maternal functional class, cyanosis, myocardial dysfunction, left heart obstruction, prior arrhythmia, and prior cardiac events are all predictive of maternal cardiac complications. In 1 study, maternal heart failure, arrhythmia, or stroke occurred in 18% of completed pregnancies, and neonatal complications (death, respiratory distress syndrome, intraventricular hemorrhage, premature birth, and small-for-gestational-age birth weight) occurred in 17% (Circ 1997;96:2789).

16.6 Prevention

Reduced exercise capacity in asymptomatic women is a stronger independent predictor of CV death than in men (Circ 2003;108:1554). Higher folate intake is associated with reduction in risk of HT (Jama 2005;293:320).

Vigorous exercise is reported to facilitate short- and longer-term smoking cessation in women when combined with a cognitive-behavioral smoking cessation program and delayed weight gain following smoking cessation (Arch IM 1999;159:1229). Prospective data indicate that brisk walking and vigorous exercise are associated with substantial and similar reductions in the incidence of coronary events among women (Nejm 1999;341:650).

Among women, adherence to lifestyle guidelines involving diet, exercise, and abstinence from smoking is associated with a very low risk of CAD (Nejm 2000;343:16).

Nurses' Health Study: Low levels of HDL are a major contributor to risk of CAD events in postmenopausal women (Circ 2004;110:2824). Moderate alcohol consumption is associated with reduced CHD risk in women with diabetes (Circ 2000;102:494).

A dietary source of a partial estrogen agonist are the phytoestrogens. Epidemiologic data indicate that women ingesting high amounts of phytoestrogens—particularly as isoflavones in soy products—have less cardiac and vascular disease, breast and uterine cancer, and menopausal symptoms than those eating Western diets. Clinical studies have found that isoflavones have lipid-lowering effects and an ability to inhibit LDL oxidation (J Am Coll Cardiol 2000;35:1403).

In 27,939 healthy women followed for 8 yr, hsCRP was a stronger predictor of CV events than were serum LDL levels (Nejm 2002; 347:1557).

In older women with CV disease, a linear relationship exists between systolic BP and risk of events (Circ 2004;109:623). In these pts, antioxidant vitamin supplements provided no CV benefit (Jama 2002;288:2432).

AHA recommendations: See Jama 2004;291:2243.

Chapter 17

Prevention and Assessment

17.1 Prevention of CAD

See also **ASHD.**

Circ 1999;100:988

Risk Assessment

See Table 17.1 and Figures 17.1 and 17.2 for assessment.

Smoking

Compared with other preventive interventions, smoking cessation is extremely cost-effective. The more intensive the intervention, the lower the cost. Intensive counseling and the nicotine patch are particularly useful (Jama 1997;278:1759).

AHCPR recommendations: Every person who smokes should be offered smoking cessation treatment at every office visit. Cessation treatments even as brief as 3 min per visit are effective. More intense treatment is more effective in producing long-term abstinence. Three treatment elements, in particular, are effective, and one or more of these elements should be included in smoking cessation treatment: (1) nicotine replacement therapy (nicotine patches or gum), (2) social support (clinician-provided encouragement and assistance), and (3) skills training/problem solving (techniques on achieving and maintaining abstinence).

Table 17.1 Categories of Risk Factors for CAD
Causative Risk Factors
Cigarette smoking
Elevated blood pressure
Elevated serum cholesterol (or LDL cholesterol)
Alternative: elevated apolipoprotein B
Low HDL cholesterol
Diabetes mellitus
Coronary plaque burden as a risk factor
Age
Nonspecific ST-segment changes on resting EKG
Conditional Risk Factors
Triglycerides[1]
Small LDL particles[1]
Lp(a)[1]
Homocysteine[1]
Coagulation factors[1]
Plasminogen activating factor inhibitor-1
Fibrinogen
C-reactive protein
Predisposing Risk Factors
Overweight and obesity (especially abdominal obesity)[2]
Physical inactivity[2]
Male sex
Family h/o premature CHD
Socioeconomic factors
Behavioral factors (eg, mental depression)
Insulin resistance
Susceptibility risk factor
Left ventricular hypertrophy

[1]These factors are considered conditional risk factors when serum levels are abnormally high.
[2]Obesity and physical inactivity are counted as major risk factors by the AHA.
(Circ 2000;101:111)

Age	Points
20-34	−9
35-39	−4
40-44	0
45-49	3
50-54	6
55-59	8
60-64	10
65-69	11
70-74	12
75-79	13

Total Cholesterol	Points				
	Age 20-39	Age 40-49	Age 50-59	Age 60-69	Age 70-79
< 160	0	0	0	0	0
160-199	4	3	2	1	0
200-239	7	5	3	1	0
240-279	9	6	4	2	1
≥ 280	11	8	5	3	1

	Points				
	Age 20-39	Age 40-49	Age 50-59	Age 60-69	Age 70-79
Nonsmoker	0	0	0	0	0
Smoker	8	5	3	1	1

HDL (mg/dL)	Points
≥ 60	−1
50-59	0
40-49	1
< 40	2

Systolic BP (mm Hg)	If Untreated	If Treated
< 120	0	0
120-129	0	1
130-139	1	2
140-159	1	2
≥ 160	2	3

Figure 17.1 Calculation of CAD risk in men (ATP-III). (NIH)

Continues

PREVENTION AND ASSESSMENT

Point Total	10-Year Risk %
< 0	< 1
0	1
1	1
2	1
3	1
4	1
5	2
6	2
7	3
8	4
9	5
10	6
11	8
12	10
13	12
14	16
15	20
16	25
≥ 17	≥ 30

Figure 17.1 continued

Substantial evidence exists for risk factor clustering in smokers. Smokers are more likely than nonsmokers to have elevated lipids and HT (Circ 1997;96:3243).

Post-CABG, smokers 1 yr after surgery had more than twice the risk for MI and reoperation compared with pts who stopped smoking. Pts who were still smoking at 5 yr after surgery had even more elevated risks for MI, reoperation, and increased risk for angina. Pts who started to smoke again within 5 yr after surgery had increased risks for reoperation and angina. No differences in outcome were found between pts who stopped smoking since surgery and nonsmokers (Circ 1996;93:42).

Age	Points
20-34	−7
35-39	−3
40-44	0
45-49	3
50-54	6
55-59	8
60-64	10
65-69	12
70-74	14
75-79	16

Total Cholesterol	Points				
	Age 20-39	Age 40-49	Age 50-59	Age 60-69	Age 70-79
< 160	0	0	0	0	0
160-199	4	3	2	1	1
200-239	8	6	4	2	1
240-279	11	8	5	3	2
≥ 280	13	10	7	4	2

	Points				
	Age 20-39	Age 40-49	Age 50-59	Age 60-69	Age 70-79
Nonsmoker	0	0	0	0	0
Smoker	9	7	4	2	1

HDL (mg/dL)	Points
≥ 60	−1
50-59	0
40-49	1
< 40	2

Systolic BP (mm Hg)	If Untreated	If Treated
< 120	0	0
120-129	1	3
130-139	2	4
140-159	3	5
≥ 160	4	6

Figure 17.2 Calculation of CAD risk in women (ATP-III). (NIH)

Point Total	10-Year Risk %
< 9	< 1
9	1
10	1
11	1
12	1
13	2
14	2
15	3
16	4
17	5
18	6
19	8
20	11
21	14
22	17
23	22
24	27
≥ 25	≥ 30

Figure 17.2 continued

Data on exposure to passive smoking as assessed by self-report suggest that regular exposure increases risk of CAD among non-smoking women (Circ 1997;95:237).

Data on smokeless tobacco are inconclusive: Adverse CV effects are less than those caused by smoking but are greater than those found in non-tobacco users (Arch IM 2004;164:1845).

BP

HCTZ, atenolol, captopril, clonidine, diltiazem, and prazosin have no long-term adverse effects on plasma lipids. Previously reported short-term adverse effects from using HCTZ are limited to nonresponders (Arch IM 1999;159:551).

MRFIT (7-yr multifactor intervention program for lowering BP and serum cholesterol and for smoking cessation among high-risk men): At 16 yr, the intervention group had an 11.4% lower CAD mortality rate and a 20.4% lower rate for acute MI (Circ 1996; 94:946).

Lipids

The risk/benefit ratio supports use of statins in CAD. Elevated hepatic enzyme or CK levels < 10× nl require close monitoring but do not automatially mandate cessation of rx (Circ 2002;40:567).

In a study of 1017 young men followed 27-42 yr, the risk of developing CV disease in midlife correlated with earliest serum cholesterol levels (J Am Coll Cardiol 2002;40:2122; Nejm 1993;328:313). Statin therapy appears to be safe and effective in children with homozygous familial hyperlipidemia (Circ 2002;106:2231).

In pts at high risk for development of CAD, LDL goal of < 70 mg/dL is a therapeutic option (J Am Coll Cardiol 2004;44:720).

In elderly pts (4736 pts with mean age 72), baseline total, non-HDL, and LDL cholesterol levels and ratios of total, non-HDL, and LDL to HDL cholesterol are significantly related to CAD incidence. HDL cholesterol and triglycerides were not significant (SHEP program) (Circ 1996;94:2381).

In a small controlled study, cholesterol lowering with lovastatin produced a significant reduction in the number of episodes of ST-segment depression on AECG in pts with known ASHD (Circ 1997;95:324).

In middle-aged/elderly white men, a high level of fasting triglycerides is an independent risk factor for ASHD (Circ 1998;97:1029).

In a 5-yr prospective follow-up study of 2156 French Canadian men, Lp(a) was not an independent risk factor for ASHD but increased risk when associated with other lipid risk factors (J Am Coll Cardiol 1998;31:519).

Although current guidelines target reduction of LDL as the primary goal, rx of pts with low HDL has been shown to reduce future event risk (Circ 2003;109:1809).

In all populations studied, pts who were prescribed lipid-lowering drugs remained without filled prescriptions for over 1/3 of the study year. After 5 yr, ~50% of the surviving cohort had stopped using lipid-lowering rx altogether (Jama 1998;279:1458).

Activity

In a study of 25,714 adult men age 44 ± 10 yrs, low cardiorespiratory fitness was an independent predictor of CVD and all-cause mortality (Jama 1999;282:1547). In previously sedentary healthy adults, lifestyle and physical activity intervention was as effective as a structured exercise program in improving cardiorespiratory fitness and BP (Jama 1999;281:327). In the Physicians' Health Study, habitual vigorous exercise reduced the risk of sudden death during exercise (Nejm 2000;343:1355).

In older (mean age 68 ± 5 yr) pts s/p MI, CABG, peak aerobic capacity improves with aerobic conditioning. The mechanism appears to be associated with peripheral skeletal muscle adaptations with no discernible improvements in CO (Circ 1996;94:323).

Regular weekly exercise can improve lipid profile independent of weight loss (Nejm 2002;347:1483). Walking and vigorous exercise are associated with a reduction in the incidence of CV events in postmenopausal women (Nejm 2002;347:716).

In a study of men with known ASHD who were enrolled in a program of physical exercise and low-fat diet, coronary stenoses progressed at a significantly slower rate than in the control group. Angiographic changes appeared to be largely due to chronic physical exercise (Circ 1997;96:2534).

Women with heart disease participating in a cardiac rehab program showed a 38% decrease in total cholesterol/HDL cholesterol over 5 yr (14% decrease in men). Total cholesterol decreased 20% in women and 8% in men, and LDL cholesterol decreased 34% in women and 15% in men (Circ 1995;92:773).

In a Finnish twin cohort study, leisure-time physical activity was associated with reduced mortality even after genetic and other familial factors were taken into account (Jama 1998;279:440).

Ornish: Intensive lifestyle changes may lead to regression of coronary atherosclerosis after 1 yr. More regression occurred after 5 yr than after 1 yr in an experimental group, while coronary atherosclerosis continued to progress and more than twice as many cardiac events occurred in controls (Jama 1998;280:2001).

Exercise Prescription

If an individual is < 40 yr old and asymptomatic, no further workup is needed. If an individual is > 40 yr old, an exercise test is recommended if vigorous exercise is planned. If test is normal, no further restrictions are needed. If test is abnormal, the individual should be treated as if he/she has CAD. If the pt has no known CVD but major risk factors or sx that suggest CAD, an exercise test is needed.

In the absence of ischemia/significant arrhythmias, exercise intensity should approximate 50-80% of VO_{2max}, as ascertained by exercise test (use target of 20 beat/min above resting HR until test performed); target HR is 50-75% of heart rate reserve:

$$\text{Resting HR} + (0.5 \textit{ or } 0.75) \times (\text{max HR} - \text{resting HR})$$

Target work intensity: Achieve training HR after 5-10 min of steady-state workload, expressed in METs. For walking on a level surface, activity can be prescribed as the step rate found on a treadmill to generate the desired HR.

Can also judge intensity of exercise as a rating of perceived exertion, which can be equated to desirable HR during laboratory exercise. A value < 12 correlates with light exercise (40-60% of max), 12-14 correlates with somewhat hard exercise (60-75% of max), and 14-16 correlates with hard exercise (75-90% of max).

The appropriate initial intensity of training is 50-60% of VO_{2max} or a rating of perceived exertion of 12-13 on a scale of 6-20. Increase duration in 5-min increments q 1 wk or as HR response to exercise decreases with conditioning.

In the presence of ischemia/arrhythmia, an exercise test is essential. Recommended training HR is 10 beat/min less than that associated with abnormal findings.

For *apparently healthy* individuals, there is no evidence of increased cardiovascular risk for exercise. EKG, BP monitoring, and exercise supervision are not required.

For individuals with *known, stable cardiovascular disease with low risk for vigorous exercise* (NYHA class 1 or 2, exercise capacity > 6 METs, no evidence of CHF, free of ischemia/angina at rest or on exercise test at 6 METs, appropriate rise in systolic BP during exercise, no sequential PVCs), moderate activity is not believed to be associated with increased risk. Monitor EKG and BP during the early prescription phase of training. Provide medical supervision during prescription sessions, and nonmedical supervision for other exercise sessions until the pt understands how to monitor activity.

For individuals at *moderate/high risk for cardiac complications during exercise* (pts with ≥ 2 MIs, NYHA class 3 or greater, exercise capacity < 6 METs, ischemic horizontal or downsloping ST depression ≥ 4 mm or angina during exercise, fall in systolic BP with exercise, previous episode of primary cardiac arrest, VT at workload < 6 METs, cardiomyopathy, valvular heart disease, exercise test abnormalities not directly related to ischemia, previous episode of VF/cardiac arrest, complex ventricular arrhythmias uncontrolled at mild/moderate work intensities with medication, 3-vessel disease or left main disease, EF < 30%), continuous EKG and BP monitoring and medical supervision are required during exercise sessions until their safety is established.

For individuals with *unstable disease with activity restriction* (unstable ischemia, uncompensated CHF, uncontrolled arrhythmias, severe and symptomatic AS), no activity is recommended for conditioning purposes.

Weight/Diet

Obesity is defined as weight > 30% above desirable, BMI ≥ 30, or waist circumference > 40 in. in men or > 35 in. in women (Figure 17.3) and is an independent risk factor for CAD mortality among men and contributes to risk of CAD among women. Part of the risk is mediated through other known cardiovascular risk factors (Circ 1996;93:1372). Risk of death from cardiovascular disease increases throughout the range of moderate and severe overweight for both men and women in all age groups (Nejm 1999;341:1097). Offspring of parents with early CAD were overweight beginning in childhood and developed an adverse cardiovascular risk factor profile at an increased rate (Jama 1997;278:1749).

After 1 yr, moderate restriction of dietary fat intake produces sustained LDL-C reductions in hypercholesterolemic pts; more extreme restriction of fat intake offers little further advantage (Jama 1997; 278:1509).

High Na^+ intake is strongly associated with increased risk of CVD and all-cause mortality in overweight persons (Jama 1999; 282:2027).

In a dietary study of 43,757 U.S. male health professionals, cereal fiber was most strongly associated with a reduced risk of total MI, independent of fat intake (Jama 1996;275:447).

Nurses Health Study: Consumption of fruits and vegetables—particularly cruciferous and green leafy vegetables and citrus fruit and juice—may reduce ischemic stroke risk (Jama 1999;282:1233).

Dietary fish consumption and omega-3 fatty acid intake are not associated with reduced risk of MI, nonsudden cardiac death, or total cardiovascular mortality. Fish consumption is associated with significantly reduced risk of total mortality (Jama 1998;279:23).

A population study of 22,043 adults in Greece reported an association between adherence to the Mediterranean diet and reduction in total mortality (Nejm 2003;348:2599). The Lyon Diet Heart Study demonstrated a reduction in CV events after first MI in pts who followed a Mediterranean-type diet (Circ 1999;99:779).

Locate the height of interest in the leftmost column and read across the row for that height to the weight of interest. Follow the column of the weight up to the top row that lists the BMI. BMI of 19-24 is the healthy weight range, BMI of 25-29 is the overweight range, and BMI of 30 and above in the obese range.

Height — Weight in Pounds

BMI	19	20	21	22	23	24	25	26	27	28	29	30	31	32	33	34	35
4′10″	91	96	100	105	110	115	119	124	129	134	138	143	148	153	158	162	167
4′11″	94	99	104	109	114	119	124	128	133	138	143	148	153	158	163	168	173
5′	97	102	107	112	118	123	128	133	138	143	148	153	158	163	168	174	179
5′1″	100	106	111	116	122	127	132	137	143	148	153	158	164	169	174	180	185
5′2″	104	109	115	120	126	131	136	142	147	153	158	164	169	175	180	186	191
5′3″	107	113	118	124	130	135	141	146	152	158	163	169	175	180	186	191	197
5′4″	110	116	122	128	134	140	145	151	157	163	169	174	180	186	192	197	204
5′5″	114	120	126	132	138	144	150	156	162	168	174	180	186	192	198	204	210
5′6″	118	124	130	136	142	148	155	161	167	173	179	186	192	198	204	210	216
5′7″	121	127	134	140	146	153	159	166	172	178	185	191	198	204	211	217	223
5′8″	125	131	138	144	151	158	164	171	177	184	190	197	203	210	216	223	230
5′9″	128	135	142	149	155	162	169	176	182	189	196	203	209	216	223	230	236
5′10″	132	139	146	153	160	167	174	181	188	195	202	209	216	222	229	236	243
5′11″	136	143	150	157	165	172	179	186	193	200	208	215	222	229	236	243	250
6′	140	147	154	162	169	177	184	191	199	206	213	221	228	235	242	250	258
6′1″	144	151	159	166	174	182	189	197	204	212	219	227	235	242	250	257	265
6′2″	148	155	163	171	179	186	194	202	210	218	225	233	241	249	256	264	272
6′3″	152	160	168	176	184	192	200	208	216	224	232	240	248	256	264	272	279

Healthy Weight (BMI 19–24) | Overweight (BMI 25–29) | Obese (BMI 30–35)

Figure 17.3 Adult BMI chart. (NHLBI Clinical Guidelines on Obesity in Adults, 1998)

Multivariable analyses showed a significant, inverse relationship between tea intake and severe aortic atherosclerosis (Arch IM 1999;159:2170).

In eastern France, moderate wine drinking was associated with lower all-cause mortality; drinking both wine and beer reduced risk of cardiovascular death (Arch IM 1999;159:1865). Men who consumed light-to-moderate amounts of alcohol (2-6 drinks/wk) had a reduced risk of sudden cardiac death compared with those who rarely or never consumed alcohol (Circ 1999;100:944).

Soy protein may lower total and HDL cholesterol levels and triglycerides and is recommended for inclusion in diet by AHA (Circ 2000;102;2555; Nejm 1995;333:276).

Here is the consensus in nutrient recommendations from several different organizations:

- Saturated fat: < 10% of calories
- Total fat: 30% of total calories
- Polyunsaturated fat: 10% of total calories
- Monounsaturated fat: 15% of total calories
- Cholesterol: 300 mg/dL
- Carbohydrates: 55% of total calories
- Total calories: to achieve and maintain desirable weight
- Salt intake: < 6 gm/dL (Circ 1999;100:450)
- Weight: See Figure 17.3

Metabolic Syndrome

Circ 2003;108:1422,1537; 2002;106:286

Components include

- Abdominal obesity (waist circumference ≥ 40 in. in men, ≥ 35 in. in women)
- Atherogenic dyslipidemia (triglycerides ≥ 150 mg/dL, HDL ≤ 40 mg/dL in men and ≤ 50 mg/dL in women)
- BP ≥ 130/≥ 85 mm Hg
- Insulin resistance ± glucose intolerance (FBS ≥ 110 mg/dL) (ATP III)

WHO clinical criteria:

- NIDDM, impaired fasting glucose, or impaired glucose tolerance plus any of the following:
- Antihypertensive rx and/or BP $\geq$ 140/$\geq$ 90 mm Hg
- Plasma triglycerides $\geq$ 150 mg/dL
- HDL $\leq$ 35 mg/dL in men or $\leq$ 39 mg/dL in women
- BMI $\geq$ 30 kg/m^2
- Urinary albumin excretion rate $\geq$ 20 μgm/min or albumin: creatinine ratio $\geq$ 30 mg/gm

Framingham Study: metabolic syndrome predicted ~25% of all new CVD (Circ 2004;109:433). NHANES: Syndrome was associated with increased MI and CVA risk in both men and women (Circ 2004;110:1245; 2004;109:42).

First-line rx is lifestyle modification, 7-10% reduction of body weight in obese persons over 6-12 mon, minimum of 30 min of exercise qd (Circ 2004;109:551).

Drugs/Supplements

ASA use: Absolute risk reduction of 137 events/10,000 persons in MI, 39 events/10,000 persons in ischemic stroke, absolute risk increase of 12 events/10,000 persons in hemorrhagic stroke; overall benefit may outweigh adverse effects in most populations (Jama 1998;280:1930).

Long-term vitamin E supplementation improves endothelium-dependent relaxation in forearm resistance vessels of hypercholesterolemic smokers (J Am Coll Cardiol 1999;33:499). However, in pts at high risk for cardiovascular events, rx with vitamin E for a mean of 4.5 yr had no apparent effect on cardiovascular outcomes (Nejm 2000;342:154) and may increase the risk of CHF in pts with vascular disease or renal failure (Jama 2005;293:1338).

Supplementation with α-tocopherol was associated with only a minor decrease in angina incidence. β-Carotene has no preventive effect and was associated with an slight increase in angina (Jama

1996;275:693). Antioxidant vitamin use does not reduce 5-yr mortality from CVD (Lancet 2002;360:23).

Ingestion of plant sterols/stanols appears to be safe and reduces LDL levels by ~10% (Mayo Clin Proc 2003;78:965).

Homocysteine concentrations > 80th percentile, red cell folate concentrations < 10th percentile, and vitamin B_6 concentrations < 20th percentile are associated with an increased risk of vascular disease independent of traditional risk factors (Circ 1998;97:437). In 35 human studies, homocysteine levels were consistently higher in pts with ASHD ($n = 4338$) than in controls ($n = 22,593$) (Arch IM 1997;157:2299). Elevated nonfasting homocysteine levels were independently associated with increased rates of all-cause and CVD mortality in the elderly (Arch IM 1999;159:1077). The association between homocysteine levels and CVD is generally strong but data from prospective studies are less consistent; epidemiologic observations of association do not prove the existence of a causal relationship (Ann IM 1999;131:363). Hypothyroidism may be a treatable cause of hyperhomocysteinemia (Ann IM 1999;131:348).

Estrogens: See Chapter 16.

Psych

J Am Coll Cardiol 2005;45:637

In an observational study of 1190 male medical students followed 40 yr, clinical depression was an independent risk factor for incident CAD for several decades after the onset of the clinical depression (Arch IM 1998;158:1422). In a community sample of 6676 initially stroke-free adults, depressive sx were associated with increased risk of stroke mortality (Arch IM 1998;158:1133). In Glostrup, Denmark, depressive sx were associated with increased risks of MI and mortality. This risk factor is best viewed as a continuous variable that represents a chronic psychological characteristic (Circ 1996;93:1976).

The association between psychotropic medication use and MI is probably a reflection of the primary relationship between depression and MI (Circ 1996;94:3123).

The Northridge, California, earthquake was a significant trigger of sudden death due to cardiac causes, independently of physical exertion. This finding suggests that emotional stress may precipitate cardiac events in people predisposed to such events (Nejm 1996;334:413).

Mental stress during daily life can more than double the risk of myocardial ischemia in the subsequent hour (Jama 1997; 277:1521). The presence of mental stress-induced ischemia was associated with higher rates of subsequent fatal/nonfatal cardiac events, independent of age, baseline LVEF, previous MI, and predicted events over and above exercise-induced ischemia (Jama 1996;275:1651).

CAD risk is related to 5 specific psychosocial domains: (1) depression, (2) anxiety, (3) personality factors and character traits, (4) social isolation, and (5) chronic life stress. Psychosocial conditions can contribute to adverse health behaviors as well as to neuroendocrine and platelet activation (J Am Coll Cardiol 2005;45:637; Circ 1999;99:2192).

Mechanisms: Mental stress-induced myocardial ischemia is associated with a significant increase in SVR and minor increase in HR and rate-pressure product compared with ischemia induced by exercise (Circ 1996;94:2402). Mental stress in the laboratory results in a substantial sympathetic response in normal middle-aged and older men and women, but EF commonly falls because of a concomitant rise in afterload (Circ 1996;94:2768). Abnormal PVR responses to mental stress and exercise are observed in patients with a mental stress-induced fall in LVEF (J Am Coll Cardiol 1998;31:1314).

Hypertensive but not hypercholesterolemic patients have impaired NO-dependent vasodilation during mental stress (J Am Coll Cardiol 1998;32:1207).

PIMI: Pts with daily-life ischemia exhibit a heightened generalized response to mental stress. ST-segment depression in response to mental or exercise stress is predictive of ST-segment depression during routine daily activities (J Am Coll Cardiol 1999;33:1476).

In pts with prior positive exercise stress tests, mental stress-induced ischemia, as defined by new wall motion abnormalities, predicts daily ischemia independent of exercise-induced ischemia (Circ 1995;92:2102). Both nifedipine and atenolol are effective in preventing mental stress-induced wall-motion abnormalities (mechanisms of prevention may be different) (J Am Coll Cardiol 1998;32:1680).

Mental stress alters VT cycle length and could contribute to sudden death through the facilitation of lethal ventricular arrhythmias (Circ 2000;101:158).

17.2 Perioperative Assessment and Management

Circ 2002;105:1257

Clinical Predictors of Increased Perioperative Cardiovascular Risk

Major: Unstable coronary syndromes such as recent MI with evidence of important ischemic risk and unstable or severe angina; decompensated CHF, significant arrhythmias (high-grade AV block, symptomatic arrhythmias in the presence of underlying heart disease, supraventricular arrhythmias with uncontrolled ventricular rate), severe valvular disease

Intermediate: Mild angina pectoris, prior MI, compensated or prior CHF, DM

Minor: Advanced age, abnormal EKG, rhythm other than sinus, low functional capacity, h/o stroke, uncontrolled systemic HT

Surgery Risk

High-Risk Surgery: Major emergency surgery, particularly in elderly pts; aortic and other major vascular surgery; peripheral vascular surgery; anticipated prolonged procedures associated with large fluid shifts and/or blood loss

Intermediate-Risk Procedures: Carotid endarterectomy, head and neck surgery, intraperitoneal and intrathoracic, orthopedic, and prostate surgery

Low-Risk Procedures: Endoscopic and superficial procedures, cataract surgery, breast surgery

Energy Expenditure

Eating, dressing, walking around the house, dishwashing: 1-4 METs

Climbing 1 flight of stairs, walking on level ground at 6.4 km/hr, running a short distance, scrubbing floors, or playing a game of golf: 4-10 METs

Strenuous sports (swimming, singles tennis, football): > 10 METs

Self-reported exercise tolerance can be used to predict in-hospital perioperative risk (Arch IM 1999;159:2185).

Steps for Pre-op Evaluation of Pts for Noncardiac Surgery (AHA)

Is surgery emergent? Emergencies may not allow time for preoperative cardiac evaluation.

Coronary revascularization in past 5 yr? If so and clinically stable, further cardiac testing is generally not necessary.

Coronary evaluation in past 2 yr? If findings are favorable, repeat testing is usually not necessary unless pt is experiencing changed/new sx.

Unstable coronary syndrome or major clinical predictor of risk? Defer elective surgery.

Intermediate predictor of risk plus moderate/excellent functional capacity? Intermediate-risk surgery carries little likelihood of perioperative death/MI; poor functional capacity or moderate functional capacity and planned higher-risk surgery mandate further testing, especially for pts with ≥ 2 intermediate predictors.

Noncardiac surgery is generally safe for pts with no major/intermediate predictors and moderate/excellent functional capacity (≥ 4 METs). Pts without clinical markers but poor functional capacity who are facing higher-risk operations may need further testing.

The absence of severe coronary stenoses can be predicted with 96% positive predictive value for pts with no h/o diabetes, prior angina, previous MI, or h/o CHF and with 94% positive predictive value for those with no prior angina, previous MI, or h/o CHF (Circ 1996;94:1561).

Pts with h/o MI or stress-induced ischemia on dobutamine echo have a high risk of fatal/nonfatal cardiac events after vascular surgery. Pts with both a h/o MI and extensive stress-induced ischemia are at especially high risk (Circ 1997;95:53).

Renal function: H/o prior heart surgery, presence of cardiomegaly, pt's pre-op functional class, h/o PVD, and need for IABP increase the risk of post-op acute renal failure in pts undergoing bypass or valve surgery (Circ 1997;95:878).

Anticoagulation and Surgery

INR will fall to 1.5 4 days after warfarin is stopped. After warfarin is restarted, it takes ~3 days for INR to reach 2.0. Once the INR reaches 1.5, surgery can be safely performed. Therefore, if warfarin is withheld before surgery and restarted asap after surgery, pts can be expected to have a subtherapeutic INR for ~2 days before and 2 days after surgery.

Elective surgery should be avoided in the 1st month after arterial embolism. If surgery is essential, preoperative iv heparin should be administered; post-op heparin is recommended only if the risk of post-op bleeding is low.

In all other pts who receive anticoagulants to prevent arterial embolism (mechanical heart valves, h/o nonvalvular Afib), the risk of embolism is not high enough to warrant pre-op or post-op iv heparin. Sc low-dose heparin or LMW heparin is recommended for hospitalized pts whose risk of arterial embolism does not justify the use of iv heparin. Administration of sc heparin to outpts does not appear to be justified.

Noncardiac surgery performed within 6 wk of carotid stenting is associated with increased risk of AMI, stent thrombosis, major bleeding, or death (Am J Cardiol 2005;95:755).

17.3 Screening of Athletes

Circ 2004;109:2807; 1998;97:2294; Nejm 2003;349:1064

Screening (AHA)

Preparticipation cardiovascular screening for high school and collegiate athletes should include complete personal and family hx, and physical exam before participation in organized high school (repeat q 2 yr) and collegiate sports (interim hx and BP q 1 yr).

Key findings in hx: Prior occurrence of exertional chest pain/discomfort, syncope/near-syncope, excessive/unexpected/unexplained shortness of breath or fatigue associated with exercise; past detection of heart murmur or increased BP; family h/o premature death (sudden or otherwise), or significant disability from CVD in close relative(s) < age 50; specific knowledge of the occurrence of hypertrophic cardiomyopathy, dilated cardiomyopathy, long QT syndrome, Marfan syndrome, or clinically important arrhythmias

Physical exam must include precordial auscultation in both the supine and standing positions to identify, in particular, heart murmurs consistent with dynamic left ventricular outflow obstruction; assessment of the femoral artery pulses to exclude coarctation of the aorta;

recognition of the physical stigmata of Marfan syndrome; and brachial blood pressure measurement in the sitting position (Circ 1998;97:2294).

In 1 study, abnormal EKG patterns occurred in 40% of athletes. False-positive EKGs represent a potential limitation to routine EKG testing as part of preparticipation screening (Circ 2000;102:278).

Sudden Cardiac Death

Risk ≈ 1 in 200,000/yr in high school student athletes; higher in male athletes (J Am Coll Cardiol 1998;32:1881)

Sudden death in young competitive athletes is usually precipitated by physical activity. Structural CVD identified at autopsy as the primary cause of death in one study included hypertrophic cardiomyopathy (36%), anomalous coronary artery origin (19%), increased cardiac mass (10%), ruptured aorta (5%), tunneled LAD CAD (5%), AS (4%), myocarditis (3%), dilated cardiomyopathy (3%), arrhythmogenic RV dysplasia (3%), MVP (2%), CAD (2%), and other CVD (6%) (Jama 1996;276:199).

In another study, the most common causes of sudden death in athletes were arrhythmogenic RV cardiomyopathy (22%), coronary atherosclerosis (18%), and anomalous coronary artery origin (12%). Hypertrophic cardiomyopathy was detected in only 0.07% but accounted for 3.5% of cardiovascular reasons for disqualification. None of the disqualified athletes with hypertrophic cardiomyopathy died during a mean follow-up period of 8.2 ± 5 yr (Nejm 1998;339:364).

A third study found hypertrophic cardiomyopathy in 26%, commotio cordis in 20%, coronary anomalies in 14%, LVH in 8%, myocarditis in 5%, ruptured aortic aneurysm in 3%, arrhythmogenic RV cardiomyopathy in 3%, coronary artery bridging in 3%, AS in 3%, ASHD in 3%, dilated cardiomyopathy in 2%, and mitral valve disease in 2%.

The incidence of congenital coronary anomalies is uncertain (perhaps 0.3-1%). They may be responsible for > 12% of deaths in

U.S. high school and college athletes. The optimal sports-related screening approach has not yet been identified (Circ 2002;105:2449). In screening for congenital coronary artery anomalies of "wrong" aortic sinus origin in young competitive athletes, rest/exercise EKGs are unlikely to provide clinical evidence of myocardial ischemia. Because premonitory cardiac sx occur shortly before sudden death, a h/o exertional syncope or chest pain requires assessment (J Am Coll Cardiol 2000;35:1493).

Frequent and complex ventricular tachyarrhythmias are common in trained athletes and are usually not associated with underlying CV abnormalities or with adverse clinical outcomes (J Am Coll Cardiol 2002;40:446).

LV Dimensions

In a sample of highly trained athletes, LV cavity dimension increased to a degree compatible with primary dilated cardiomyopathy in ~15% of participants. In the absence of systolic dysfunction, cavity dilatation is likely to be a physiologic adaptation to intensive conditioning. The long-term consequences and significance of such remodeling are unknown (Ann IM 1999;130:23).

Commotio Cordis

Sudden death related to impact to chest and not associated with traumatic injury is probably due to ventricular dysrhythmia induced by an abrupt, blunt precordial blow delivered at an electrically vulnerable phase of ventricular excitability. In pigs, impacts occurring 15-30 ms before the peak of the T wave produced Vfib (Nejm 1995;333:337; 1998;338:1805).

Chapter 18

Cardiac Medications

18.1 Angiotensin-Converting Enzyme Inhibitors

Nejm 2000;342:210; 1999;341:577

Drugs of this type: Benazepril (Lotensin), captopril (Capoten), enalapril (Vasotec), fosinopril (Monopril), lisinopril (Prinivil, Zestril), moexipril (Univasc), perindopril (Aceon), quinapril (Accupril), ramipril (Altace), trandolapril (Mavik)

Pharmacology: Prevent conversion of angiotensin I to angiotensin II (potent vasoconstrictor); decrease aldosterone secretion; increase bradykinin levels and thus stimulate prostaglandin synthesis; reduce peripheral vascular resistance; increase renal blood flow

Pharmacokinetics: See Table 18.1.

Uses: HT; CHF; AMI

Effects on other organs: Trandolapril and ramipril are secreted in breast milk; whether other ACEIs are also secreted in milk is not known

Precautions and contraindications: Pts with renal artery stenosis may develop renal failure when treated with ACEIs.

0.5-5% of pts with HT and/or CHF are reported to develop hyperkalemia with ACEIs.

ACEI use in the 2nd and 3rd trimesters of pregnancy is associated with fetal and neonatal injury and death.

Neutropenia developed in 0.2% of pts with impaired renal function and no collagen vascular disease treated with captopril

Table 18.1 Pharmacokinetics of ACE Inhibitors

Agent	Protein Binding	Half-life[1]	Elimination (24 hr)
Benazepril (Lotensin)	96%	10-11 hr	11-12% (bile)
Captopril (Capoten)	25-30%	< 2 hr	> 95% (urine)
Enalapril (Vasotec)	No data available	1.3 hr po; 11 hr iv	94% (urine, feces)
Fosinopril (Monopril)	99%	12 hr	50% urine, 50% feces
Lisinopril (Prinivil, Zestril)	No data available	12 hr	100% (urine)
Moexipril (Univasc)	50%	2-9 hr	13% urine, 53% feces
Perindopril (Aceon)	60%	0.8-1 hr	100% (urine)
Quinapril (Accupril)	97%	2 hr	60% urine, 37% feces
Ramipril (Altace)	73%	13-17 hr	60% urine, 40% feces
Trandolapril (Mavik)	80%	5 hr	33% urine, 56% feces

1. ACE inhibitors may be administered bid if effects appear to dissipate with qd dosing.

and in 3.7% of pts with both impaired renal function and collagen vascular disease.

The dose of most ACEIs needs to be reduced in pts with impaired renal function.

Adverse effects: Cough is the most commonly reported side effect (presumably due to decreased bradykinin degradation). Angioedema is reported in 0.1-0.5% of pts treated with ACEIs.

Drug interactions: ACEIs increase serum digoxin and Li levels; administration of antacids decreases the bioavailability of ACEIs, and indomethacin reduces their hypotensive effects; phenothiazines increase their pharmacologic effects.

The effects of ACEIs are potentiated by the addition of thiazide diuretics.

Dosage and administration:

Benazepril (Lotensin): tablets 5 mg, 10 mg, 20 mg, 40 mg; HT: initial dose 10 mg qd, maximum dose 40-80 mg qd

Captopril (Capoten): tablets 12.5 mg, 25 mg, 50 mg, 100 mg; HT: initial dose 25 mg tid, maximum dose 150 mg tid; CHF: initial dose 6.25 mg tid, usual dose 50-100 mg tid; LV dysfunction post-MI: single dose 6.25 mg, if tolerated start 12.5 mg tid and titrate to target dose of 50 mg tid over several weeks; diabetic nephropathy: target dose 25 mg tid

Enalapril (Vasotec): tablets 2.5 mg, 5 mg, 10 mg, 20 mg; injection (enalaprilat) 1.25 mg/mL; HT: initial dose 5 mg qd, maximum dose 40 mg/day, iv dose 1.25 mg q 6 hr; CHF: initial dose 2.5 mg bid, maximum dose 20 mg bid

Fosinopril (Monopril): tablets 10 mg, 20 mg, 40 mg; HT: initial dose 10 mg qd, maximum dose 40-80 mg qd; CHF: initial dose 5-10 mg qd, maximum dose 40 mg qd

Lisinopril (Prinivil, Zestril): tablets 2.5 mg, 5 mg, 10 mg, 20 mg, 40 mg; HT: initial dose 10 mg qd, maximum dose 80 mg qd; CHF: initial dose 5 mg qd, usual dose range 5-20 mg qd; AMI: 2.5-5 mg within 24 hr of onset, 5 mg after 48 hr, then 10 mg qd

Moexipril (Univasc): tablets 7.5 mg, 15 mg; HT: initial dose 7.5 mg qd ac, maximum dose 30 mg/d

Perindopril (Aceon): tablets 2 mg, 4 mg, 8 mg; HT: initial dose 4 mg qd, maximum dose 16 mg qd

Quinapril (Accupril): tablets 5 mg, 10 mg, 20 mg, 40 mg; initial dose 10 mg qd; maximum dose 80 mg/d; CHF: initial dose 5 mg bid, usual dose 10-20 mg bid

Ramipril (Altace): capsules 1.25 mg, 2.5 mg, 5 mg, 10 mg; HT: initial dose 2.5 mg qd, maximum dose 20 mg/d; CHF: initial dose 1.25 mg qd or bid, target dose 5 mg bid

Trandolapril (Mavik): tablets 1 mg, 2 mg, 4 mg; HT: initial dose 1 mg qd, maximum dose 8 mg/d; CHF: initial dose 1 mg qd, target dose 4 mg/d

18.2 Aldosterone-Blocking Agents

Nejm 2003;348:1309

Drugs of this type: Eplerenone (Inspra)

Pharmacology: Binds to mineralocorticoid receptor and blocks binding of aldosterone

Pharmacokinetics: Bioavailability is unknown; 50% protein bound; metabolized by cytochrome P450 3A45; half-life is 4-6 hr

Uses: Rx of CHF post-MI; HT

Precautions and contraindications: Contraindicated in pts with serum $K^+ > 5.5$ mEq/L, creatinine clearance < 30 mL/min, pts receiving other cytochrome P450 inhibitors such as ketoconazole, itraconozole, clarithromycin, retonavir, nelfinavir. In rx of HT, contraindicated in pts with NIDDM and microalbuminuria, creatinine > 1.8 mg/dL, use of K^+ supplements or potassium-sparing diuretics. Safety in pregnancy, children unknown.

Adverse effects: Hyperkalemia; elevations of triglyceride levels

Dosage and administration: Eplerenone (Inspra) 25 mg, 50 mg tablets; starting dose in CHF is 25 mg qd; may be increased to 50 mg qd within 4 wk if serum K^+ levels permit. Dose for HT is 50 mg qd.

18.3 Angiotensin II Receptor Antagonists

Nejm 1996;334:1649

Drugs of this type: Candesartan (Atacand); irbesartan (Avapro); losartan (Cozaar, Hyzaar); olmesartan (Benicar); telmisartan (Micardis); valsartan (Diovan)

Pharmacology: Bind selectively to AT_1 receptor to block vasoconstrictor and aldosterone-secreting effects of angiotensin II

Pharmacokinetics: See Table 18.2.

Use: HT

Table 18.2 Pharmacokinetics of Angiotensin II Receptor Antagonists

Agent	Plasma Binding	Food Effect	Oral Bioavailability	Conversion to Metabolites	Terminal Half-life
Candesartan (Atacand)	> 99%	None	15%	Minor	9 hrs
Irbesartan (Avapro)	90%	None	60-80%	< 20%	11-15 hrs
Losartan (Cozaar, Hyzaar)	98.7%	Decreased 10-14%	33%	14%	2 hrs
Olmesartan (Benicar)	99%	None	26%	None	13 hrs
Telmisartan (Micardis)	> 99%	Decreased 6-20%	42-58%	11%	24 hrs
Valsartan (Diovan)	95%	Decreased 40-50%	25%	20%	6 hrs

Effects on other organs: Decreased hgb reported

Precautions and contraindications: May cause hypotension in NaCl/volume-depleted pts; may produce/worsen renal failure in pts with renal artery stenosis

Contraindicated in 2nd and 3rd trimesters of pregnancy

Adverse effects: Effects of some agents reported to be less in blacks

Drug interactions: Telmisartan may increase serum digoxin levels

Dosage and administration:

Candesartan (Atacand): 4 mg, 8 mg, 16 mg, 32 mg tablets; usual dose 16 mg qd; maximum dose 32 mg qd

Irbesartan (Avapro): 75 mg, 150 mg, 300 mg tablets; usual dose 150 mg qd; maximum dose 300 mg qd

Losartan (Cozaar, Hyzaar): 25 mg, 50 mg, 100 mg tablets; usual dose 50 mg qd; maximum dose 100 mg qd

Olmesartan (Benicar): 20 mg, 40 mg tablets; starting dose 20 mg po qd; maximum dose 40 mg qd

Telmisartan (Micardis): 40 mg, 80 mg tablets; usual dose 40 mg qd; maximum dose 80 mg qd

Valsartan (Diovan): 80 mg, 160 mg capsules; usual dose 80 mg qd; maximum dose 320 mg qd

Addition of a thiazide diuretic may increase efficacy of all agents

18.4 α_1 Adrenergic-Blocking Agents

Labetolol and carvediolol have both α- and β-blocker activity and are discussed in the section on β-blockers.

Drugs of this type: Doxazosin (Cardura), prazosin (Minipres), terazosin (Hytrin)

Pharmacology: Block postsynaptic α_1 receptors, causing dilation of arterioles and veins

Pharmacokinetics: See Table 18.3.

Table 18.3 Pharmacokinetics of α_1 Adrenergic Blockers

	Doxazosin	Prazosin	Terazosin
Oral bioavailability	65%	48-68%	90%
Time to peak level	2-3 hr	1-3 hr	1-2 hr
Protein binding	98%	92-97%	90-94%
Half-life	22 hr	2-3 hr	9-12 hr
Excretion: bile/feces	63%	$<$ 90%	60%
Excretion: urine	9%	$<$ 10%	40%

Uses: HT; BPH

Precautions and contraindications: First-dose effect: hypotension, postural hypotension, syncope with first few doses or with change in dose; administer at bedtime when initiating rx

Adverse effects: Palpitations (2-5%), nausea (3-5%), dizziness (10-20%), headache (8-16%)

Drug interactions: May reduce antihypertensive effect of clonidine

Dosage and administration:

Doxazosin (Cardura): 1 mg, 2 mg, 4 mg, 8 mg tablets: initial dose 1 mg po qhs; maximum dose 16 mg/d; titrate dose q 2 wk

Prazosin (Minipres): 1 mg, 2 mg, 5 mg capsules; initial dose 1 mg po bid-tid; maximum dose 15 mg/d; titrate dose q 2 wk

Terazosin (Hytrin): 1 mg, 2 mg, 5 mg, 10 mg caplets; initial dose 1 mg po qhs; maximum dose 20 mg/d

18.5 Antiarrhythmic Agents

Nejm 1999;340:1910; 1998;338:35

Overview

Vaughn Williams classification (based on effect on action potential)

Class I: Local anesthetics of membrane-stabilizing agents; depress phase 0 (rapid depolarization)

- Class IA (quinidine, procainamide, disopyramide): Depress phase 0; prolong action potential
- Class IB (lidocaine, tocainide, mexiletine, phenytoin): Depress phase 0 slightly; may shorten action potential duration
- Class IC (flecanide, propafenone): Depress phase 0 markedly; slight effect on repolarization

Note: Moricizine shares characteristics of Class IA, IB, and IC agents

Class II (propranolol, esmolol, acebutolol): β-Blockers; depress phase 4 (diastolic depolarization)

Class III (sotalol, bretylium, amiodarone, ibutilide): Prolong phase 3 (final rapid repolarization)

Class IV (verapamil): Depresses phase 4 depolarization; prolongs phase 1 (early rapid repolarization) and phase 2 (plateau)

Adenosine

Nejm 1991;325:1621

Drugs of this type: Adenosine (Adenocard)

Pharmacology: Slows conduction through AV node; interrupts reentrant pathways

Pharmacokinetics: Rapid uptake by erythrocytes, vascular endothelial cells; half-life < 10 sec

Uses: Conversion of PSVT, including those involving accessory bypass tracts (WPW syndrome); *not* effective in converting Aflut, Afib, but resulting transient AV block may facilitate diagnosis

Precautions and contraindications: May produce transient high-degree AV block

Adverse effects: Flushing (18%); headache (2%)

Drug interactions: Activity blocked by methylxanthines (theophylline, caffeine); potentiated by dipyridamole; carbamazepine also increases AV block

Dosage and administration: Initial dose 6 mg iv bolus; may repeat with 12 mg iv bolus

Class 1A Antiarrhythmic Agents

Nejm 1997;337:1383

Drugs of this type: Quinidine (Quinidex, Quinaglute); procainamide (Pronestyl, Procanbid); disopyramide (Norpace)

Pharmacology: Depress myocardial excitability and conduction velocity; prolong effective refractory period

Pharmacokinetics: See Table 18.4.

Uses: Treatment of paroxysmal SV tachycardia, Aflut, Afib (including maintenance rx after cardioversion); PSVT (see precautions)

Effects on other organs: All 3 agents cross the placenta and are excreted in breast milk.

Precautions and contraindications: Contraindicated in myasthenia gravis, digitalis toxicity, complete heart block, long QT syndrome or pts with h/o drug-related torsades de pointes, or in pts who develop QRS or QT prolongation; administration in Aflut may decrease AV block and produce rapid ventricular response; pretreatment with digitalis recommended; may produce complete heart block in pts with lesser degrees of conduction disturbance

Disopyramide has a significant negative inotropic effect and is contraindicated in CHF

Adverse effects: Thrombocytopenia, hemolytic anemia, hepatotoxicity, and fever reported with quinidine, and periodic CBC, liver studies recommended; most common side effects are gi

Procainamide: Agranulocytosis, neutropenia, thrombocytopenia seen in ~0.5% of pts; usually occurs within first 12 wk.

Table 18.4 Pharmacokinetics of Antiarrhythmic Agents

Agent	Protein Binding	Half-life	Duration of Action
Quinidine (Quinadex, Quinaglute)	80-90%	6-7 hr	6-8 hr
Procainamide (Pronestyl, Procanbid)	14-23%	2.5-4.7 hr	3 hr
Disopyramide (Norpace)	20-60%; concentration dependent	4-10 hr	6-7 hr
Lidocaine (Xylocaine)	40-80%	1-2 hr	10-15 min
Tocainide (Tonocard)	10-20%	Terminal elimination phase, 11-23 hr	—
Mexiletine (Mexitil)	50-60%	10-12 hr	—
Flecainide (Tambocor)	40%	Terminal elimination phase, 11-23 hr	—
Propafenone (Rhythmol)	97%	2-10 hr; 6-36 hr in poor metabolizers	—
Moricizine (Ethmozine)	95%	1.5-3.5 hr	10-24 hr
Bretylium (Bretylol)	0-8%	5-10 hr	6-8 hr
Amiodarone (Cordarone, Pacerone)	96%	26-107 d	Months

Procainamide can produce a positive ANA test and lupus-like sx and is contraindicated in pts with lupus.

Disopyramide: Dry mouth (32%), headache (3-9%), urinary hesitancy (14%), constipation (9%), muscle discomfort (3-9%)

Drug interactions: Amiodarone, antacids, cimetidine, and verapamil may increase serum quinidine levels. Hydantoins, nifedipine, rifampine, and sucralfate may reduce serum quinidine levels. Quinidine may potentiate effects of warfarin, digoxin, propafenone, and succinylcholine.

Cimetidine and ranitidine increase procainamide bioavailability. Trimethoprim increases serum procainamide levels.

Erythromycin increases disopyramide levels. Hydantoins and rifampin decrease disopyramide levels.

Dosage and administration:

Quinidine sulfate: 200 mg, 300 mg; quinidine gluconate: 324 mg; maintenance rx: 300-600 mg po q 8 hr; may administer 200 mg po as test dose

Procainamide: 250 mg, 375 mg, 500 mg tablets; 500 mg, 750 mg, 1000 mg sustained-release tablets; 100 mg/mL, 500 mg/mL injection; initial po dose up to 50 mg/kg/d in divided doses (q 4 hr standard formulation, q 6-12 hr timed-release formulation); initial iv dose 500 mg at infusion rate < 50 mg/min

Disopyramide: 100 mg, 150 mg capsules; 100 mg, 150 mg extended-release capsules: 400-800 mg qd q 6 hr (q 12 hr for extended-release formulation); in renal failure, dose is 100 mg q 8-24 hr

Class IB Antiarrhythmic Agents

Drugs of this type: Lidocaine (Xylocaine); tocainide (Tonocard); mexiletine (Mexitil)

Pharmacokinetics: See Table 18.4.

Uses:

Lidocaine: Acute short-term management of ventricular arrhythmias

Tocainide and mexiletine: Treatment of documented life-threatening ventricular arrhythmias

Effects on other organs: Lidocaine crosses the placenta. Mexiletine crosses the placenta and is excreted in breast milk.

Precautions and contraindications: Lidocaine is contraindicated in WPW syndrome, severe SA node or AV node block, or Stokes-Adams attacks. Mexiletine is contraindicated in cardiogenic shock, preexisting 2nd- or 3rd-degree AV block.

Adverse effects: CNS effects are seen in lidocaine toxicity.

Blood dyscrasias, pulmonary fibrosis, and interstitial fibrosis have been reported with tocainide and usually occur 3-18 wk after initiation of therapy. Vertigo (15%), nausea (15%), parasthesias (9%), and tremor (8%) have also been reported. Mexiletine may cause liver enzyme abnormalities, palpitations (7.5%), dizziness (26%), tremor (13%), coordination abnormalities (10%), and gi upset (40%).

Drug interactions: β-Blockers and cimetidine may increase serum lidocaine levels. Rifampin and cimetidine decrease bioavailability of tocainide. Antacids slow and metoclopramide increases mexiletine absorption. Hydantoins and rifampin increase mexiletine clearance. Mexiletine can increase serum theophylline levels.

Dosage and administration:

Lidocaine: 1 mg/kg iv bolus; may repeat in 5-15 min; 1-4 mg/min continuous iv infusion

Tocainide: 400 mg, 600 mg tablets; initial dose 400 mg po q 8 hr

Mexiletine: 150 mg, 200 mg, 250 mg capsules; initial dose 200 mg po q 8 hr; increase dose 50-100 mg q 3-5 d; maximum dose 1200 mg/d; may use bid dosing in stable pts

When transferring pts to mexiletine, initial dose is 200 mg po 3-6 hr after last dose of procainamide, 6-12 hr after last dose of quinidine or disopyramide, 8-12 hr after last dose of tocainide

Class IC Antiarrhythmic Agents

Drugs of this type: Flecanide (Tambocor); propafenone (Rhythmol)

Pharmacokinetics: See Table 18.4.

Uses: PSVT; Afib; documented life-threatening ventricular arrhythmias

Effects on other organs: Flecanide is excreted in breast milk.

Precautions and contraindications:

Flecanide: preexisting 2nd- or 3rd-degree AV block; bifascicular block; cardiogenic shock; sick sinus syndrome; CHF; recent MI (CAST study: 5.1% mortality/nonfatal VF rate)

Propafenone: Above plus bronchospasm; may cause positive ANA titer

Both drugs may increase pacing threshold. Both have negative inotropic effects and should be used with caution in combination with other negative inotropic agents.

Adverse effects:

Flecanide: Dizziness (19%); dyspnea (10%); nausea (9%); fatigue (8%); palpitations (6%); chest pain, asthenia, fever (5%)

Propafenone: Unusual taste (7%); dizziness (7%); 1st-degree AV block (4.5%); headache (4.5%); constipation (4%)

Drug interactions: Cimetidine increases flecanide and propafenone bioavailabilty. Flecanide and propafenone increase digoxin levels. Propafenone increases warfarin, β-blocker, and cyclosporine blood levels.

Dosage and administration:

Flecanide: 50 mg, 100 mg, 150 mg tablets; SVT/Afib: initial dose 50 mg po q 12 hr, maximum 300 mg/d; VT: initial dose 100 mg po q 12 hr; maximum dose 400 mg/d; reduce dosage to q 24 hr in renal failure

Propafenone: 150 mg, 225 mg, 300 mg tablets; initial dose 150 mg po q 8 hr; maximum dose 900 mg/d

For both agents, dosage should not be increased more rapidly than q 4 d.

Moricizine

Drugs of this type: Moricizine (Ethmozine)

Pharmacology: Class I antiarrhythmic; has characteristics of Class IA, IB, and IC drugs; prolongs PR interval, AV nodal, and His-Purkinje conduction time; prolongs QRS interval, and QTc slightly

Pharmacokinetics: See Table 18.4.

Uses: Ventricular arrhythmias

Effects on other organs: Moricizine does not have negative inotropic effects; excreted in breast milk; no adequate studies on use in pregnancy

Precautions and contraindications: Contraindicated in pts with 2nd- or 3rd-degree AV block, bifascicular block, cardiogenic shock; use with caution in sick sinus syndrome; has proarrhythmic potential; CAST study failed to demonstrate definite benefit and adverse trend in use with MI pts

Adverse effects: Dizziness (15%); nausea (10%); headache (8%); fatigue (6%); dyspnea (6%); palpitations (6%); proarrhythmia (3.7%)

Drug interactions: Cimetidine increases moricizine plasma levels. Digoxin produces increased PR prolongation. Moricizine decreases theophylline half-life.

Dosage and administration: Moricizine (Ethmozine): 200 mg, 250 mg, 300 mg tablets; starting dose 200 mg q 8 hr; usual dose 600-900 mg/d; if pts well controlled, may change to q 12 hr dosing; reduce dosage in pts with impaired hepatic function. When changing from another agent, start moricizine 6-12 hr after last dose of quinidine or disopyramide; 3-6 hr after last dose of procainamide; 12-24 hr after last dose of flecanide; 8-12 hr after last dose of tocainide, propafenone, or mexiletine.

Class II Antiarrhythmic Agents

See β-blockers.

Class III Antiarrhythmic Agents

Drugs of this type: Bretylium (Bretylol), amiodarone (Cordarone, Pacerone), ibutilide (Corvert); dofetilide (Tikosyn)

Sotalol (Betapace) also has class III antiarrhythmic properties.

Pharmacology: Bretylium inhibits norepinephrine release.

Pharmacokinetics: See Table 18.4.

Uses: Life-threatening ventricular arrhythmias (bretylium, amiodarone, sotalol); treatment of Aflut/Afib and PSVT (amiodarone, sotalol); conversion of Aflut/Afib (ibutilide)

Effects on other organs: Amiodarone can produce pneumonitis, liver disease, optic neuropathy, and corneal microdeposits, and it blocks peripheral conversion of T_4 to T_3. It may cause hyper- or hypothyroidism. CXR, PFTs, ophthamologic exam, and thyroid and liver function studies are required before initiation and periodically thereafter.

Precautions and contraindications: Amiodarone: Severe sinus node dysfunction or marked sinus bradycardia, 2nd- or 3rd-degree AV block

1.7% of pts receiving ibutilide developed sustained and 2.7% developed nonsustained polymorphic VT.

Adverse effects:

Bretylium: Postural hypotension (50%), transient HT, vomiting with rapid iv administration

Amiodarone: Above plus neurologic (20-40%) and gi (25%) complaints; 10% of pts develop photosensitivity

Because of the risk of life-threatening arrhythmias, dofetilide requires 3-d hospitalization for initiation of rx by a certified practitioner with reevaluation at 3 mon based on QTc interval and renal function.

Drug interactions: Amiodarone increases levels of digoxin, warfarin, cyclosporine, hydantoins, methotrexate, quinidine, procainamide, and theophylline.

Dosage and administration:

Bretylium: 2 mg/mL, 4 mg/mL, 50 mg/mL injection; 5-10 mg iv loading dose over 10 min (rapid injection possible but may produce vomiting), 1-2 mg/min maintenance infusion

Amiodarone: 200 mg tablets, 50 mg/mL injection; loading dose 400-800 mg po bid pc for 1-3 wk, then 600-800 mg/d for 1 mon, then 200-400 mg po qd; for iv loading, give 150 mg over 10 min, then 360 mg/6 hr (1 mg/min), then 540 mg/18 hr (0.5 mg/min), then 0.5 mg/min maintenance infusion

Iv amiodarone is incompatible with aminophyline, cefazolin, cefamandole, heparin, $NaHCO_3$

Ibutilide: 1 mg iv (0.01 mg/kg if wt $<$ 60 kg) over 10 min; 2nd dose may be administered 10 min after completion of 1st dose

Class IV Antiarrhythmic Agents

See Ca^{++}-channel blockers.

18.6 Anticoagulants

Warfarin

Nejm 1991;324:1865

Drugs of this type: Warfarin (Coumadin)

Pharmacokinetics: 97-99% protein bound; half-life 1-2.5 d

Uses: Treatment and prophylaxis of thrombosis and thromboembolic complications

Precautions and contraindications: Contraindicated in pregnancy, hemophilia, h/o bleeding diathesis, thrombocytopenic purpura, leukemia, major active bleeding, recent major surgery or trauma, cerebral or dissecting aortic aneurysm, hemorrhagic CVA, pericarditis, severe HT, severe renal or hepatic disease, infectious endocarditis

Adverse effects: Hemorrhage, "purple toe syndrome" (systemic cholesterol microembolization)

Drug interactions: Anticoagulant effect increased by acetaminophen, aminoglycosides, amiodarone, androgens, β-blockers, cephalosporins, chloral hydrate, chloramphenicol, chlorpropamide, cimetidine, cyclophosphamide, D-thyroxine, disulfiram, erythromycin, fluconazole, gemfibrozil, glucagon, hydantoins, influenza vaccine, INH, ketoconazole, loop diuretics, metronidazole, miconazole, moricizine, omperazole, NSAIDs, penicillins, propafenone, propoxyphene, quinine and quinidine, quinolones, salicylates, SMX-TMP, streptokinase, sulfinpyrazone, sulfonamides, tamoxifen, tetracyclines, thyroid hormone, urokinase, vitamin E

Anticoagulant effect decreased by ascorbic acid, barbiturates, carbamezepine, cholestyramine, dicloxacillin, estrogens, ETOH, gluthethimide, griseofulvin, nafcillin, rifampin, spironolactone, sucralfate, thiazide diuretics, trazodone, vitamin K

Dosage and administration: Warfarin (Coumadin): 1 mg, 2 mg, 2.5 mg, 3, mg, 4 mg, 5 mg, 6 mg, 7.5 mg, 10 mg tablets; dosage must be individualized

Heparin and Low-Molecular-Weight Heparin

Nejm 1997;337:668

Drugs of this type: Heparin, dalteparin (Fragmin), enoxaparin (Lovenox)

Pharmacology: LMW heparins obtained by depolymerization of unfractionated heparin

Pharmacokinetics: Average half-life of heparin is 0.5-3 hr; terminal half-life is 3-5 hr for dalteparin, 4.5 hr for enoxaparin

Uses: Rx and prophylaxis of thrombosis

Effects on other organs: May induce lipoprotein lipase and increase serum free fatty acid levels

Precautions and contraindications: Active major bleeding, thrombocytopenia

Adverse effects: Bleeding; thrombocytopenia

Drug interactions: Use with caution in conjunction with platelet inhibitors

Dosage and administration:

Heparin: Prophylaxis: 5,000 U sc q 12 hr; continuous infusion: 3,000-5,000 U iv bolus and then 1000 U/hr; target PTT 55-85 sec for DVT (see Table 18.5), 55-70 sec with thrombolytics

1 mg protamine (1% solution) neutralizes ~100 U heparin

Dalteprin (Fragmin): Systemic anticoagulation: 100 U/kg sc q 12 hr; hip replacement surgery: 2,500 U sc 2 hr before surgery, 2500 U sc after surgery, 5000 U sc qd thereafter; unstable coronary artery syndrome: 120 U/kg (maximum 10,000 U) sc q 12 hr for 5-8 d with ASA 81-160 mg qd

Enoxaparin (Lovenox): Recommended dose is 1 mg/kg sc q 12 hr for all indications

Table 18.5 Sample Dosage Adjustment Chart for DVT

PTT (sec)	Action	Rate Change
< 45	5000 U iv bolus	Increase by 250 U/hr
45-54		Increase by 150 U/hr
55-85		No change
86-110	Stop infusion for 1 hr	Decrease by 150 U/hr
> 110	Stop infusion for 1 hr	Decrease by 250 U/hr

18.7 FACTOR Xa INHIBITORS

ARIXTRA (fondaparinux sodium) Injection Prescribing Information 2005

Drugs of this type: Fondaparinux (Arixtra)

Pharmacology: Fondaparinux selectively binds to antithrombin III and potentates the innate neutralization of Factor Xa by antithrombin III. It does not inactivate thrombin and has no effect on platelets.

Pharmacokinetics: Absolute bioavailability after SC injection is 100%; steady-state plasma concentration is reached ~3 hr post-dose. Fondaparinux is highly bound to antithrombin III and does not bind significantly to other plasma proteins or red cells. It is eliminated in urine mainly as unchanged drug; elimination half-life is 17-21 hr. Elimination time is prolonged in the elderly and in pts with renal impairment.

Uses: Prophylaxis of thromboembolic events following knee and hip replacement surgery (including extended prophylaxis), and abdominal surgery, as well as, for the treatment of deep vein thrombosis and acute pulmonary embolism (in conjunction with warfarin sodium when initial therapy is administered in the hospital).

Precautions and Contraindications: Agents that may enhance the risk of hemorrhage should be discontinued prior to initiation of treatment. Fondaparinux should be discontinued before initiation of epidural/spinal anesthesia.

Use with caution in pts who weigh less than 50 kg (prophylaxis only) and in those with moderate renal impairment. The drug should be discontinued immediately in patients who develop severe renal impairment.

Use with extreme caution in conditions with increased risk of hemorrhage (congenital/acquired bleeding disorders, active ulcerative and angiodysplastic disease, hemorrhagic CVA, recent brain, spinal, or ophthalmological surgery, pts treated concomitantly with platelet inhibitors).

Fondapurinax is contraindicated in pts with active major bleeding or bacterial endocarditis.

PT and PTT are insensitive measures of activity. No monitoring is required with fondaparinux.

Adverse effects: Risk of hemorrhage.

Drug interactions: None known.

Dosage and administration: Fondaparinux (Arixtra) 2.5 mg, 5 mg, 7.5 mg, 10 mg pre-filled syringes; recommended dose for DVT prophylaxis is 2.5 mg SC QD.

For acute DVT and acute PE, the recommended dose is 5 mg (body weight <50 kg), 7.5 mg (body weight 50-100 kg) or 10 mg (body weight >100 kg) SC QD.

18.8 Antiplatelet Agents

Aggregation Inhibitors

Circ 2000 101:1206; 1999;100:437; Nejm 1997;337:1383

Drugs of this type: Aspirin; cilostazol (Pletal); clopidogrel (Plavix), ticlodipine (Ticlid)

Pharmacology: Cilostazol inhibits phosphodiesterase (increasing levels of cAMP) and reversibly inhibits platelet aggregation; clopidogrel and ticlodipine inhibit glycoprotein IIb/IIIa complex to inhibit platelet aggregation; ASA inhibits prostaglandin A_2 and irreversibly inhibits platelet aggregation

Pharmacokinetics: ASA half-life ≈ 15-20 min and is 90% protein bound; cilostazol is 95-98% protein bound with elimination half-life of 11-13 hr, 74% excreted in urine and 20% in feces; clopidogrel is 98% protein bound, has elimination half-life of 8 hr; 50% is excreted in urine and 46% in feces; ticlodipine is 98% protein bound, has half-life of 13 hr with single dose and 4-5 d with repeat dosing, with 60% eliminated in urine and 24% in feces

Uses: Intermittent claudication (cilostazol); reduction of atherosclerotic events (ASA, clopidogrel); reduction in risk of thrombotic stroke (ticlodipine)

Effects on other organs: Ticlodipine increases cholesterol levels 8-10%

Precautions and contraindications: All contraindicated in active bleeding; cilostazol contraindicated in CHF; ticlodipine contraindicated in pts with TTP, can cause neutropenia/agranulocytosis

Adverse effects:

Cilostazol: Headache (27-34%), diarrhea (12-19%), dizziness (9-10%), palpitations (5-10%)
Clopidogrel: Headache (8%), arthralgia (6%), gi sx (27%)
Ticlodipine: Diarrhea (12.5%), nausea or dyspepsia (7%)

Drug interactions: Cilostazol is metabolized by cytochrome P450 enzymes, which are inhibited by fluconazole, sertraline, diltiazem, erythromycin, and grapefruit juice.

Ticlodipine increases digoxin and phenytoin blood levels and prolongs theophylline half-life. Antacids decrease ticlodipine blood levels, while cimetidine reduces clearance of ticlodipine.

Dosage and administration:

Cilostazol (Pletal): 50 mg, 100 mg tablets; usual dose is 100 mg po bid
Clopidogrel (Plavix): 75 mg tablet; usual dose is 75 mg po qd
Ticlodipine (Ticlid): 250 mg tablet; usual dose is 250 mg po bid

Glycoprotein IIB/IIIa Inhibitors

Nejm 1998;339:436; 1998;338:1488; 1995;332:1553

Drugs of this type: Abciximab (ReoPro), eptifibatide (Itegrilin), tirofiban (Aggrastat)

Pharmacology: Antagonists of platelet glycoprotein IIb/IIIa receptor; prevent binding of fibrinogen and von Willebrandt factor to platelets to inhibit platelet aggregation

Pharmacokinetics: Half-life for abciximab is 10-30 min, ~2.5 hr for eptifibatide, 2 hr for tirofiban; low levels of inhibition present for up to 10 d following acbiximab infusion

Uses: Abciximab is used as an adjunct to PTCA or atherectomy. Eptifibatide and tirofiban are also indicated for use in unstable angina/non–Q-wave MI.

Precautions and contraindications: Active internal bleeding, h/o CVA major surgery or trauma in past 30 d, h/o hemorrhagic CVA, severe hypotension, intracranial hemorrhage or neoplasm, AV malformation or aneurysm, aortic dissection, acute pericarditis, platelet count < 100,000/mm^3, renal failure

Adverse effects: Bleeding; hypotension (abciximab)

Drug interactions: Use with caution in conjunction with other antiplatelet agents

Dosage and administration:

Abciximab (ReoPro): 2 mg/mL injection; usual dose 0.15-0.3 mg/kg bolus or 0.25 mg/kg bolus followed by 10 μgm/min iv infusion

Eptifibatide (Itegrilin): 0.75 mg/mL, 2 mg/mL injection; acute coronary syndrome: 180 μgm/kg bolus followed by 2 μgm/kg/min infusion for up to 72 hr; PTCA: 135 mg/kg bolus and 0.5 μgm/kg/min infusion for up to 24 hr

Tirofiban (Aggrastat): 50 μgm/mL, 250 μgm/mL injection; usual dose 0.4 μgm/kg/min infusion for 30 min, then 0.1 μgm/kg/min infusion; reduce dose by half for pts with creatinine clearance < 30 mL/min

18.9 β-Adrenergic-Blocking Agents

Nejm 1998;339:1759; 1996;34:1396

Drugs of this type: Acebutolol (Sectral), atenolol (Tenormin), betaxolol (Kerlone), bisoprolol (Zebeta), carvedilol (Coreg), esmolol (Brevibloc), labetolol (Normodyne, Trandate), metoprolol (Lopressor, Toprol XL), nadolol (Corgard), pindolol (Visken), propranolol (Inderal), sotalol (Betapace), timolol (Blocadren)

Pharmacology: Competitive inhibition of β-adrenergic agonists at both β_1 (cardiac muscle) and β_2 (bronchial and vascular smooth muscle) receptor sites (nadolol, pindolol, propranolol, sotalol, timolol, labetolol) or at β_1 sites (acebutolol, atenolol, betaxolol, bisoprolol, esmolol, metoprolol) preferentially, producing inhibition of positive inotropic, chronotropic, and vasodilator response to β-adrenergic stimulation; results in decreased heart rate and BP, slowed AV conduction, decreased myocardial contractility, decreased myocardial automaticity (β_1), and passive bronchial constriction (β_2)

Propranolol, acebutolol, betaxolol, and pindolol also have quinidine-like membrane-stabilizing effects. Pindolol and acebutolol have intrinsic sympathomimetic (ISA) or partial agonist activity.

Carvedilol also has selective β_1-adrenergic-blocking activity, which reduces peripheral vascular resistance.

Pharmacokinetics: See Table 18.6.

Chemistry: Esmolol not compatible with 5% $NaHCO_3$ injection

Iv labetolol not compatible with 5% $NaHCO_3$ injection, iv furosemide, alkaline solutions

Uses: Angina pectoris; MI; HT; cardiac arrhythmias, including PSVT, rate control in Afib, Aflut, arrhythmias associated with thyrotoxicosis and digitalis toxicity, PVCs; hypertrophic cardiomyopathy; (no agent has an indication for all uses)

Metoprolol and carvedilol are also used in rx of CHF.

Esmolol is designated for rapid short-term control of SVT.

Effects on other organs: As a result of altered renal hemodynamics, Na^+ reabsorption increases and GFR may be reduced; hepatic blood flow may similarly be reduced.

β-Blockers also inhibit glycogenolysis in skeletal muscle and can block the release of insulin that usually results from adrenergic stimulation. They can blunt si/sx of hypoglycemia and interfere with GTT.

β-Blockers may mask clinical signs of developing hyperthyroidism.

β-Blockers may increase serum lipid levels, but data are inconsistent and clinical significance is uncertain.

Sx of peripheral vascular disease may increase with use of β-blockers due to both decrease in CO and reduction in peripheral β_2 stimulation.

Most β-blockers are excreted in breast milk, but propranolol and metoprolol are excreted only in small quantities.

Precautions and contraindications: Contraindicated in significant sinus bradycardia, 2nd- and 3rd-degree AV block, hypotension, cardiogenic shock. Nonselective β-blockers are contraindicated in pts with reactive airway disease; agents with relative β_1 selectivity may be used cautiously.

Sotalol has proarrhythmic effects, is contraindicated in congenital or acquired long QT syndrome, and may be associated with an excess of sudden deaths when used at high doses in pts post-MI; the risk of torsades de pointes increases with dose of drug, hypokalemia, hypomagnesemia, and h/o sustained VT or CHF.

The existence of β-blocker withdrawal syndrome with hypersensitivity to catecholamines has been reported but is controversial.

Dosage adjustments may be necessary in pts with impaired hepatic function. Nadolol, sotolol, and atenolol are excreted primarily by kidney, and acebutolol and esmolol have active

Table 18.6 Pharmacokinetics of β-Blockers

Agent	Receptor-Blocking Activity	Protein Binding	Lipid Solubility	Oral Bioavailability	Half-life
Acebutolol (Sectral)	β_1; β_2 at high doses	26%	Low	20-60%	3-4 hr
Atenolol (Tenormin)	β_1; β_2 at high doses	6-16%	Low	50-60%	6-9 hr
Betaxolol (Kerlone)	β_1; β_2 at high doses	50%	Low	89%	14-22 hr
Bisoprolol (Zebeta)	β_1; β_2 at high doses	30%	Low	80%	9-12 hr
Esmolol (Brevibloc)	β_1; β_2 at high doses	55%	Low	Iv only	10 min
Labetolol (Normodyne, Trandate)	β_1; β_2; α_1	50%	Moderate	30-40%	5.5-8 hr
Metoprolol (Lopressor, Toprol XL)	β_1; β_2 at high doses	12%	Moderate	40-50%; 77% for long-acting forms	3-7 hr
Nadolol (Corgard)	β_1; β_2	30%	Low	30-50%	20-24 hr
Pindolol (Visken)	β_1; β_2; also has ISA	40%	Moderate	100%	3-4 hr
Propranolol (Inderal)	β_1; β_2	90%	High	30%; 9-18% for long-acting forms	3-5 hr; 8-11 hr for long-acting forms
Sotalol (Betapace)	β_1; β_2	0%	Low	90-100%	12 hr
Timolol (Blocadren)	β_1; β_2	10%	Low/moderate	75%	4 hr

metabolites excreted by kidney, so dosage adjustment is necessary in pts with impaired renal function.

Safety for use of β-blockers in pregnancy is not established; avoid use of in the 1st trimester.

Pts receiving β-blockers for treatment of CHF (metoprolol, carvedilol) may experience worsening symptoms initially.

Adverse effects: Fatigue, lethargy, insomnia, sleep disturbances, nightmares, mood change, sexual dysfunction

Drug interactions: Bioavailability is decreased by aluminum and Ca^{++} salts, barbiturates, cholesyramine and colstipol, NSAIDs, penicillin, rifampin, salicylates, and sulfinpyrazone. Bioavailability may be increased by oral contraceptives, flecanide, haloperidol, and phenothiazines. β-Blockers may increase serum lidocaine levels.

Dosage and administration:

Acebutolol (Sectral): 200 mg, 400 mg capsules; HT, PVCs: initial dose 400 mg qd or 200 mg po bid, maximum dose 1200 mg/d, usual dose range 400-800 mg/d, reduce dose by 50% if creatinine clearance < 50 mL/min

Atenolol (Tenormin): 25 mg, 50 mg, 100 mg tablets; 5 mg/10 mL injection; angina, HT, acute MI: initial dose 25-50 mg qd, maximum dose 200 mg/d; AMI: iv dose 5 mg over 5 min, repeat in 10 min, 50 mg po bid thereafter

Betaxolol (Kerlone): 10 mg, 20 mg tablets; HT: starting dose 5-10 mg qd, maximum effective dose 20 mg/d, titrate dose q 7-14 d

Bisoprolol (Zebeta): 5 mg, 10 mg tablets; HT: starting dose 2.5-5 mg qd, maximum dose 20 mg/d

Carvedilol (Coreg): 3.125 mg, 6.25 mg, 12.5 mg, 25 mg tablets; HT, CHF: initial dose 3.125 mg bid, maximum dose 25-50 mg bid, monitor BP 1 hr after administration, titrate dose q 14 d, may need to increase dose slowly in pts with CHF

Esmolol (Brevibloc): 10 gm/mL, 250 mg/mL injection; arrhythmias: loading dose 500 μgm/kg/min for 1 min followed by

50 μgm/kg/min infusion for 4 min; if no response in 5 min, repeat loading dose and increase maintenance dose to 100 μgm/kg/min; titrate q 5-10 min, repeating loading dose and increasing maintenance dose by 50 μgm increments to 200 μgm/kg/min until desired HR attained or BP limits reached; usual dilution is 5 gm in 500 cc (10 mg/mL)

Labetolol (Normodyne, Trandate): 100 mg, 200 mg, 300 mg tablets; 5 mg/mL injection; HT: initial po dose 100 mg po bid, maximum dose 400 mg/d, titrate dose q 3 d; iv dose 20 mg bolus over 2 min, 40-80 mg q 10 min to maximum dose of 300 mg *or* continuous infusion starting at 2 mg/min and titrate infusion rate

Metoprolol (Lopressor, Toprol XL): 50 mg, 100 mg tablets; 50 mg, 100 mg, 200 mg extended-release tablets; 1 mg/mL injection; HT, angina, AMI: initial dose 50-100 mg qd in divided doses or extended-release form, maximum dose 400 mg/d; iv dose in AMI is 5 mg q 5 min for 3 doses, followed by 50 mg po q 6 hr or 100 mg po bid

Nadolol (Corgard): 20 mg, 40 mg, 80 mg, 120 mg, 160 mg tablets; angina, HT: starting dose 40 mg qd, maximum dose 240 mg/d, titrate q 3-7 d, adjust dose or dosing interval in renal failure

Table 18.7 Recommended Doses of Propranolol

Indication	Initial Dose	Usual Range	Maximum Dose
Arrhythmia		10-30 mg tid or qid	
Hypertension	40 mg bid	120-240 mg/d	640 mg/d
Angina	80 mg/d	160 mg/d	320 mg/d
AMI		180-240 mg/d	240 mg/d
Hypertrophic cardiomyopathy		20-40 mg tid or qid	
Pheochromocytoma		60 mg/day for 3 d pre-op	

CARDIAC MEDICATIONS

Pindolol (Visken): 5 mg, 10 mg tablets; HT: starting dose 5 mg po bid, maximum dose 60 mg/d, titrate dose q 3-4 wk

Propranolol (Inderal): 10 mg, 20 mg, 40 mg, 60 mg; 80 mg tablets; 60 mg, 80 mg, 120 mg, 160 mg timed-release capsules; 1 mg/mL injection; angina, AMI, HT, arrhythmias, hypertrophic cardiomyopathy: see Table 18.7

Sotalol (Betapace): 80 mg, 120 mg, 160 mg, 240 mg tablets; ventricular arrhythmias: starting dose 80 mg po bid, usual dose up to 320 mg/d although doses as high as 640 mg/d have been employed, titrate dose q 3 d, monitor QR interval, withdraw other antiarrhythmic rx for minimum of 2-3 half-lives; increase dosing interval to q 24 hr for creatinine clearance of 30-60 mL/min, q 36-48 hr for creatinine clearance of 10-30 mL/min

Timolol (Blocadren): 5 mg, 10 mg, 20 mg tablets; HT, AMI: initial dose 10 mg po bid, maximum dose 60 mg/d, titrate dose q 7 d

18.10 Calcium-Channel Blockers

Dihydropyridines

Drugs of this type: Amlodipine (Norvasc, Caduet), felodipine (Plendil), isradipine (DynaCirc), nicardipine (Cardene), nifedipine (Procardia, Adalat), nisoldipine (Sular)

Pharmacology: Inhibit movement of Ca^{++} ions across cell membranes through slow (calcium) channels; do not change serum Ca^{++} concentration; inhibit contraction of cardiac and smooth muscle, producing dilation of coronary and systemic arteries; little effect on SA or AV node conduction; little negative inotropic effect seen in vivo

Pharmacokinetics: Typically 90+% oral absorption but variable effective bioavailability because of extensive first-pass effects; onset of action 20 min for nifedipine, nicardipine; 120 min for isradipine, felodipine; protein binding 92-98%

Half-life: amlodipine, 50 hr; felodipine, 11-16 hr; isradipine, 8 hr; nicardipine and nifedipine, 2-5 hr; nisoldipine, 7-12 hr; 10% of amlodipine dose is excreted unchanged in urine; for others only ~1% is excreted unchanged

Uses: Chronic stable angina; vasospastic angina; essential HT (not all agents have FDA approval for all 3 indications)

Effects on other organs: No well-controlled studies on use in pregnancy; however, nifedipine has been used in pregnancy-associated HT with no reported adverse effects on fetus; nicardipine is excreted in breast milk

Precautions and contraindications: Should be used with caution in hypotension (systolic BP < 90 mm Hg), severe AS

Because dihydropyridines are heavily metabolized by liver, they must be used with caution and/or in decreased dosage in pts with impaired hepatic function.

Ca^{++}-channel blockers may inhibit platelet function.

Oral/sl nifedipine is no longer recommended for use in hypertensive crisis.

Adverse effects: 10% of pts develop mild/moderate edema with nifedipine; edema with felodipine is dose and age dependent

Short-acting nifedipine is not recommended for use in pts with CAD.

Drug interactions: Felodipine: Barbituates, hydantoins, and carbamazepine may decrease bioavailability; erythromycin increases pharmacologic effect. Felodipine can decrease serum theophylline levels slightly, and may increase serum digoxin levels.

Cimetidine increases the bioavailability of felodipine, nifedipine, and nicardipine.

Nicardipine can increase cyclosporine levels.

Neuromuscular blockade and hypotension have been reported with concomitant administration of nifedipine and parenteral $MgSO_4$, hypotension with concomitant use of nifedipine and fentanyl.

Nifedipine may increase theophylline effects and may decrease serum quinidine levels.

Grapefruit juice and ETOH may increase the bioavailability of nifedipine and other dihydropyridines.

Dosage and administration:

Amlodipine (Norvasc): 2.5 mg, 5 mg, 10 mg tablets; starting dose 2.5-5 me po qd; maximum dose 10 mg qd; titrate dose q 7-14 d

Felodipine (Plendil): 2.5 mg, 5 mg, 10 mg extended-release tablets; starting dose 2.5-5 mg po qd; maximum dose 10 mg qd; titrate dose q 14 d

Isradipine (DynaCirc): 2.5 mg, 5 mg capsules; 5 mg, 10 mg extended-release tablets; initial dose 2.5 mg po bid; maximum dose 20 mg/d, although most pts show little additional effect above 10 mg/d; titrate dose q 14-28 d

Nicardipine (Cardene): 20 mg, 30 mg capsules; 30 mg, 45 mg, 60 mg; 2.5 mg/mL injection; initial dose 20 mg po tid or 30 mg po bid for sustained-release form; titrate dose q 3 d; usual effective dose 60-120 mg/d (see Table 18.8)

Nifedipine (Procardia, Adalat): 10 mg, 20 mg capsules; 30 mg, 60 mg, 90 mg sustained-release tablets; initial dose 30 mg total qd; maximum recommended dose 120 mg qd; titrate dose over 7-14 d

Nisoldipine (Sular): 10 mg, 20 mg, 30 mg, 40 mg extended-release tablets; usual initial dose 20 mg qd (10 mg qd in elderly pts); maximum dose 60 mg qd; titrate dose q 7 d

Bepridil

Drugs of this type: Bepridil (Vascor)

Pharmacology: Same as other Ca^{++}-channel blockers; also inhibits fast Na^{+} channels and has Class I antiarrhythmic properties

Pharmacokinetics: 100% oral absorption; 59% effective bioavailability; onset of action 60 min; protein binding 99%; half-life 24 hr

Chemistry: Diarylaminopropylamine derivative structurally unrelated to other Ca^{++}-channel blockers

Uses: Chronic stable angina; not considered first-line agent because of arrhythmia potential

Effects on other organs: 2 cases of agranulocytosis reported; bepridil is excreted in breast milk

Precautions and contraindications: Bepridil is contraindicated in pts with h/o arrhythmias, congenital prolonged QT syndrome, or in conjunction with other drugs that prolong QT interval. It has prorhythmic effects seen with other Class I antiarrhythmics, including torsades de pointes and VT/VF; QT interval and rhythm must therefore be monitored.

Active metabolites of bepridil are excreted primarily in urine. Dosage may need to be adjusted in pts with hepatic dysfunction, and possibly in pts with renal dysfunction.

Drug interactions: No definite interaction with digoxin documented

Dosage and administration: Bepridil: 200 mg, 300 mg, 400 mg tablets; usual adult dose 200 mg qd; maximum dose 400 mg qd; doses should not be increased more frequently than q 10 d

Table 18.8 Equivalent Oral and Iv Infusion Doses of Nicardipine

Oral Dose	Iv Infusion Rate
20 mg po q 8 hr	0.5 mg/hr
30 mg po q 8 hr	1.2 mg/hr
40 mg po q 8 hr	2.2 mg/hr

Diltiazem

Drugs of this type: Diltiazem (Cardizem, Dilacor-XT, Dilacor-XR, Tiazac)

Pharmacology: Effects on influx of extracellular Ca^{++} transport through slow channels similar to other Ca^{++}-channel blockers. In addition, diltiazem prolongs intranodal AV conduction and refractory period (prolonged AH interval) with little effect on His-Purkinje conduction; the effect is frequency dependent.

Diltiazem does not prolong the refractory period of the accessory pathway in WPW syndrome.

No negative inotropic effect is seen clinically in vivo.

Pharmacokinetics: Absorption 80-90%; effective bioavailability 40-60% due to first-pass effect; oral bioavailability increases disproportionately with increasing dosage; protein binding 70-80%; onset of action 30-60 min with po sustained-release dose; half-life is 2-11 hr after oral administration (oral metabolites may have half-life of 20 hr), 3.4 hr after single iv injection, 4-5 hr with continuous infusion (7 hr in Afib)

Chemistry: Benzothiazepine derivative structurally unrelated to other Ca^{++}-channel blockers

Iv solution is physically incompatible with many other drugs, including acetazolamide, acyclovir, aminophylline, ampicillin, cefamadole, diazepam, furosemide, heparin, hydrocortisone, insulin, methylprednisolone, nafcillin, phenytoin, $NaHCO_3$

Lipophylic; extensively distributed in body tissue

Uses: Chronic stable angina; vasospastic angina; HT; SVT; Afib; 86-88% of pts with PSVT convert to NSR within 2-3 min of administration of iv diltiazem; iv diltiazem produces > 20% reduction in ventricular response rate in Afib, Aflut; > 80% of pts sustain rate reduction with continuous iv infusion but < 10% of pts convert to NSR

Effects on other organs: Diltiazem is excreted in breast milk.

Precautions and contraindications: Caution is required in pts with hypotension, sick sinus syndrome, 2nd- or 3rd-degree AV block, hepatic dysfunction, or CHF. Negative inotropic and chronotropic effects of diltiazem and β-blockers are additive.

Iv diltiazem should not be administered to pts with Afib and WPW syndrome because very rapid ventricular response and VT/Vfib may result.

Adverse effects: Edema (2.5- 9%); headache (1.5-7%); blurred vision or dysequilibrium (2-12%)

Drug interactions: Cimetidine or ranitidine may increase the bioavailability of diltiazem. Data on diltiazem-digoxin interactions are conflicting. Diltiazem increases cyclosporine and carbamazepine levels.

Dosage and administration: Diltiazem: 30 mg, 60 mg, 90 mg, 120 mg tablets; 120 mg, 180 mg, 240 mg, 300 mg, 360 mg sustained-release tablets/capsules; 5 mg/mL injection; initial dose 120 mg qd; maximum dose up to 480 mg/d for angina, 540 mg/d for HT

Iv for conversion of PSVT or rate control in Afib, Aflut: 0.25 mg/kg iv bolus over 2 min; may repeat 2nd bolus 0.35 mg/kg in 15 min; continuous infusion 5-15 mg/hr iv; infusion > 24 hr not recommended

Verapamil

Drugs of this type: Verapamil (Calan, Isoptin, Verelan, Covera HS)

Pharmacology: Pharmacologic actions on Ca^{++} influx through slow channels similar to other Ca^{++}-channel blockers; also has Class IV antiarrhythmic properties; slows conduction and prolongs refractory period of AV node; does not prolong QT interval; minimal effects on conduction through accessory pathways; may impair intraatrial conduction in diseased tissue; has negative inotropic properties

Pharmacokinetics: Absorption 90%; effective bioavailability 20-35% due to first-pass effects; onset of action 30 min po, 2-3 min iv; protein binding 83-92%; half-life 2-8 hr after single dose, 4.5-12 hr after multiple doses, 14-16 hr in pts with cirrhosis; almost completely metabolized by liver; 70% of dose excreted as metabolites in urine; norverapamil (metabolite) has ~20% of cardiovascular activity of verapamil

Chemistry: Phenylalkylamine derivative structurally unrelated to other Ca^{++}-channel blockers; solution has pH 4-6.5 and is chemically compatible with parenteral solutions with pH 3-6; precipitates at higher pH; not compatible with iv albumin, amphotericin B, hydralazine

Uses: Classic angina pectoris; vasospastic angina; HT; PSVT; Afib; Aflut; MAT; hypertrophic cardiomyopathy

60-100% of pts with PSVT convert to NSR with iv verapamil. It is more effective in prevention of PSVT due to AV nodal reentry than PSVT associated with a concealed accessory pathway.

70% of pts with Afib/Aflut have a slower rate with verapamil but conversion to NSR is uncommon. Verapamil is more effective in controlling the ventricular response rate during exercise. It should not be used in pts with Afib and WPW syndrome.

Verapamil may improve symptoms in pts with hypertrophic cardiomypathy without necessarily altering the degree of hypertrophy.

Effects on other organs: Crosses placenta; present in breast milk

Precautions and contraindications: Use with caution in pts with systolic dysfunction; contraindicated in pts with EF < 30%, systolic BP < 90 mm Hg, 2nd- or 3rd-degree block, sick sinus syndrome, or pts with AV conduction abnormalities who are taking β-blockers, or in pts with Afib/Aflut and WPW syndrome; reduce dose in pts with renal or hepatic dysfunction

Adverse effects: Constipation (9%); other gi sx (3%); headache (4%)

Drug interactions: Negative inotropic, chronotropic, and dromotropic effects additive with β-blockers; may increase serum digoxin levels 50-75%; reported to produce hypotension when administered with quinidine to pts with hypertrophic cardiomyopathy; increases plasma levels of carbamezapine, prazosin, and theophylline; may decrease serum Li levels

Rifampin may reduce the bioavailability of po verapamil. Vitamin D may reduce its efficacy.

Hyperkalemia has been reported when verapamil is administered with dantrolene.

Verapamil may enhance the muscle relaxant effects of nondepolarizing muscle relaxants.

Use with caution in pts receiving other highly protein-bound drugs (eg, warfarin, hydantoins, sulfonamides, sulfonureas).

Dosage and administration: Verapamil: 40 mg, 80 mg, 120 mg tablets; 120 mg, 180 mg, 240 mg, 360 mg extended-release tablets/capsules; 2.5 mg/mL injection; individualize po doses; maximum 480 mg/d; iv dose for SV arrhythmias 5-10 mg bolus over 2-3 min, may repeat in 30 min

18.11 Cholesterol-Lowering Agents

Circ 2000;101:207; Nejm 1999;341:410

HMG-COA Reductase Inhibitors

Drugs of this type: Atorvastatin (Lipitor, Caduet), fluvastatin (Lescol), lovastatin (Mevacor, Advicor), pravastatin (Pravacol), simvastatin (Zocor, Vytorin), rosuvastatin (Crestor)

Pharmacology: Inhibit rate-limiting step in cholesterol synthesis; increase HDL and decrease LDL, VLDL, and total cholesterol levels, apolipoprotein B, and serum triglyceride levels

HMG-COA reductase inhibitors are less effective in pts with homozygous familial hypercholesterolemia.

Pharmacokinetics: All agents except rosuvastatin have extensive first-pass metabolism; 60-98% excretion in feces; half-life varies from $<$ 1 hr (fluvastatin) to 19 hr (rosuvastatin); pravastatin is $\sim$ 50% protein bound, others are 88-95% protein bound; atorvastatin, fluvastatin, pravastatin, and simvastatin levels are increased with impaired hepatic function; cerivastatin, lovastatin, simvastatin, and rosuvastatin levels are increased in severe renal failure

Uses: Treatment of hyperlipidemia

Effects on other organs: Most agents are excreted in breast milk; nursing mothers should discontinue the drug.

Precautions and contraindications: Acute liver disease or unexplained transaminase elevation are contraindications to use. Liver function testing is recommended before initiating therapy, at 6 and 12 wk, and semi-annually thereafter.

HMG-COA reductase inhibitors are contraindicated in pregnancy.

Adverse effects: Headache, nausea, diarrhea, abdominal pain, constipation, arthralgias; myalgias

Rhabdomyolysis with renal failure; risk is increased in pts receiving cyclosporine, erythromycin, gemfibrizol, antifungals, niacin

Lovastatin and simvastatin are reported to cause insomnia.

Drug interactions: May increase protime in pts on warfarin

Dosage and administration:

Atorvastatin (Lipitor): 10 mg, 20 mg, 40 mg tablets; initial dose 10 mg qd; maximum dose 80 mg/d

Fluvastatin (Lescol): 20 mg, 40 mg capsules; initial dose 20 mg qhs; maximum dose 80 mg/d

Lovastatin (Mevacor): 10 mg, 20 mg, 40 mg tablets; initial dose 20 mg qhs; maximum dose 80 mg/d; titrate dose q 4 wk

Pravastatin (Pravacol): 10 mg, 20 mg, 40 mg tablets; initial dose 10-20 mg qhs

Rosuvastatin (Crestor): 5 mg, 10 mg, 20 mg, 40 mg; initial dose 5-10 mg qhs

Simvastatin (Zocor): 5 mg, 10 mg, 20 mg, 40 mg, 80 mg tablets; initial dose 5-10 mg qhs

Bile Acid Sequestrants

Drugs of this type: Cholestyramine (Questran, Prevalite), colestipol (Colestid), colesevelam (WelChol)

Pharmacology: Bind bile acids in intestine, removing them from enterohepatic circulation and increasing oxidation of cholesterol to bile acids

Pharmacokinetics: Resin is not absorbed from gi tract

Uses: Reduction of LDL cholesterol level

Effects on other organs: Hyperchloremic acidosis has been reported

Precautions and contraindications: Complete biliary obstruction

Resins may interfere with fat adsorption. Supplementation of fat-soluble vitamins and folic acid may be needed.

Adverse effects: Constipation; abdominal cramping, bloating

Drug interactions: May decrease effect of administered warfarin, thyroid hormone, fat-soluble vitamins

Dosage and administration:

Cholestyramine: 4 gm in liquid bid; maximum dose 24 gm/d; increase dose at intervals > 4 wk

Colestipol: initial dose 5 gm qd bid po in liquid; maximum dose 30 gm qd; increase dose at intervals > 4 wk

Colesevelam: 625 mg; 3 tabs po bid

Fibric Acid Derivatives

Drugs of this type: Fenofibrate (Tricor, Antara), gemfibrozil (Lopid)

Pharmacology: Decrease triglycerides and VLDL cholesterol levels

Pharmacokinetics:

Fenofibrate: Absorption increased with food; 99% protein bound; elimination half-life 20 hr; 60% of active metabolites excreted in urine, 25% in feces

Gemfibrozil: Plasma half-life 1.5 hr but biological half-life longer due to enterohepatic circulation and reabsorption; excretion 70% in urine

Uses: Rx of hypertriglyceridemia (type IV, type V hyperlipidemia)

Effects on other organs: Decreased hgb/hct, wbc count reported

Precautions and contraindications: Abnormal liver enzymes, hepatic or severe renal dysfunction, primary biliary cirrhosis, gallbladder disease (may increase cholesterol excretion into bile); can also be associated with rhabdomyolysis, myoglobinuria, myositis, liver enzyme elevations; gemfibrozil has hyperglycemia effect

Adverse effects:

Fenofibrate: Rash, dyspepsia

Gemfibozil: Dyspepsia (20%), abdominal pain (10%), diarrhea (7%), fatigue (4%)

Drug interactions: Increased risk of rhabdomyolysis when administered with HMG-COA reductase inhibitors; may enhance effects of oral anticoagulants

Dosage and administration:

Fenofibrate: Tricor: 48 mg, 145 mg capsules, maximum dose 160 mg/d with meals; Antara: 43 mg, 87 mg, 130 mg capsules, maximum dose 130 mg po qd, initiate rx with lowest dose in elderly or pts with impaired renal function

Gemfibrozil (Lopid): 600 mg tablets, 600 mg po bid 30 min before meals

Cholesterol Absorption Inhibitors

Drugs of this type: Ezetimibe (Zetia, Vytorin)

Pharmacology: Selective inhibition of intestinal absorption of cholesterol by ~54%

Pharmacokinetics: Extensively conjugated to active glucuronide; bioavailabilty is undetermined; > 90% bound to plasma proteins; plasma half-life ≈ 22 hr; 78% excretion in feces

Uses: Rx of hyperlipidemia; as monotherapy, reduces total cholesterol levels by 12%, LDL levels by 18%, triglyceride levels by 8%; with statin reduces total cholesterol levels by 15-46%, LDL levels by 20-61%, triglyceride levels by 11-40%

Effects on other organs: Effects in pts with hepatic insufficiency are unknown

Precautions and contraindications: Contraindicated in pts with active liver disease, in pregnancy

Adverse effects: Abdominal pain, diarrhea, arthralgia, back pain: all < 5%

Drug interactions: Gemfibrozil, fenofibrate, and cyclosporine may increase ezetimibe bioavailability; cholestyramine decreases serum levels

Dosage and administration: Ezetimibe: 10 mg tablets, 1 po qd

Other Antihyperlipidemic Agents

Ann IM 1996;125:529

Drugs of this type: Niacin (Niacin, Niaspan, Advicor)

Pharmacology: Uncertain

Pharmacokinetics: 50-76% oral absorption; complex first-pass metabolism; 60-76% excretion in urine as niacin and metabolites

Uses: Rx of hyperlipidemia: reduces total cholesterol levels by 2-17%, LDL levels by 3-17%, triglyceride levels by 10-29%; increases HDL levels by 10-26%

Effects on other organs: Abnormal liver tests; rare cases of hepatic necrosis in pts using sustained-release preparation; potential increase in risk of myopathy when administered with statins; small reductions in platelet count and serum phosphorus levels have been reported

Precautions and contraindications: Contraindicated in pts with active liver disease; use in pregnancy untested; may be excreted in milk

Adverse effects: Flushing, itching, diarrhea; sx usually improve with continued administration, use of extended-release preparations, administration of ASA 325 mg po 30 min before taking niacin, ingestion with low-fat snacks (especially those containg apple pectin)

Drug interactions: ASA may decrease metabolic clearance of niacin; niacin binding with colestipol

Dosage and administration: Niaspan: 500 mg, 750 mg, 1000 mg tablets; initial dose 500 mg qhs, may increase in 200 mg increments every 4 wk; usual maximum dose 2000 mg qd

18.12 Diuretics

Nejm 1998;339:387

Loop Diuretics

Drugs of this type: Bumetanide (Bumex), furosemide (Lasix), torsemide (Demadex)

Pharmacology: Furosemide inhibits reabsorption of Na^+ and Cl^- from proximal and distal tubules and the loop of Henle. Bumetanide is more chloruretic than naturetic and does not act on distal tubules. Torsemide works in the ascending limb of the loop of Henle.

Pharmacokinetics:

Bioavailability after oral dose: bumetanide, 72-96%; furosemide, 60-64%; torsemide, ~80%

Duration of action: bumetanide, 4-6 hr; furosemide and torsemide, 6-8 hr

Relative potency: bumetanide > torsemide > furosemide

Uses: Edema; CHF; HT

Effects on other organs: In pts with cirrhosis, sudden electrolyte shifts can precipitate hepatic coma. Loop diuretics may exacerbate systemic lupus erythematosis.

Precautions and contraindications: Contraindicated in anuria, sulfonurea sensitivity, hepatic coma, severe electrolyte depletion; monitor renal function and electrolytes carefully

Adverse effects: Hyperuricemia, hyperglycemia, elevation of serum LDL levels, photosensitivity, diarrhea

Drug interactions: May enhance effects of anticoagulants; may increase serum Li levels; synergistic effects with thiazide diuretics

Dosage and administration:

Bumetanide (Bumex): 0.5 mg, 1 mg, 2 mg tablets; 0.25 mg/mL injection; usual dose 0.5-2 mg po qd

Furosemide (Lasix): 20 mg, 40 mg, 80 mg tablets; 10 mg/mL injection: usual dose 20-80 mg qd po; do not mix iv furosemide with solutions having pH < 5.5

Torsemide (Demadex): 5 mg, 10 mg, 20 mg, 100 mg tablets; 10 mg/mL injection; usual dose 10-20 mg po qd (5 mg qd for HT and cirrhosis), maximum dose 200 mg qd

Thiazide Diuretics

Drugs of this type: Chlorthalidone (Hygroton), chlorthiazide (Diuril), HCTZ (Esidrix, Oretic), indapamide (Lozol), methyclothiazide (Enduron), metolazone (Zaroxolyn)

Pharmacology: Decrease Na^+ and H_2O reabsorption in loop of Henle; increase K^+ and HCO_3^- excretion

Pharmacokinetics: See Table 18.9.

Uses: Edema, HT, nephrogenic diabetes insipidus

Effects on other organs: Thiazides are excreted in breast milk.

Precautions and contraindications: Contraindicated in anuria, renal decompensation

Adverse effects: Hyponatremia; hypokalemia; hypochloremic alkylosis; hyperuricemia; hypercalcemia; hyperglycemia; increased total cholesterol, LDL cholesterol, and triglyceride levels

Drug interactions: Thiazides decrease renal clearance of lithium, enhance the effects of vitamin D, and potentiate the effects of loop diuretics. Cholestyramine and colestipol reduce gi absorption of thiazide diuretics.

Table 18.9 Pharmacokinetics of Oral Thiazide Diuretics

Diuretic	Absorption (%)	Duration of Action	Half-life	Equivalent Dose
Chlorthalidone (Hygroton)	64%; bioavailability is dose dependent	24-72 hr	40 hr	50 mg
Chlorthiazide (Diuril)	10-21%; bioavailability is dose dependent	6-12 hr	0.75-2 hr	500 mg
Hydrochlorthiazide (Esidrix, Oretic, Hydrodiuril)	65-75%	6-12 hr	5.5-15 hr	50 mg
Indapamide (Lozol)	93%	36 hr	14 hr	2.5 mg
Methyclothiazide (Enduron)	No data available	24 hr	No data available	5 mg
Metolazone (Zaroxolyn)	65%	12-24 hr	No data available	5 mg

Dosage and administration:

Chlorthalidone (Hygroton): 25 mg, 50 mg, 100 mg tablets; 50-100 mg po qd

Chlorthiazide (Diuril): 250 mg, 500 mg tablets; 0.5-1 gm po qd-bid

Hydrochlorthiazide (Esidrix, Oretic): 25 mg, 50 mg, 100 mg tablets; 25-100 mg po qd; lower doses (12.5 mg qd) effective in combination with ACEIs and angiotensin II blockers

Indapamide (Lozol): 1.25 mg, 2.5 mg tablets; initial dose 1.25 mg po qd for HT, 2.5 mg po qd for edema; increase dose q 1 wk for edema, q 4 wk for HT; maximum dose 5 mg qd

Methyclothiazide (Enduron): 2.5 mg, 5 mg tablets, 2.5-10 mg po qd

Metolazone (Zaroxolyn): 2.5 mg, 5 mg, 10 mg tablets; 2.5-20 mg qd

K^+ Sparing Diuretics

Drugs of this type: Amiloride (Midamor, Moduretic), spironolactone (Aldactone), triamterene (Dyrenium, Dyazide, Maxide)

Pharmacology: Interfere with Na^+ reabsorption in distal tubules and decrease K^+ secretion. Spironolactone competitively inhibits the effect of aldosterone on distal tubules. Amiloride and triamterene act directly on distal renal tubules.

Pharmacokinetics:

Bioavailability: Amiloride, 15-25%; spironolactone, > 90%; triamterene, 30-70%

Protein binding: Amiloride, 23%; spironolactone, > 98%; triamterene, 50-67%

Half-life: Amiloride, 6-9 hr; spironolactone, 20 hr; triamterene, 3 hr

Uses: CHF, edema, HT, hypokalemia; spironolactone also indicated in primary hyperaldosteronism

Effects on other organs: Spironolactone may cause gynecomastia.

Precautions and contraindications: May cause hyperkalemia. Use with caution in pts with metabolic/respiratory acidosis, or renal or hepatic failure. Triamterene is a weak folic acid antagonist and may raise glucose levels in pts with NIDDM.

Adverse effects: Headache, vomiting, gi upset

Drug interactions: Use with caution in pts receiving K^+ supplements or ACEIs. NSAIDs may reduce the effect of amiloride. ASA may reduce the diuretic effect of spironolactone. Cimetidine may increase triamterene levels. Concomitant administration of triamterene and indomethacin can produce acute renal failure.

Dosage and administration:

Amiloride (Midamor): 5 mg tablet; starting dose 5 mg po qd; maximum dose 20 mg qd

Spironolactone (Aldactone): 25 mg, 50 mg, 100 mg tablets; usual dose 25-100 mg po qd

Triamterene (Dyrenium): 50 mg, 100 mg capsules; usual dose 100 mg po bid pc; maximum dose 300 mg/d

18.13 Drugs for Hypertensive Emergencies

Drugs of this type: Diazoxide (Hyperstat), nitroprusside (Nipride)

Pharmacology: Diazoxide relaxes smooth muscle in resistance arterioles. Nitroprusside relaxes both arteriolar and venous smooth muscle.

Pharmacokinetics:

Diazoxide: > 90% protein bound; plasma half-life of 20-36 hr; onset of effect within 1 min; maximum effect 2-5 min

Nitroprusside: circulatory half-life of 2 min; onset of action 1-2 min

Uses: Severe HT, hypertensive crisis; nitroprusside also used for pre- and afterload reduction in acute CHF

Effects on other organs: Diazoxide can stop uterine contractions during labor.

Precautions and contraindications: Diazoxide is ineffective in pts with pheochromocytoma.

Nitroprusside can produce dangerous levels of cyanide ion and cyanmethemoglobin. Cyanide accumulation is present at infusion rates > 2 μgm/kg/min. Free cyanide ion is eliminated as thiocyanate (half-life, 3 d). Cyanide is metabolized by the liver, so cyanide toxicity is a greater risk in pts with hepatic disease.

Adverse effects: Diazoxide frequently causes transient hyperglycemia, Na^+ retention, and can cause hypotension (7%), nausea/vomiting (4%), or dizziness (2%).

Drug interactions: Diazoxide may displace other protein-bound drugs and decreases the serum dilantin level.

Dosage and administration:

Dyazoxide: 15 mg/mL injection; bolus injection 1-3 mg/kg iv (150 mg maximum); repeat q 5-15 min until BP lowered and then q 4-24 hr

Nitroprusside (Nipride): 50 mg/2 mL, 50 mg/5 mL solution; must be diluted for use; dose 0.3-10 μgm/kg/min infusion; protect from light

18.14 Human B-Type Natriuretic Peptide

Drugs of this type: Nesiritide (Natrecor)

Pharmacology: Increases intracellular cyclic GMP levels; dilates both veins and arteries

Pharmacokinetics: Elimination half-life is 18 min. Elimination is through cell uptake, proteolytic cleavage, and renal filtration.

Uses: Acute CHF

Effects on other organs: Hypotension; possible risk of worsening renal function

Precautions and contraindications: Contraindicated in cardiogenic shock, systolic BP < 90 mm Hg, severe AS, restrictive or obstructive cardiomyopathy, constrictive pericarditis, pericardial tamponade

Adverse effects: Hypotension, VT, headache, nausea

Drug interactions: Incompatible with iv heparin, insulin, bumetamide, enalaprilat, hydralazine, furosemide

Dosage and administration: 2 μgm/kg iv bolus followed by continuous iv infusion at 0.01 μgm/kg/min; continue up to 48 hr

18.15 Inotropic Agents

Circ 1999;99:1265; Nejm 1998;339:1848; 1997;336:525

Digoxin

Drugs of this type: Digoxin (Digitek, Lanoxicaps, Lanoxin)

Pharmacology: Inhibits Na^+-K^+-activated ATPase, augments Ca^{++} influx, and enhances excitation-contraction coupling. As a result, digoxin increases the force and velocity of systolic contraction. CO is increased in pts with CHF, producing a subsequent reflex reduction in sympathetic tone and peripheral vascular resistance (PVR). In normal subjects, CO remains unchanged and PVR increases due to a direct effect on smooth muscle and CNS-mediated increase in sympathetic tone. Baroreceptor sensitization also increases carotid sinus nerve activity.

AV node conduction velocity is decreased and the effective refractory period is increased primarily through increased vagal tone. A direct effect on the AV node is apparent at higher doses. High (toxic) doses depress SA node automaticity and increase spontaneous diastolic depolarization of other cardiac tissue.

Pharmacokinetics: Absorbed from small intestine not affected by gastric pH, subtotal gastrectomy, jejunoileal bypass; absorption is 60-85% of po tablet, 90-100% of po caplet, 80% of im injection; crosses blood-brain barrier and placenta

Onset of action is 30-120 min after oral administration, 5-30 min after iv administration. Peak action is 6-8 hr after po dose, 1-5 hr after iv dose. Therapeutic range (6-8 hr post-administration) is 0.5-2 ng/mL; 20-30% binding to plasma proteins.

Elimination half-time is 33-44 hr with normal renal function, > 4.5 d in anephric pts. Steady-state plasma concentrations (without loading dose) are attained by 7 d.

50-75% of digoxin is excreted in urine unchanged by kidneys. Elimination times are prolonged by renal failure or hypothyroidism; ~30% of total body digoxin is eliminated qd with normal renal function, ~14% qd in anuric pts. Digoxin is not removed by hemodialysis or exchange transfusion.

Chemistry: Insoluble in water; iv injection at pH 6.6-7.4; compatible with most iv fluids

Uses: In CHF, digoxin usually produces measurable hemodynamic effects, and it may improve sx (exercise capacity, hospitalization rates), but has no apparent effect on overall mortality. Effects are additive with those of ACEIs and diuretics. Digoxin is less effective in rx of "high-output" failure (fever, hyperthyroidism, AV fistula, thiamine deficiency, Paget's disease), cor pulmonale, and myocarditis.

In Afib, digoxin may control the ventricular response rate but has not been shown to produce conversion to NSR. Because the effect on the AV node is mediated through vagal tone, HR may increase markedly with exercise.

In Aflut, digoxin slows ventricular response by increasing AV block; conversion to NSR or Afib may occur

Effects on other organs: Digoxin crosses the placenta; fetal serum concentrations are typically 50-80% of maternal serum concentration. Its safety in pregnancy has not been established. Breast milk concentration is 60-90% of the plasma level.

Precautions and contraindications: Pts with AMI, severe carditis, advanced COPD, or severe CHF may have increased sensitivity to digoxin.

Digoxin use should be avoided in pts with WPW syndrome because it can enhance conduction through the accessory pathway and produce very rapid ventricular response rates and/or Vfib in Afib.

SV arrhythmias associated with hypermetabolic states are generally resistant to rx with digoxin.

Digoxin may worsen outflow obstruction in hypertrophic cardiomyopathy due to its positive inotropic effect.

Pts with constrictive pericarditis, restrictive cardiomyopathy, and acute cor pulmonale are particularly susceptible to digoxin toxicity.

The role of digoxin in cardiogenic shock (if any) has not been established.

Pts with sick sinus syndrome may develop worsening SA or AV node dysfunction with digoxin.

Adverse effects: Lethal dose is 20-50 times the usual daily maintenance dose. The toxic dose range is notoriously variable and difficult to predict, especially in elderly pts.

Common si/sx of toxicity include anorexia, nausea, bradycardia, AV conduction disturbances, AV dissociation, nonparoxysmal junctional tachycardia, PAT with variable AV block, and multifocal PVCs. Digoxin toxicity may simulate virtually any arrhythmia.

Toxicity is more likely in the setting of hypokalemia, hypomagnesemia, or hypercalcemia. Rapid Ca^{++} administration may precipitate arrhythmias in digitalized pts.

Estrogen-like effects have been reported with chronic administration, especially in elderly pts.

Treatment of toxicity includes correction of electrolyte imbalances; atropine for bradycardia; phenytoin (50-100 mg q 5 min; 600 mg maximum); digoxin immune FAB.

Drug interactions:

Reported to *increase* serum digoxin levels: alprazolam, amiodarone, benzodiazepines, captopril, cyclosporine, dilatizem, erythromycin, esmolol, felodipine, flecanide, ibuprofen, indomethacin, nifedipine, omperazole, propafenone, quinidine, tolbutamide, verapamil

Reported to *decrease* serum digoxin levels: oral aminoglycosides, ASA, antacids, antihistamines, barbiturates, bleomycin, cholestyramine, colstipol, cyclophosphamide, doxorubicin, hydantoins, kaolin/pectin, methotrexate, metoclopramide, neomycin, rifampin, sucralfate, sulfasalazine, vincristine

Succinylcholine may increase digoxin toxicity.

Dosage and administration: Digoxin: 0.125, 0.25, 0.5 mg tablets; 0.05, 0.1, 0.5 mg liquid-filled capsules; 0.05 mg/mL elixir; 0.1 mg/mL, 0.25 mg/mL injection; digitalizing dose in adults with normal renal function is 10-15 μgm/kg po, 8-12 μgm/kg iv; maintenance dose is 25-35% of loading dose; reduce dose in renal failure

Iv Inotropic Agents

Drugs of this type: Amrinone (Inocor), milrinone (Primacor)

Pharmacology: Non-β-adrenergic-mediated positive inotropic and vasodilator effect; increase cellular levels of cAMP; reduces pre- and afterload through direct relaxant effect on vascular smooth muscle

Pharmacokinetics:

Amrinone: 10-49% protein bound; mean elimination half-life ≈3.6 hr, 5.8 hr in pts with CHF; native drug and metabolites excreted in urine

Milrinone: ~70% protein bound; mean elimination half-life-2.4 hr; 83% of drug excreted unmetabolized in urine

Uses: Short-term management of CHF

Effects on other organs: Amrinone may produce a dose-related thrombocytopenia; platelet count < 100,000/mm^3 reported in 2.4% of pts

Precautions and contraindications: Severe pulmonary or aortic valve disease

Adverse effects:

Amrinone: Arrhythmia (3%), nausea (1.7%), hypotension (1.3%), vomiting (0.9%)

Milrinone: Ventricular arrhythmias (12%), hypotension (2.9%), headache (2.9%)

Dosage and administration:

Amrinone: 5 mg/mL injection; initial dose 0.75 μgm/kg iv bolus over 2-3 min, followed by 5-10 μgm/kg/min iv infusion; maximum dose 10 mg/d; dilute in NS, **not** dextrose solutions; incompatible with iv furosemide

Milrinone: 1 mg/mL injection; loading dose 50 μgm/kg iv bolus over 10 min, followed by 0.375-0.75 μgm/kg/min iv infusion; maximum dose 1.13 mg/kg/d; dilute in 0.45% NaCl, 0.9% Nacl, D_5W; incompatible with iv furosemide

Table 18.10 Milrinone Infusion Rates in Renal Failure

Creatinine Clearance	Iv Rate (μgm/kg/min)
50	0.43
40	0.38
30	0.33
20	0.28
10	0.23
5	0.20

18.16 Nitrates

Nejm 1998;338:520

Drugs of this type: Nitroglycerin, isosorbide dinitrate (Isordil, Dilatrate SR), isosorbide mononitrate (Ismo, Imdur, Monoket)

Pharmacology: Stimulates intracellular production of GMP to produce relaxation of smooth muscle; has a greater effect on venous than on arteriolar beds; hence, reduction in preload is greater than reduction in afterload

Pharmacokinetics: TNG has a half-life of 1-4 min and is 60% protein bound. The sl/spray form has a duration of action up to 30 min; the sustained-release oral form, 3-8 hr; topical ointments, 2-12 hr; transdermal patch, up to 24 hr, although tolerance may develop after 12 hr.

ISDN has a duration of action of 4-6 hr in oral form, and 6-8 hr in sustained release form. No data are available for ISMN.

Uses: Treatment of angina and CHF

Effects on other organs: May increase intraocular pressure; use with caution in pts with glaucoma

Precautions and contraindications: Can produce postural hypotension; nitrate tolerance develops with continuous administration

Iv TNG is absorbed by many plastics; may need to use glass or selected plastic containers

Adverse effects: Headache; tachycardia

Drug interactions: Alcohol and ASA can increase serum nitrate concentrations.

Dosage and administration:

Nitroglycerin: 0.3 mg, 0.4 mg, 0.6 mg tablets; oral spray: 1 sl prn, 0.5 mg/mL; 5 mg/mL injection: initial dose μgm/min iv infusion, titrate dose q 3-5 min by 5-10 μgm/min increments; monitor BP, HR, sx

Isosorbide dinitrate: 5 mg, 10 mg, 20 mg, 40 mg tablets; 40 mg sustained-release tablets: 5-40 mg po q 6 hr with nitrate-free period qd, or sustained-release form 2× d 7 hr apart; sl and chewable forms also available

Isosorbide mononitrate: Ismo: 20 mg tablets, 2 po qd, 7 hr apart; Imdur: 30, 60, 120 mg tablets, 1 po qd

18.17 Other Antihypertensive Agents

Drugs of this type:

Centrally acting: Clonidine (Catapres), guanabenz (Wytensin), guanfacine (Tenex), methyldopa (Aldomet)

Peripherally acting: Guanethidine (Ismelin), reserpine, hydralazine

Pharmacology: Stimulate α-adrenergic receptors centrally to decrease sympathetic stimulation and peripheral vascular resistance. Reserpine depletes catecholamine stores, guanethidine inhibits release of norepinephrine at sympathetic junction, and hydralazine is a direct arterial dilator.

Pharmacokinetics:

Clonidine: Elimination half-life is 6-24 hr; 50% elimination in urine and 50% metabolized by liver

Guanabenz: 75% oral availability; half-life is 6 hr; metabolism not determined

Guanethidine: 3-50% oral availability; half-life is 4-8 d

Guanfacine: 80% oral bioavailability; 70% protein bound; elimination half-life is 10-30 hr; excreted in urine

Methyldopa: 50% bioavailability; elimination half-life is 1.8 hr; 70% of po dose excreted in urine

Reserpine: 50% oral bioavailability; 97% protein bound; mean half-life is 33 hr; metabolism not studied

Hydralazine: 20% bioavailabilty; 87% protein bound; duration of action is 6-8 hr; extensive and individually variable hepatic metabolism

Use: HT

Effects on other organs: Methyldopa and clonidine cross the placenta. Reserpine crosses the placenta and is secreted in breast milk. Guanethidine is excreted in breast milk.

Precautions and contraindications: Rebound HT can occur with discontinuation of centrally acting agents.

Guanethidine is contraindicated in pheochromocytoma. Withdraw 2 wk prior to general anesthesia. Avoid use in pts with renal insufficiency, asthma recent MI, or CHF. It can cause severe orthostatic hypotension.

Methyldopa is contraindicated in active hepatic disease and in pts receiving MAO inhibitors (metabolites stimulate the release of catecholamines). 10-20% of pts develop positive direct Coombs test. Fever, eosinophilia, and abnormal liver studies are also noted.

Reserpine may cause depression, sometimes severe, and peptic ulcer disease.

Adverse effects:

Clonidine: Dry mouth (40%), drowsiness (33%), dizziness (16%), constipation (10%)

Guanabenz: Sedation (20-39%), dry mouth (28-38%), dizziness (12-17%), weakness (10%)

Guanethidine: Fluid retention, fatigue, nausea, inhibition of ejaculation

Guanfacine: Sedation (5-13%), dry mouth (10-42%)

Hydralazine: Headache, nausea, palpitations, lupus syndrome

Drug interactions: Prazosin, β-blockers, and TCAs block the effects of clonidine.

Haldoperidol, pheonthiazines, and TCAs inhibit the effects of guanethidine. Guanethidine potentiates the effects of sympathomimetics.

Methyldopa potentiates the effects of haldoperidol, can elevate BP when coadministered with phenothiazines, and may precipitate lithium toxicity. Its effects are reduced by TCAs.

Reserpine should not be used with MAO inhibitors, and it may increase the risk of arrhythmia when used with digoxin or quinidine.

NSAIDs may decrease the hemodynamic effects of hydralazine.

Dosage and administration:

Clonidine (Catapres): 0.1 mg, 0.2 mg, 0.3 mg tablets and patches; initial dose 0.1-0.2 mg po bid; usual dose 0.2-0.6 mg/d; dosing for patch is q wk rather than qd

Guanabenz (Wytensin): 4 mg, 8 mg tablets; initial dose 4 mg po bid; increment by 4-8 mg/d q 2 wk; maximum dose 32 mg bid

Guanethidine (Ismelin): 10 mg, 25 mg tablets; initial dose 10 mg po qd; increase dose q wk; average dose 25-50 mg qd; check BP lying, standing, and after exercise

Guanfacine (Tenex): 1 mg, 2 mg tablets; initial dose 1 mg po qhs; increase to 2 mg in 3-4 wk if needed

Methyldopa (Aldomet): 125 mg, 250 mg, 500 mg tablets; 50 mg/mL injection; initial dose 250 mg po bid-tid; maintenance 500-2000 mg/d; iv 250-500 mg iv q 6 hr administered over 30-60 min

Reserpine: 0.1 mg, 0.25 mg tablets; initial dose 0.5 mg po qd for 1-2 wk; 0.1-0.25 mg po qd maintenance

Hydralazine: 10 mg, 25 mg, 50 mg, 100 mg tablets; initial dose 10 mg po qid for 2-4 d, then 25 mg po qid; maximum dose 50 mg po qid

18.18 Thrombolytic Agents

Drugs of this type: Alteplase (Activase), reteplase (Retavase), streptokinase, tenecteplase (TNKase)

Pharmacology: Alteplase and reteplase are tissue-type plasminogen activators produced by recombinant DNA. Streptokinase is produced by group C β-hemolytic streptococci. All catalyze conversion of plasminogen to plasmin, which in turn degrades the fibrin matrix of a thrombus.

Pharmacokinetics: 80% of the alteplase dose in plasma is cleared in 10 min. Reteplase has an effective half-life of 13-16 min. The metabolism of streptokinase is very complex.

Uses: Rx of acute transmural MI; alteplase is also indicated in treatment of acute ischemic stroke and massive PE

Precautions and contraindications: Active internal bleeding, CVA in past 2 mon, intracranial hemorrhage, trauma or neoplasm, known bleeding diathesis, AV malformation, uncontrolled severe HT. Use with caution in pts with major surgery, trauma, gi or gu hemorrhage in past 10 days, cerebrovascular disease, HT, suspected pericarditis or endocarditis, liver dysfunction, pregnancy, diabetic retinopathy, and pts on warfarin or > 75 yr old.

Adverse effects: Bleeding: gi (2-9%), gu (1-10%), ecchymosis (1%), CNS (0.7%)

Drug interactions: Bleeding risks increased in pts on warfarin, heparin, ASA, dipyridamole, abciximab

Dosage and administration: See also sections on MI and CVA.

Alteplase: AMI: 15 mg bolus iv, 50 mg iv (0.75 mg/kg for pts < 67 kg) over 30 min, 35 mg iv (0.5 mg/kg for pts < 67 kg)

CARDIAC MEDICATIONS

Table 18.11 Tenecteplase Dosing

Pt Weight	Dose
< 132 lb (< 60 kg)	6000 U (30 mg or 6 mL)
133-153 lb (61-69 kg)	7000 U (35 mg or 7 mL)
154-175 lb (70-79 kg)	8000 U (40 mg or 8 mL)
176-197 lb (80-89 kg)	9000 U (45 mg or 9 mL)
> 197 lb (> 89 kg)	10,000 U (50 mg or 10 mL)

over 60 min; CVA: total dose 0.9 mg/kg (90 mg maximum) with 10% of total dose administered as iv bolus over 1 min; PE: 100 mg iv over 2 hr

Reteplase: Double bolus: 10 units each iv over 2 min with 2nd bolus administered 30 min after initiation of 1st bolus

Streptokinase: AMI: 1.5 million U iv over 60 min; DVT or arterial thrombosis: 250,000 U iv over 30 min and 100,000 U/hr for 72 hr

Tenecteplase: Administer as single iv dose over 5-10 sec based on pt weight (see Table 18.11); maximum dose 10,000 U (50 mg)

18.19 Vasopressors

Drugs of this type: Dobutamine (Dobutrex), dopamine, epinephrine, isoproterenol (Isuprel), norepinephrine Levophed)

Pharmacology: See Table 18.12. α-Adrenergic stimulation produces vasoconstriction; β_1 stimulation increases HR and myocardial contractility; β_2 stimulation produces peripheral vasodilation.

Dopamine also dilates renal, mesenteric, cerebral, and coronary vascular beds (dopaminergic receptors).

Uses: Shock; cardiac arrest (epinephrine, norepinephrine, isoproterenol); cardiac decompensation

Precautions and contraindications: Dobutamine may produce hypotension and is contraindicated in hypertrophic cardiomyopathy with obstruction.

Dopamine is contraindicated in tachyarrhythmias and pheochromocytoma.

Epinephrine is contraindicated in narrow-angle glaucoma.

Isoproterenol is contraindicated in pts with tachyarrhythmias, angina, and hyperthyroidism; it increases myocardial O_2 requirements.

Norepinephrine is contraindicated in pts with mesenteric or peripheral vascular thrombosis.

Table 18.12 Effects of Vasopressors

Agent	Myocardial Contractility	HR	Vaso-constriction	Vaso-dilation	Renal Perfusion	CO	Vascular Resistance	BP
Dobutamine	+++	0/+[1]	0/+[1]	+	0	↑	↓	↑
Dopamine	+++	+/++[1]	+/+++[1]	0/+	↑ at low dose	↑	↑ at high doses	0/↑
Epinephrine	+++	+++	+++[1]	++[1]	↓	↑	↓	Systolic ↑; diastolic ↓
Isoproterenol	+++	+++	0	+++	↓; ↑ in shock	↑	↓	Systolic ↑; diastolic ↓
Norepinephrine	++	++[2]	+++	0	↓	0/↓	↑	↑

1. Effects are dose dependent.
2. Reflex mechanisms may slow heart rate.

Iv volume depletion should be corrected in all pts.

Adverse effects: Tachycardia, HT, hypotension, angina, flushing

Drug interactions: Bretylium and TCAs potentiate the effects of vasopressors on adrenergic receptors but decrease the effects of mixed-acting vasopressors such as dopamine.

Dosage and administration: Usual infusion rates: dobutamine, 2.5-15 μgm/kg/min; dopamine, 2.5-20 μgm/kg/min; isoproterenol, 5 μgm/min; norepinephrine, initial rate 8-12 μgm/min and maintenance rate 2-4 μgm/min

Dobutamine is incompatible with $NaHCO_3$ and alkaline solutions, cefazolin, cephalothin, cefamandole, penicillin, hydrocortisone, and heparin. It may be coadministered with dopamine, lidocaine, tobramycin, verapamil, nitroprusside, and KCl.

Dopamine is incompatible with alkaline solutions.

To prevent necrosis after extravasation of dopamine or norepinephrine, infuse the area with 5-10 mg phentolamine in 10-15 mL NS.

Index

INDEX

A

B

C

D

I

K

L

M

Q

R

S

T

U

V

W

INDEX